The Psychology
of Flavour

The Psychology of Flavour

Richard J. Stevenson

Associate Professor of Experimental Psychology,
Macquarie University

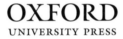

OXFORD
UNIVERSITY PRESS

OXFORD
UNIVERSITY PRESS

Great Clarendon Street, Oxford OX2 6DP

Oxford University Press is a department of the University of Oxford.
It furthers the University's objective of excellence in research, scholarship,
and education by publishing worldwide in

Oxford New York

Auckland Cape Town Dar es Salaam Hong Kong Karachi
Kuala Lumpur Madrid Melbourne Mexico City Nairobi
New Delhi Shanghai Taipei Toronto

With offices in

Argentina Austria Brazil Chile Czech Republic France Greece
Guatemala Hungary Italy Japan Poland Portugal Singapore
South Korea Switzerland Thailand Turkey Ukraine Vietnam

Oxford is a registered trade mark of Oxford University Press
in the UK and in certain other countries

Published in the United States
by Oxford University Press Inc., New York

© Oxford University Press, 2009

British Library Cataloguing in Publication Data

Data available

Library of Congress Cataloging in Publication Data

Data available

Typeset in Minion by Cepha Imaging Private Ltd., Bangalore, India
Printed in Great Britain
on acid-free paper by
The MPG Books Group

ISBN 978-0-19-953-9352 (hbk.)

10 9 8 7 6 5 4 3 2 1

Contents

Preface

This book concerns flavour – what we experience when we eat and drink – and more broadly, the flavour system, that is all of the senses and related processes that contribute to successful food choice in humans. The book approaches flavour and the flavour system from a psychological standpoint, with reference to underlying neural processes where relevant. The book is organized around three themes. First, to provide an overview of the literature. This has not been attempted before on this sort of scale, and so the book brings together many diverse streams of research into one place for the first time. Second, to provide a theoretical overview of flavour and the flavour system, with special attention paid to learning and memory, multisensory processing and binding. Third, throughout the book, attempts have been made to focus on function, especially as it relates to ingestive behaviour. Hopefully, the book will fill a much-needed gap in the broader literature on human ingestive behaviour as well as stimulating further study in flavour psychology and neuroscience.

In writing this book, I would like to start by thanking my old school for initially igniting my interest in food. The meals provided were so singularly revolting that even a quarter of century later thinking about them is sufficient to induce disgust. More importantly, I would like to thank: my colleagues Dr Trevor Case, Prof Martin Yeomans, Prof Bob Boakes, Prof Don Wilson, Dr Laurie Miller, Dr John Prescott, Dr Megan Oaten and Dr Caroline Tomiczek for their help and support at different times; the Australian Research Council for their financial support for much of my work on flavour; Dolly Mittal for helping me with the references; and of course my family, Caroline, Lucy, Harry and Gemma – and Chris and Mike Thomas – who have had to put up with a very distracted person over the last year. Finally, I would like to thank all the people at OUP who have made this book possible, especially Martin Baum, Carol Maxwell and Helen Hill, and the team at CEPHA Imaging Private Ltd.

Chapter 1

Introduction

Flavour and its function in omnivores

There are many potential sources of nutrients available in the environment. Some are harmful, even lethal, and whilst others may be harmless, they can vary markedly in nutrient content. Under the strong selection pressure imposed by making poor dietary choices, omnivores have evolved a powerful series of interlocking mechanisms to guide this process. Here, these mechanisms are referred to as the flavour system. The flavour system is composed of all of the senses and processes that are directed at the overarching goal of optimizing food choice.

The exteroceptive senses of vision, audition, and orthonasal (via sniffing) olfaction form part of the flavour system. These senses are instrumental in locating and identifying food in the environment and in determining its likely post-ingestive consequences. Once a decision has been made to place a food in the mouth, the interoceptive senses of taste, oral somatosensation (including touch, temperature, and irritation) and retronasal (via the nasopharynx) olfaction, come to the fore. Taste and somatosensation are capable of detecting particularly harmful features of a food, notably bitter tastes (poisons), certain textures (choking hazards), and pain (tissue damage). Information from these three interoreceptive senses are combined to form an emergent property—flavour—and unfamiliar flavours are learned. As consumption of a food progresses, its flavour becomes less appealing, promoting dietary variety as well as regulating intake prior to the onset of gut-based satiety signals. After eating is complete, the delayed consequences of a meal—its satiating value (if it was energy dense) or the nausea and vomiting it produced (if it was a poison)—may become associated with the food's flavour. This learning, of both the flavour itself and of its delayed consequences, is utilized by the exteroceptive senses in future ingestive decisions. Further food intake following a meal is then regulated, in part, by the state of repletion, which can temporarily reduce the appeal of food and its flavour. This summary encapsulates the various functions of the flavour system, all of which contribute to optimizing the intake of safe and nutritious food. Understanding the nature of this flavour system in humans, and especially its psychological basis, is the principal aim of this book.

Themes and organization of the book

The interoceptive and exteroceptive senses that contribute to the flavour system do not function independently. For example, colour can affect the way participants perceive flavour; the sound that accompanies eating certain foods can alter perception of texture; and certain odourants can affect participants' perception of taste and vice versa. Such interactions are important for two reasons. First, of all areas of flavour psychology, interactions within and between the flavour senses have been studied in the most depth (see Delwiche 2004, Keast *et al.* 2004), so this forms a logical starting point for the book. Second, and more importantly, examining these interactions reveals much about the flavour system, with respect to function, learning, and the cognitive penetrability of flavour and its component senses. For these reasons Chapter 2 reviews this literature, focussing on interactions both within and between the senses that compose the flavour system, and, where possible, partitioning interaction effects into those with a central/psychological cause and those with a peripheral basis (e.g. receptor-based interactions, etc).

The distal and proximal causal basis of the centrally based interactions identified in Chapter 2, are the focus of Chapter 3. A key conclusion of Chapter 3 is that several forms of interaction are a *side effect* of prior flavour learning— learning that is directed towards two specific goals. The primary goal is *future* food selection and this can manifest in two ways. First, the exteroceptive olfactory system recovers flavour memories, so aiding detection and recognition of nutritious and safe food in the environment. This is a perceptual process that allows the orthonasal olfactory system to predict, based upon past flavour experiences, what something will probably 'taste' like if it were to be placed into the mouth. Second, the visual system draws upon semantic memory to identify food and its likely flavour. This recollective process can lead to the formation of, often overt, expectancies about the likely flavour a food will have. A further (and, as will become apparent, a related) goal is to enable the brain to recognize *departures* from prior experience with a particular flavour (e.g. an off-taste, a slightly different flavour, etc), when it is experienced in the mouth. All of these processes can, under appropriate circumstances, produce interactions of the sort described in Chapter 2.

Chapter 4 examines the apparent duality of flavour perception. Flavour appears to be an example of a preservative emergent property (see Kubovy & Van Valkenburg 2001). That is, flavour can be experienced as a unitary percept (e.g. Auvray & Spence 2008, Lawless 1995, Small & Prescott 2000) or as a series of parts. Encoding flavour as a unitary percept is important because the *whole* flavour can then be accessed by the orthonasal olfactory system to assess the likely palatability and flavour of a food *before* placing it in the mouth. This represents a key functional benefit of generating a unitary percept. However, putting food in the mouth affords the last chance to reject it prior to it entering the body proper. From a functional perspective, there are good biological reasons for maintaining an ability to detect the parts of a flavour—notably tastes and textures. Indeed, there is good evidence that even naïve participants can readily extract taste and somatosensory information from flavour. The ability to extract olfactory components is rather different, and this results from smell's reliance on pattern recognition as a perceptual processing strategy.

Chapter 4 also examines a related issue, namely the nature of expertise within particular flavour domains, as it applies to wine and beer, and the sensory evaluation of food by trained panels. An important conclusion here is that flavour expertise, irrespective of domain, requires three things: semantic knowledge about the domain, perceptual knowledge accrued through experience with that domain, and extensive cross-linking between these two forms of knowledge. This can be viewed as an extension of the processes that all humans require to make successful food choices.

Arguably, the most salient feature of the flavour system is its capacity to generate affective states, and this is examined in Chapter 5. The hedonic aspects of flavour can be readily integrated into the broader flavour system outlined above. A key component of flavour hedonics is plasticity. From infancy onwards, humans acquire a steadily growing body of knowledge about food—both semantic and perceptual/affective (note the parallel to 'expertise' above). This knowledge informs our hedonic reactions to food when it is detected and examined by the exteroceptive senses of vision and olfaction. Whilst we retain innate hedonic reactions to certain taste and somatosensory stimuli, even these can be heavily influenced by experience, allowing us to enjoy, e.g. the burning sensation produced by chilli pepper.

Flavour can also become associated with pleasant or unpleasant affective states. These states may be delayed—such as sickness from food poisoning or the state of pleasant repleteness following a large meal—or immediate, such as the pleasant sweetness of sugar or an unpleasantly bitter taste. The information acquired by this hedonic learning is again utilized in future ingestive decision making. Finally, flavour hedonics plays a role in regulating food intake, via homeostatic and non-homeostatic mechanisms.

It is possible to conceive of flavour in several ways; as a multimodal object, a sensory system, a unique sense in and of itself, and a set of discrete senses bound together by centrally mediated processes. Chapter 6 deals with these, and related theoretical issues, whilst also providing a more detailed, functional overview of flavour as a sensory system. Flavour is clearly multimodal, but where does one draw the boundary? After all, visual and auditory stimuli influence flavour perception, so are they part of a flavour sense? One way of navigating around these issues is to regard all of the senses that contribute to flavour, as part of the flavour system (as done so far…), but to retain the term 'flavour' for the stimulus experienced in the mouth.

For flavour psychology, a problem of central interest is that of binding or multisensory integration. That is, how do the mind and brain take anatomically discrete sensory input and generate the unitary experience of flavour? Not only is this a central problem for the study of flavour, it is a central problem for psychology and neuroscience in general, and all of the data from earlier chapters are brought to bear on this problem. This is not the only binding problem. An additional one, and one unique to flavour, is the ability of the orthonasal olfactory system to recover and integrate a currently experienced smell, with the flavour it was once a part of (this is termed redintegration). Not only is this a unique binding problem, in that taste and somatosensory experience can become attributed to the olfactory system, it also has similarities to the rare neurodevelopmental synaesthesiae (e.g. seeing the stimulus A and experiencing A). A central component of both of these binding problems is the distinction between orthonasal and retronasal olfaction. The nature of this distinction—again unique amongst the sensory systems—and its role in binding are examined in Chapter 6.

Two additional conceptual problems are also examined here. The first of these concerns flavour perception in the mouth as a form of multisensory processing. At first glance, flavour would appear to be a paradigmatic case of the latter, until one starts to question the functional benefit of multisensory processing in this *context*. As argued in Chapter 6, the functional benefits of multisensory processing of flavour occur primarily in the future (with two notable exceptions discussed in Chapter 3: creaminess and auditory–tactile interactions), not in the present as is typically the case (i.e. where multisensory processing assists identification or detection, or facilitates appropriate responding, *now*). A second problem concerns that of regarding a food's flavour as a multisensory object. Based upon contemporary definitions of objecthood, namely figure–ground discrimination, it would appear that flavour does not readily fit this definition. The implications of this are examined.

Chapter 7 explores some of the broader theoretical and practical implications that arise from this book. Key theoretical issues concern flavour hedonics, and the concepts of wanting and liking, as well as the implications of orthonasal flavour redintegration for the study of neurodevelopmental synaesthesia and vice versa. Two related issues concerning the functional goal of multisensory processing and the orthonasal/retronasal distinction, especially as it applies to the two binding problems examined in Chapter 6, are also discussed. Practical implications concerning the role of the flavour system in obesity, malnutrition in the elderly, and the optimization of flavour expertise are also reviewed, alongside recent methodological advances that may be important for future developments in the field. The final part of Chapter 7 explores some of the future directions that flavour research in psychology and the neurosciences might take, focussing on interactions between the senses, the role of attention, the nature of binding, and the orthonasal/retronasal distinction and hedonics.

Before getting started, the remainder of this chapter provides a brief introduction to three areas that form a necessary background for what is to follow. The first concerns the nature of the stimulus—food and drink. Whilst many readers will have a background in biology, chemistry, or food science, many will not and so a brief introduction to some basic concepts in relation to the 'flavour' stimulus is included. A similar consideration led to the incorporation of two further introductory sections. One provides a summary of basic oral anatomy, and the processes involved in mastication and swallowing. The other provides a brief overview of the sensory physiology and psychology of each of the interoceptive flavour senses—smell, taste, and somatosensation.

The flavour stimulus—food and drink

Food and drink have two basic features. These are their chemical composition and their bulk properties (i.e. the physical characteristics of the food as a whole). Looking first at chemical composition, this can be considered to have three important aspects. The first concerns chemical components that are volatile, typically organic in nature, which can be detected by the human olfactory system. Such volatile agents usually have an atomic mass less than 300 Da, as well as being sufficiently soluble to diffuse across the olfactory mucosa (Ohloff *et al.* 1991). These volatiles are principally drawn from nine functional groups of organic molecule, as detailed in Table 1.1.

An important characteristic of most foods is that they have a very large number of different volatile components. Whilst a small subset may be sufficient to capture something approximating the original 'natural' food aroma, the whole combination is typically necessary to produce a well-rounded flavour (i.e. referring here, of course, to the olfactory component of flavour). Table 1.2 provides some examples, taken from Maarse (1991), that illustrate the typical chemical complexity of food and drink—even those with an

Table 1.1 Main functional groups from which detectable volatile chemicals are drawn, including examples and the foods in which they occur

Functional group	Example	Characteristic food flavour
Alcohols	Menthol	Peppermints
Lactones	Gamma decalactone	Peach
Aldehydes	Benzaldehyde	Almonds
Terpenes	Thymol	Thyme
Thiols	Grapefruit mercaptan	Grapefruit
Amines	Trimethylamine	Fish
Esters	Isoamyl acetate	Banana
Ethers	Eugenol	Cloves
Ketones	Acetyl pyrroline	Fresh bread

apparently 'simple' flavour. Whilst many component volatiles occur at low concentrations, even this does not rule out their contribution to flavour, as many such agents may combine together to produce a detectable odour even if the individual constituents are below the threshold of detection (e.g. Laska & Hudson 1991). An additional source of complexity is provided by the interactions that may occur between these multiple chemical constituents on the olfactory epithelium and at the receptor level too.

Table 1.2 Number of different volatile chemicals identified in several foods (data obtained from Maarse 1991)

Food	Number of different volatile chemicals
Coffee	790
Tea	541
Baked potato	259
Bread	296
Crispbread	90
Tomato	385
Banana	225
Chicken (cooked & heated)	381
Cheddar cheese	213
White wine	644

A second aspect of the chemical composition of foods is the non-volatile components. These include most of the agents that are perceived as tastes. Whilst they represent a relatively limited *perceptual* set (bitter, sour, sweet, salty, proteinaceous [umami], and possibly, some others), they reflect a much larger group of potentially taste-inducing chemicals. A further class here are the agents that activate the somatosensory system, namely certain chemical irritants. Of course, many volatile agents (i.e. detectable by the olfactory system) are also irritants (e.g. menthol in Table 1.1), but several that are important commercially, such as capsaicin (from the chilli pepper), are not (or at least are not detectable by the olfactory system).

The third chemical aspect of food concerns its nutritional components. These can be subdivided into the macro- and micronutrients, the latter including certain elements required for normal bodily functions (e.g. sodium, chlorine, calcium, etc) as well as the vitamins. Turning to the macronutrients, the flavour system has been shaped to detect certain characteristic macronutrients (and, of course, the key micronutrients sodium and chlorine, as salt [and possibly calcium, too]). There are three main chemical groups of macronutrients: fats, carbohydrates, and proteins. Fats are the most energy-dense chemical nutrient, in that they contain more energy per gram (38 KJ/g), than carbohydrates or proteins (both at 17 KJ/g). Ethanol might also be included here as an additional energy source at 30 KJ/g, but it is not usually consumed for this purpose. Fats come in several forms. The two principal types of dietary fats are the saturated (typically solid at room temperature) and the unsaturated (typically liquid at room temperature).

The most important energy source for the body is the carbohydrates. These also come in two principal forms, the simple (namely various forms of sugar) and the complex (of which the starches are the most important). Humans can not digest some forms of complex carbohydrates that are used as energy sources by other animals (e.g. herbivores), notably cellulose, but this still is of some dietary significance as 'roughage'. The final macronutrient group are the proteins, some of which must be provided in the diet, and some of which can be synthesized by the body. The macronutrients serve to provide the body with energy—all three can fulfil this role, although carbohydrates can be regarded as the primary energy source, with fats second. Fats and proteins fulfil a much large range of functions, all of which are essential for routine maintenance of the body.

The bulk properties of food can be categorized at a most basic level by whether the food is solid, semi-solid, or liquid. Perhaps, the most important property of liquid foods, and to some extent semi-liquid foods, is their viscosity (Kokini 1985). Viscosity can be loosely defined as the thickness of a liquid food; honey and porridge being highly viscous, soy sauce, milk, and water, being, in contrast, of low viscosity. Viscous foods resist being stirred or put more formally, sheered. In fact, the viscosity of a food that is *being sheered* will often change, and very few foods demonstrate consistent viscosity with increasing sheer rate—so-called Newtonian behaviour (examples of the latter include milk, sucrose solution, alcohol, and tea). Most liquid foods demonstrate sheer thinning—where the fluid becomes less viscous following shaking or stirring. Tomato ketchup and whipped cream are two such examples. Many semi-liquid foods behave in a similar manner.

Solid foods have a number of important physical properties, the key ones of which are illustrated in Figure 1.1 (see Lucas *et al.* 2002 for review). Here, the effect of force (applied by the teeth) results in varying degrees of deformation that is dictated by the stiffness of the food. A food's hardness reflects the force necessary to start it cracking, either completely, resulting in the formation of two parts, or intermittently and progressively, as with more brittle food. The area under the force/defamation line (delimited by the point of breakage, indicating the food's hardness) represents how 'tough' the food is.

A final feature, of all foods—but particularly liquid and semiliquid ones—is consistency, which can vary between smooth and granular, depending upon the size and presence of particulate matter (e.g. Engelen *et al.* 2005). Consistency

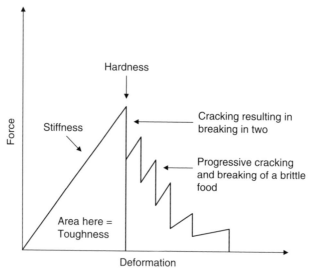

Fig. 1.1 Key bulk properties of solid foods (adapted from Dobraszczyk & Vincent 1999).

can also vary by its homogeneity (e.g. ice cream containing brittle chunks of chocolate or biscuit). Studies of terms used to describe the physical characteristics of foods (Kokini 1985, Szczesniak 2002) suggest three basic dimensions to food texture that approximately match the properties described above: mechanical-related (notably hardness), geometrical-related (notably grittiness), and chemical-related (notably fattiness). Interestingly, these also correspond with the three psychophysical dimensions of soft–hard, rough–smooth, and elastic–inelastic, derived from somatosensory qualities of objects felt by the hand (Hollins *et al.* 1993).

Oral anatomy, mastication, and swallowing

Active ingestion starts with the placing of food into the mouth or by biting a piece off with the incisors (sculpting). Food, if solid, is moved by the tongue to the teeth, small items being dealt with by the incisors. As the food fragments, it is rhythmically chewed by the molars, further reducing particle size. During this process, saliva is secreted into the mouth from three main sources; the sublingual glands under the tongue, the submandibular glands near the angle of the lower jaw, and the parotid glands beneath each ear (Wilkinson *et al.* 2000). Saliva has several functions, including lubrication, facilitating taste perception, initial digestive functions for fats and starches, antimicrobial activity, and buffering against the acidity generated by oral microorganisms. There are considerable individual differences in both salivary volume and masticatory behaviour.

The secretion of saliva also acts to assist—at least for solid food—the formation of a bolus, this being shaped by the tongue (Heath & Prinz 1999). The series of events, which then leads to a swallow, starts to unfold. This is very carefully orchestrated, as the close proximity of the opening of the trachea and oesophagus carries significant risks for choking (e.g. recall President G.W. Bush and the pretzel). Indeed, Wilkinson *et al.* (2000) suggest that the dislike for stringy, doughy, and slimy food (pretzels aside) may be a consequence of the greater risk they pose for choking.

The stages involved in swallowing food involve both voluntary and involuntary components. Outside of eating and drinking, most swallowing (which occurs about once per minute) is involuntary. During eating, the decision to *start* the swallowing process is voluntary, but once the food bolus is moved to the back of the mouth the process comes under involuntary control (Dodds 1989). The first stage is velopharyngeal closure (see Figure 1.2), preventing the bolus from lodging in the posterior nares. Pharyngeal peristalsis then moves the bolus to the top of the oesophagus, after which the larynx closes (see Figure 1.2). The sphincter at the top of the oesophagus then opens

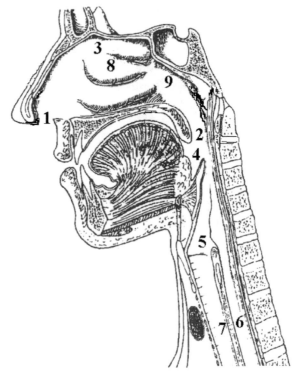

Fig. 1.2 Gross anatomy of the head in the sagittal plain, showing; 1. Anterior nares, 2. Posterior nares and velum (left) 3. Olfactory epithelium (right), 4. Epiglottis (right), 5. Larynx, 6. Oesophagus, 7. Trachea, 8. Nasal conchae and, 9. Nasopharynx (adapted from Buettner *et al.* 2001, Figure 2).

and oesophageal peristalsis propels the bolus to the stomach. This is then followed by an exhalation of breath.

A question of considerable importance concerns the process by which volatile chemicals are presented to the olfactory epithelium via the posterior nares and nasopharynx (see Figure 1.2). Velopharyngeal closure of the posterior nares can produce an airtight seal, preventing the ascent of volatiles to the olfactory mucosa (Buettner *et al.* 2001). In the case of liquids placed in the mouth, MRI scans reveal that the only time the velopharyngeal flap opens is when the person exhales immediately following a swallow (Buettner *et al.* 2002). As other studies with liquid foods now indicate, post-swallow exhalation provides one route by which volatiles (some picked up from food deposits left in the back of the mouth after swallowing) reach the olfactory mucosa via the posterior nares (Trelea *et al.* 2008).

For solid foods, and indeed for any foods that involve some degree of mastication, there is an additional pathway that is independent of swallowing. Rhythmic chewing acts to pump volatiles out of the mouth and into the airstream generated by exhalation, providing frequent pulses of volatiles to the olfactory mucosa via the posterior nares (Hodgson *et al.* 2003). Several further points about this process are worth noting. First, there is considerable individual variation in both the patency of velopharyngeal closure and in the timing/frequency of its opening—except perhaps when the process of swallowing occurs reflexively. Second, the quantity of food in the mouth and its type (liquid or solid) may dictate both, the frequency of swallows and velopharygeal closure/opening, independent of swallowing. Third, it appears possible to learn to open or close the velopharyngeal flap. Fourth, the dynamics of this process are difficult to study naturalistically, and so it is likely that there will be further revision to the mechanics of this process, as techniques and approaches to study it are refined.

The interoceptive flavour senses—olfaction, gustation, and somatosensation

The purpose of this section is to present a brief overview of smell, taste, and oral somatosensory perception and their sensory physiology. Vision and audition also play significant roles in flavour perception, which are examined in detail in various parts of this book. For example, audition contributes to the perception of several textural attributes of food, whilst visual perception is especially important in decision making about food prior to ingestion and in deriving expectations of its likely flavour. However, it seems tangential to provide an introduction to these senses, as one can readily appreciate their role without it.

Olfaction

Chemical stimuli can reach the olfactory receptors in two ways (see Figure 1.2). First, by sniffing an odourant—orthonasal olfaction. Second, by the passage of odourants into the nasopharynx, via the posterior nares, during eating and drinking—retronasal olfaction. Whilst much will be said about the processing of these two forms of odourant delivery, for now it is sufficient to note that both result in volatile chemicals reaching the receptor cells embedded in the olfactory epithelium. Each receptor cell expresses only one type of G-protein coupled receptor, out of the 300 or so that humans are known to posses (Buck 2000). These are quite broadly tuned and responsive to a range of chemicals, so even a single agent can produce quite a complex pattern of activation across many receptor types. This activation pattern also has a significant temporal component of which more is discussed below.

The signal from olfactory receptor cells expressing the same G-protein coupled receptor converges on to broadly the same glomerulus, a structure located in the olfactory bulb. At least in mice, and also probably in humans, the number of glomeruli *broadly* reflect the number of G-protein receptor types. The glomeruli are arranged in a two-dimensional sheet. This arrangement is not random, as neighbouring glomeruli tend to have similar chemical sensitivities (note that the distribution of particular G-protein receptor types across the olfactory epithelium also shows evidence of spatial organization). The output from the glomerular layer is then composed of a spatial component, representing the pattern of activity across many different G-protein coupled receptors, and a temporal component, as these activity patterns change due to various interactions at the receptor level.

This spatio-temporal output pattern forms the input to the primary and secondary olfactory cortex. However, it is not possible to understand olfactory processing (focussing here on orthonasal olfaction) without reference to the type of stimuli that it has to deal with and a clear focus on the functional goal of this system, namely, recognizing biologically salient chemical signals. These signals are complex (often chemical blends) and they have to be recognized against a continuously shifting chemical background (again chemical blends). To successfully achieve recognition, the olfactory system relies upon two primary processes. The first is rapid adaptation to background chemical stimuli, which is a cortical phenomenon (Sobel *et al.* 2000). For example, in rats, Kadohisa and Wilson (2006) reported that cells in the olfactory bulb responded in a similar manner to two chemicals presented simultaneously, and to two chemicals presented together *after* one had already been present for some time. In contrast, for the latter case, piriform cortex cells responded *only* to the appearance of the 'new' odour against the 'old' background odour, thus adapting (filtering) out background stimulation.

The second central process involved in olfactory perception is pattern recognition (Stevenson & Boakes 2003). This is achieved by comparing the output of the processing system above to a store of previously encountered glomerular patterns. If there is a match, then this results in a discrete olfactory percept. When there is not a match, the resulting percept is vague and ill formed, and the odour is hard to discriminate from other unfamiliar odours. The olfactory system, however, is capable of rapidly learning novel inputs, so that when this particular combination is encountered again, it is recognized and thus readily discriminated from other odours. It is important to note here that the processing strategy utilized by the olfactory system may result in a significant loss of information about the component chemicals that go to make up a particular signal (e.g. see Wilson & Stevenson 2003).

Whilst the olfactory bulb and piriform cortex are particularly important in these basic perceptual processes, the olfactory system involves a far more extensive network of neural structures and functions. Uniquely amongst the senses, it projects information directly to the neocortex—to the orbitofrontal cortex—as well as having a link to the latter structure via the mediodorsal nucleus of the thalamus (Ray & Price 1992). A large number of other structures also appear to be involved in different facets of olfactory processing, including the cerebellum, amygdala, insular, and the entorhinal/hippocampal region (Savic 2001, Zald & Pardo 2000). Functionally, these structures may be involved, respectively, in coordinating sniffing (arguably the functional equivalent of directed attention in olfaction), hedonics, and memory-related roles.

Gustation

The organs of taste perception are located on the upper surface of the tongue and, to a limited extent, on the soft palate, epiglottis, and oesophagus. The organ of taste perception is the taste bud. These occur as groups of buds organized into structures called papillae. Three types of papillae are found on the tongue. The most numerous are the fungiform—each containing relatively few buds and located most densely on the front part of the tongue. A further kind is the circumvallate papillae of which there are around 12. These have an appearance similar to a fried egg, and are located towards the rear of the tongue. The third kind is the foliate papillae. These are ridge like, occurring on the right and left sides, again towards the rear of the tongue. The functional significance of these three types of papillae is not currently known, although the high density of fungiform papillae on the anterior tongue, and the high sensitivity of this area to tastants, suggests two things. First, that the tip of the tongue may be used to test food *before* placing it in the mouth and second, to assist in the *immediate* detection of taste when a food is placed within the mouth (i.e. whilst the food can still be safely rejected). Perhaps, the circumvallate papillae provide a last chance to detect and reject bitter-tasting foods by provoking reflexive gagging.

Each taste bud is composed of somewhere between 50 and 100 taste-receptor cells. The taste-receptor cells extend microvillae into a small mucus-filled pit. Chemicals from food, dissolved in saliva, pass into this pit and then interact with the various taste receptors located on the microvillae. Each taste-receptor cell may be sensitive to multiple taste stimuli (Rawson & Li 2004). Taste cells deploy three primary methods of chemoreception. G-protein coupled receptors are employed to detect stimuli that yield sweet, bitter, and umami (proteinaceous taste) percepts, (Smith & Margolskee 2001, Bellisle 1999). A combination of ion channels and paracellular pathways are utilized to detect stimuli that yield sour and salty percepts, (Rawson & Li 2004, Neta *et al.* 2007). Whilst the range of adequate stimuli for the ion channel and paracellular pathways is limited, there are a large number of stimuli that can bind to the receptors responsible for detecting sweet and bitter (and to a lesser extent, umami) tastes.

There may be only one multifaceted receptor for sweet (capable of detecting several chemically different functional groups). However, there may be as many as 30 different receptors that yield a bitter percept, reflecting the cost associated with failing to detect what may be a poison (Parry *et al.* 2004). Two further possible additions need to be considered. Studies on rodents suggest that they can detect fatty acids via taste-based receptors, and there is preliminary evidence for a similar capacity in humans (Chale-Rush *et al.* 2007). More recent animal studies also suggest the possibility of calcium detection, but there is no evidence for this in humans as yet.

Following depolarization of taste-receptor cells, signals pass to: (1) the chorda tympani and greater superior petrosal branches of the facial nerve, which innervates the front two-thirds of the tongue and the soft palate; (2) to the lingual branch of the glossopharyngeal nerve for the rear third of the tongue; and (3) to the superior laryngeal branch of vagus nerve for the epiglottis and oesophagus. Information is then relayed to the nucleus of the solitary tract in the brainstem, and then to the ventroposteromedial nucleus of the thalamus (Pritchard *et al.* 1986). From here, projections are made to primary taste cortex—the insular (Faurion *et al.* 1999), as well as to a variety of subcortical structures, the lateral hypothalamus and the amygdala (see Bermudez-Rattoni 2004, Simon *et al.* 2006).

It has been suggested that intensive processing may be based in the insular with recognition of taste quality evoking additional activity in the anteromedial temporal lobe, especially the amygdala (Small *et al.* 1997a). The insula also projects to a secondary taste area—the orbitofrontal cortex. The manner in which the brain utilizes information from receptors to generate a specific taste quality is still the subject of debate. It almost certainly involves a combination of labelled lines, i.e. neural pathways that appear to be differentially sensitive to one taste quality over another, as well as drawing upon the pattern of activity across multiple fibres. The precise way in which both of these forms of coding interact to produce the final taste percept is not currently known.

Somatosensation

Somatosensation in the mouth and related structures can be organized into three subsystems, based upon physiology and functional goals. Physiologically, this classification is imperfect because many receptors involved in different facets of somatosensation overlap (e.g. sensitivity to warm temperatures, thermal pain, low pH, and the irritant capsaicin rely upon the same receptor)— hence, the need to consider function. An additional complication is the involvement of kinaesthetic input and proprioceptive feedback in generating 'touch' (making food texture)-related sensations, i.e. the perception of food texture an explorative process. This involves integrating static and active feedback from muscles, tendons, and joints, when engaged in holding and manipulating food, with tactile-receptor input from organs located in the hard and soft palate, tongue, and gums (Christensen 1984, Brown *et al.* 1994).

The first oral somatosensory subsystem functions to detect the tactile qualities of food in the mouth. Physiologically, this involves two components (Guinard & Mazzucchelli 1996). First, there are mechanoreceptors located near the surface of the mouth, in the lips, tongue, etc. In these tissues, there are five types of mechanoreceptor that are believed to be involved in generating tactile sensation: (1) Pacinian and (2) Meissner corpuscles, both of which are rapidly adapting and thus sensitive to stimulus onset and offset—these may be responsible for signalling velocity of deformation of the soft oral tissue by food. In contrast, (3) Merkell cells and (4) Ruffini cylinders are slow to adapt and discharge for the duration of a particular stimulus. These are useful for signalling the location of stimulation in the mouth. An additional receptor, (5) the Krause end bulb, is rather specific to the mouth, and is sensitive to low-frequency vibration, whilst the Pacinian corpuscles are sensitive to higher-frequency vibration. The density of receptors in the mouth and the large area of the sensory homunculus (in the somatosensory cortex) devoted to processing this information make this area second only to the fingertips, in terms of sensitivity to tactile stimuli.

The other components to this tactile subsystem are the organs located in the muscles, tendons, and joints of the mouth, which sense the static position and dynamic movement of the jaws, tongue, and teeth. The two key receptor types here are the muscle spindles, which are sensitive to the velocity of stretching, and the Golgi tendon organs, which are responsive to changes in tension. Information from these receptors is actively used to modulate chewing (Bosman *et al.* 2004). More importantly here, it is this information, in combination with input from the five types of mechanoreceptor described above, that ultimately gives rise to oral tactile perception.

The second subsystem concerns the detection of thermal and certain types of chemical stimulation (chemaesthesis). There is considerable overlap between the ability to detect thermal and chemical stimulation and the ability to perceive thermal and chemically induced pain (Jordt *et al.* 2003). Both thermal and chemical sensitivity depend upon a further type of receptor, the free nerve ending.

These originate from either the fast-conducting A δ fibres or the slow-conducting unmyelinated C fibres. Both are distributed throughout the tissues of the mouth and especially around the base of each taste bud. Importantly, some of these free nerve endings are polymodal, whilst others contain more specialized receptors (Green 2004). An important discovery in this regard was of a family of receptors known as the transient receptor channels (these may also play a role in detecting certain cations and anions indicative of salt and acid tastants). One such receptor, known as TRPV1, has an activation threshold of around 42°C that corresponds to the onset of thermal pain. This receptor is also sensitive to the oral irritant capsaicin. Several other members of this family have also been identified, with different thermal and chemical sensitivities, including TRMP8, which responds to thermal stimuli in the 10–25°C range and to menthol.

A further class of receptor, the two-pore domain channel, may be involved in cold sensitivity. It is likely that the perception of oral chemical and thermal sensation, involves the interaction between receptors and signalling systems that are focussed on detecting tissue damage *and* in monitoring departures from thermal neutrality (i.e. body temperature). Note, however, that in Chapter 2, thermal and irritant stimuli are treated separately (in contrast perhaps to their underlying physiology), simply because they have discrete stimuli and are, typically, treated separately in the literature. There is also considerable interaction between the tactile and thermal/chemaesthetic subsystems. This has major functional significance, most notably in the attribution of thermal sensation; either to an object (e.g. picking up a hot potato) or to the skin (e.g. radiant heat). Finally, the third subsystem concerns the detection of thermal, mechanical, or chemical stimuli that produce tissue damage. This is detected by the free nerve endings and results in a distinct sensation—pain.

Transmission of neural information from receptors to the brain, for all of these subsystems, is mainly accomplished by the trigeminal nerve, with a lesser contribution from the facial, glossopharyngeal, and vagus nerves. Sensory information, from the trigeminal and the latter three nerves, converges in the main trigeminal nucleus in the brainstem, whilst pain information converges in the spinal trigeminal nucleus. Both then project to the thalamus. For sensory information, this is projected solely to the ventral posterior nucleus, whilst pain information projects to several locations in the thalamus, including the ventral posterior, ventromedial, and dorsomedial nuclei. From the thalamus, sensory information then travels to the post-central gyrus of the parietal lobe, namely, primary somatosensory cortex. Pain information also converges here, as well as to other sites including the insular and cingulate cortices. Finally, the way in which the brain utilizes the receptor information to generate a textural (thermal or pain) percept is not well understood, at least as it pertains to the mouth. It is tempting to suggest that it will likely share similarities with taste, in utilizing a combination of labelled lines and pattern-recognition approaches. Part of the reason for suggesting this is that, as detailed in Chapter 4, participants appear able to discern relatively specific parts of a somatosensory stimulus (i.e. there is a correspondence between the psychological 'parts' of texture and particular physical attributes of the stimulus)—as with taste perception, but not olfaction.

Chapter 2

Types of flavour interaction

Introduction

The aim of this chapter is to identify psychological interactions between the various senses that comprise the flavour system. The study of flavour interactions is, by far, the most extensive branch of flavour psychology (see Delwiche 2004, Keast *et al.* 2004) and so makes a good point of departure for what is to come later in the book. More importantly, the nature of the interactions have much to tell us about the functional goals of flavour processing, the mechanisms that may underpin them, and the probable limits of human flavour perception (e.g. it may never be possible to experience certain components of flavour). The approach taken here is a broad one, encompassing interactions both within and between the interoceptive flavour senses (somatosensation, taste, and smell), as well as the effect of the exteroceptive senses of vision and audition on flavour perception (i.e. the flavour system).

An interaction occurs when the response of a participant to a change in one parameter of a stimulus results in changes to their judgement of another. In other words, there is a lack of independence. Interactions may occur for stimuli that primarily affect just one sense or that involve multiple senses. The nature of the interaction can also vary, and this can be characterized as a hierarchy going from stimulus-based interactions to psychological (or centrally based) causes. Whilst stimulus-based interactions are important in their own right, they are a source of noise from the perspective of this chapter—a source that has to be understood and eliminated (or controlled for) so that psychological (or centrally based) interactions can be clearly identified.

At least three general types of peripheral interaction have been documented. First, the chemical constituents of a flavour may react with one another, either permanently forming covalent bonds, or temporarily via hydrogen bonds or van der Waals forces (van Ruth and Roozen 2002). Second, the bulk physical properties of the stimulus may affect the rate at which volatiles reach equilibrium in the airspace of the mouth or the speed with which tastants can reach receptors (de Roos 2003). Third, different chemicals may compete for the same receptor, affect the binding of other chemicals to that receptor, or otherwise influence the transduction process (e.g. Simons *et al.* 2002).

From the receptor upwards, we might identify two further classes of interaction. Both involve the central nervous system, but either with or without a conscious component. These are interchangeably referred to in this chapter as psychological or centrally based interactions.

The following section is organized, as far as possible, on a modality-by-modality basis, a logical approach that has been adopted by other comprehensive reviews of this material (Delwiche 2004, Keast *et al.* 2004). Where possible, evidence indicating the likely psychological basis of the interaction is provided, but unfortunately this has often not been fully determined. The data are organized first for each individual modality (i.e. taste, smell, somatosensation, etc.) where interactions between two or more stimuli from 'within' that modality are examined, with respect to the psychological dimensions of intensity (i.e. psychological magnitude) and quality (i.e. the type of qualia experienced). Binary combinations of flavour modalities (i.e. taste and smell, taste and somatosensation, smell and somatosensation, etc.) are then reviewed, followed by higher-order combinations. Finally, interactions involving vision and audition with the flavour modalities are examined.

Taste

It is unusual for a food to contain just one tastant. When two tastants are combined, three effects are typically observed. First, the overall intensity of the mixture will often be less than the sum of the mixture components (e.g. Bartoshuk 1975). This observation is not surprising because 'self-addition', that is doubling the concentration of a single tastant, would generally produce a similar outcome. This is because of compression, whereby increasing tastant concentration is not accompanied by an equal rate of increase in perceived intensity (i.e. an exponent of less than one in the psychophysical power function). Second, the component taste qualities of a binary mixture are often judged as less intense than when judged alone. Whilst this is broadly correct for moderate- to high-concentration mixtures, low-concentration mixtures may demonstrate enhancement (see Figure 6 of Keast and Breslin (2002) for an informative diagrammatic summary). Third, the suppressive effects within a particular mixture may be asymmetric, with one taste quality suppressed more than another (e.g. Schifferstein and Frijters 1990).

Relatively few studies have specifically explored the locus (i.e. central vs. peripheral) of interactive effects between pairs of tastants. Of those that have, the most elegant are those which make use of the split-tongue procedure (Gillan 1982, Kroeze and Bartoshuk 1985). If interaction effects are peripheral, then the intensity of the mixture applied to one side of the tongue should be different to the intensity of each component applied to a separate side of the tongue. This is because the latter condition will only reveal central effects as there can be no peripheral interaction because; (1) the two tastants are not in physical contact and (2) information from each side of the tongue does not converge until the thalamus (see Kroeze and Bartoshuk (1985) for a summary of the evidence for this claim).

Kroeze and Bartoshuk (1985) found clear evidence for both peripheral and central forms of suppression, but the findings were compound specific. That is, for quinine-salt mixtures, both peripheral and central effects combined to produce suppression of the bitter-taste intensity, whilst for quinine-sucrose mixtures central effects were dominant in accounting for suppression. A significant role for central processes has been suggested by several other investigations using alternate approaches to this problem (e.g. Bujas *et al.* 1995).

One finding that is undoubtedly clear is that, for binary mixtures of differing quality (e.g. bitter and sweet), participants generally have little trouble in judging the intensity of individual components of such mixtures (Bartoshuk 1977). This appears to be true across a range of studies using different stimuli, methodologies, and concentrations. Whilst the binary interactions noted above may act in a similar manner in the real world (e.g. adding sucrose to a lemon drink to reduce sourness) the characteristic 'qualities' of the individual components do not generally appear to be lost. They may be diminished or altered, but they are still detectable. There are, of course, exceptions to this. The presence of salt in bread would appear to be one such case in point. Bread does not taste appreciably salty, but bread without salt is very unpalatable. Salt appears to add to the overall flavour, without its own quality (saltiness) being overtly detectable.

Psychophysical studies of more complex taste mixtures are rare. Only one study has examined interactions amongst a four-component mixture of tastes, namely sweet (sucrose), sour (hydrochloric acid, HCl), bitter (quinine), and salty (salt; Bartoshuk 1975). Two findings emerged. First, these moderately intense stimuli were all judged less intense than their unmixed components, with the exception of the sour tastant, HCl. Second, whilst this suppression was clearly evident for each component—other than HCl—participants were readily able to judge the intensity of the individual components of the mixture, as Bartoshuk herself noted (Bartoshuk 1975, p.648). In sum, whilst tastes interact, often reducing each others perceived intensity, the component taste qualities are generally evident.

Smell

Odour mixtures share some broad similarities with taste mixtures. For judgements of overall intensity of binary odour mixtures, the intensity of the mixture is generally found to be less than the sum of the intensities of the parts, i.e. the mixture demonstrates hypoadditivity (e.g. Berglund and Olsson 1993, Cain *et al.* 1995). This probably occurs for a similar reason to that of taste—response compression. The specifics of this effect are, to some extent, odourant dependent, although the detail here is lacking because most investigations have used differing sets of odours.

The nature of the hypoadditivity varies, with some demonstrating what Cain and Drexler (1974) term compromise (i.e. the mixture intensity falls between the intensity of the strongest and weakest component) and others demonstrating partial addition, in which the mixture exceeds the intensity of the strongest individual component. One exception to hypoadditivity may occur when odourants, which are subthreshold alone, are presented in combination. In this case, the combination can become clearly detectable, and this either represents additivity or even hyperadditivity (Laska and Hudson 1991). Whilst this finding is somewhat peripheral to the focus here, it is worth mentioning because of its implications for the perception of ecologically valid odourants, which are typically composed of several hundred chemicals, many of which alone may not be detectable (see Chapter 1).

There have also been several studies examining the intensity of individual component qualities within binary mixtures. Typically, individual components are judged to be weaker than the intensity judgement of the single unmixed component (e.g. Moskowitz and Barbe 1977), but there are plenty of exceptions, especially where the components differ in perceived intensity (e.g. Cain and Drexler 1974). Indeed, in these cases one component may mask another. The peripheral or central nature of these effects has also been explored. There is a significant peripheral component to mixture suppression and the degree to which this occurs is probably odourant dependent (Bell *et al.* 1987, Laing and Willcox 1987). However, as with tastes, a central component has been identified for some cases of mixture component suppression (e.g. pinene and limonene). This has been observed using a procedure analogous to the split-tongue technique described above. When one component of an odour mixture is presented to the left nostril and the other to the right, simultaneously, 'some' binary mixtures still demonstrate component suppression (Laing and Willcox 1987). This effect has to be of central origin, as the left and right olfactory epithelia are not in direct physical contact.

Several investigators have examined the effect of mixtures on the perception of odour quality of each component. As with taste, the thorny issue of the nature of this perceptual experience (bluntly, whether it is analytic or synthetic) is postponed until the next chapter, where a broader evidence base is drawn upon. However, two general observations can be made about binary odour mixtures. First, as should be apparent from above (e.g. Cain *et al.* 1995, Cain and Drexler 1974, Moskowitz and Barbe 1977), individual components of similar intensity are generally detectable (there are of course exceptions, e.g. citral, a mixture of geranial and nerol, is perceived as a single entity). Second, Moskowitz and Barbe (1977) had participants' rate target and non-target qualities (e.g. (target) mintyness and (non-target) fruitiness for oil of wintergreen) for components and binary mixtures. Whilst the reported amount of the target quality decreased in nearly all cases (i.e. suppression), participants still judged the target quality to exceed non-target qualities.

Many of the conclusions above start to change as odour mixtures become more complex. Moskowitz and Barbe (1977) studied up to five component mixtures, examining overall intensity and the intensity of each target and non-target quality within the mixture. They found that hypoadditivity tended to become more marked as the number of components increased and that suppression of individual components, sometimes nearly total, became more common. Which odourant/s suppressed other odourant/s was quite idiosyncratic. Laing *et al.* (1994) conducted a similar study, but this time focussing solely on sewage-related odours. They too observed progressively greater hypoadditivity as they moved from two- to three- to four-component mixtures. Suppression of individual odourants was widespread, even though some odourants were more prone to this than others.

Somatosensory system

Interaction effects within the somatosensory system have received little attention. For oral tactile stimuli, there appears to be no psychophysical studies available, partly because of the difficulty involved in independently manipulating certain textural characteristics, the only exception being astringency. For temperature perception, the system itself is not really suitable for mixture studies 'within' this sub-modality, unless of course one subjected different parts of the mouth to different temperatures. For chemaesthetic stimuli, there has been some preliminary work, mainly for nasal pungency. Whilst there is only one study directly examining interactions between different oral irritants, there are a much larger number of studies that have examined sensitization/desensitization between irritants. The latter are informative in relation to receptor commonality (and therefore, are something to be studied with respect to neurophysiology), but they are less informative about the way that irritants interact during routine flavour perception. For this reason, they are not included in this section.

Studies of nasal pungency are complicated by the fact that most chemicals that induce nasal chemaesthesis (typically at higher concentrations) can also be detected by the olfactory system. Commetto-Muniz *et al.* (1989) reported that mixtures of ammonia and formaldehyde (which are both irritants and odourants) demonstrate hypoadditivity at low perceived intensities, additivity at moderate intensities, and possibly hyperadditivity at high intensities. They suggested that the hypoadditive component reflected the olfactory system, and that as concentration (and perceived intensity) increased the chemaesthetic system progressively cut in, producing the additive effects (and possibly hyper-additive effects) observed at higher concentrations. This interpretation was confirmed in a later study using the same stimuli, but where participants rated both, odour intensity and pungency (Cometto-Muniz and Hernandez 1990). Similar additive effects were also observed in anosmic participants, but this time for combinations of pungent odourants at threshold. Combinations of such odourants were additive, so that thresholds, e.g. for a combination of three pungent odourants, were around one-third their individual thresholds (Cometto-Muniz *et al.* 1997). Whilst all of these results pertain to the nasal cavity, it is not unreasonable to suggest that similar results for the chemaesthetic sub-modality might also be observed in the mouth.

Only one study has directly examined the effect of mixing oral irritants. Lawless and Stevens (1989) gave participants equi-intense mixtures of piperine (the pungent principle of black pepper) and capsaicin, at low, moderate, and high perceived intensities. As with nasal pungency, they observed near-perfect additivity for low and high perceived-intensity mixtures, whilst hyperadditiv-ity was observed for moderate perceived-intensity mixtures. The only other study which comes close to examining direct mixing of irritants came from the same laboratory. Participants were presented with 60-s exposure to one irritant followed by 60-s exposure to another—the irritants being capsaicin and piperine. When both irritants were matched for perceived intensity, Stevens and Lawless (1987) observed something approaching additivity, in that the second stimulus effectively added (though not perfectly) to the first. This effect was symmetrical and, as with the studies of nasal pungency, may reflect peripheral recruitment of additional receptors.

Astringency refers to a set of sensations that appear to rely primarily upon the somaesthetic sense (Breslin *et al.* 1993). Using four different astringent agents—alum, gallic acid, catechin, and citric acid (broadly representative examples of the various chemical classes that generate this sensation)—Lawless *et al.* (1994) found evidence for both, small additive and larger suppressive effects. These effects were compound specific and, at least for the suppressive effects, may have resulted from chemical reactions in the mouth between alum and gallic acid, and alum and citric acid, reducing their respective abilities to bind salivary proteins.

Taste and smell

The primary feature of unimodal interactions within taste or smell is that they are hypoadditive. That is, the reported intensity of the components almost always sums up to something less than their total. With mixtures of taste and smell, the picture is considerably less clear. Murphy *et al.* (1977) found that for mixtures of saccharin and ethyl butyrate (strawberry odour), judgements of overall intensity for retronasal smell and taste approximately summed to ratings of overall intensity. A follow-up study by Murphy and Cain (1980) obtained similar results using both—citral and sodium chloride, and citral and sucrose—suggesting that the findings from the original study did not depend upon some synergy between 'particular' taste and smell combinations. Several other studies followed. In contrast to these earlier findings, Burdach *et al.* (1984), Enns and Hornung (1985), and Hornung and Enns (1986), all observed hypoadditivity. This did not appear to result from the way the stimuli were delivered (e.g. orthonasal vs. retronasal perception), but from the form of rating used (i.e. modality specific vs. overall intensity). Overall intensity ratings of each component and the mixture resulted in additivity, and modality-specific ratings resulted in hypoadditivity (Hornung and Enns 1986). The reasons for this difference are not currently known.

The qualitative aspects of odour–taste mixtures have received extensive study, and they suggest that interactions do occur between taste and smell. This was first observed by Murphy *et al.* (1977), who reported that participants sampling citral by mouth reported significant levels of 'taste' intensity, an effect which disappeared when the nostrils were occluded preventing retronasal olfaction. A similar effect, albeit in the opposite direction, was reported by Calvino *et al.* (1990). They found that the addition of sucrose to coffee reduced participants' ratings of coffee flavour. Whilst this effect may have resulted from some interaction between sucrose (tastant) and coffee (as an odourant), the presence of caffeine (and hence bitterness) in the coffee may suggest a taste-based locus for this effect.

Several studies have reported that the presence of a tastant may affect olfactory qualities. Von Sydow *et al.* (1974) found that the addition of sucrose to fruit juice increased several attributes of the flavour that presumably have an olfactory basis (e.g. fruity, berry-like, sweet odour, aromatic, etc.), as well as suppressing others (e.g. pungent, vinegar-like, green, etc.). Similar effects of taste on olfactory qualities have also been reported, using both sucrose and citric acid (both increased the perceived fruitiness of orange; Bonnans and Noble 1993) and sucrose alone (increasing the fruitiness of peach; Cliff and Noble 1990). In all of these cases the effects were asymmetric, with the tastant affecting ratings of olfactory quality, but not the other way round.

Certain odourants also appear to influence the perception of tastants. Frank and Byram (1988) described how a mixture of sucrose and whipped cream was perceived to taste sweeter when strawberry odourant was added. This effect was odourant and tastant specific, in that adding peanut butter odourant did not affect sweetness ratings, whilst the presence of strawberry odourant did not affect saltiness ratings. Similar findings were reported by Frank et al. (1989), using water-based stimuli (rather than cream), and by Stevenson et al. (1999) and, Lavin and Lawless (1998) using many different odourants with sucrose or citric acid. Stevenson et al. (1999) also observed a qualitative suppression effect, whereby the presence of certain odourants acted to reduce participants' ratings of sourness for the tastant citric acid.

The basis for these qualitative interaction effects has attracted considerable attention. One obvious possibility is that the presence of certain tastants increases the release of volatiles from the fluid in which both the tastant and odourant are dissolved ('salting out'). Several investigators have looked for such effects and they have not been found—or at least they only occur with high concentrations of sucrose (e.g. Rabe et al. 2003—in excess of 20% sucrose). Von Sydow et al. (1974) and Murphy et al. (1977), both reported that the presence of the tastants sucrose and saccharin did not affect the quantity of volatiles present in the headspace when examined by mass spectroscopy (MS). Similarly, Pfeiffer et al. (2006) tested for the main components of strawberry odourant in all of their sucrose–acid–strawberry mixtures (using chemical ionization MS). Whilst they found no evidence of changes in volatiles as a function of the tastant present in the mixture, they observed significant effects of the tastants on the perception of strawberry flavour. Both, acids (e.g. citric acid) and sucrose, enhanced the reported strawberry flavour.

In a further study, in which volatile release was measured in a model throat, King et al. (2006) found that the chemical agents responsible for fruity/pear/candy notes—which had been enhanced by the presence of sucrose in a parallel judgement task—did not vary as a consequence of the presence of sucrose. This method was of sufficient sensitivity to predict reductions in ratings of green notes, as the model throat data suggested a physical reduction in the presence of such volatiles. Finally, Marsh et al. (2006) added sugars and acids to kiwi-fruit pulps, and examined the effects of this on the flavour profile. Sucrose increased judgements of banana notes, but it did not affect the headspace of the chemical agents responsible for this smell. It would seem unlikely, then, that physical alteration of volatile release by the presence of sugars, within the normal range used in experiments and food, is responsible for taste enhancement of olfactory qualities.

Certain odourants may be capable of stimulating taste receptors, giving them an actual taste and thus leading to (say) sweetness-taste enhancement.

This issue has also been thoroughly explored, mainly by presenting the odourant dissolved in water, by mouth, whilst the nostrils are pinched to eliminate retronasal perception. The question, then, is whether any stimulus can be detected under these conditions. Labbe *et al.* (2006) found that vanilla odourant enhanced the perceived sweetness of cocoa, but that this effect was eliminated when participants evaluated the same stimuli with a nose-clip. Almost identical findings have been reported by Murphy *et al.* (1977), Frank and Byram (1988), and Stevenson *et al.* (2000a). A related approach is to simultaneously present the odourant via the nares (i.e. orthonasally) whilst the tastant is presented to the mouth. Using vanilla and aspartame, Sakai *et al.* (2001) reported the same magnitude of sweetness-taste enhancement, irrespective of whether the odourant was presented orthonasally or retronasally. It appears that taste-enhancement effects can be obtained even when the odourant has little, if any, taste. Of course, this does not preclude the fact that certain odourants can induce taste sensations via stimulation of taste receptors, but this is clearly not a necessary condition.

A related question is whether pure tastants can smell, which might then result in enhancement of certain olfactory qualities. Pure tastants, such as sucrose, often contain small quantities of volatile contaminants, many of which can be detected by the nose (trying sniffing at a jar of ordinary white sugar after it has been sealed for several hours). These contaminants—probably present for all tastants, even those obtained after considerable purification, can be detected by purely olfactory means (Mojet *et al.* 2005) and these probably do make a small contribution to the effect of tastants on odourants. However, this is certainly not equivalent to the magnitude of the taste-induced odour-enhancement effects described above.

Based upon the discussion so far, it would appear that qualitative odour–taste interactions are a central, rather than a peripheral, phenomenon. To recap: a mixture say of strawberry odourant (with no taste) and sucrose (with no smell) may result in participants judging the sweetness of the mixture as stronger than the sweetness of an equivalent concentration of sucrose (and similarly for enhancement of fruitiness). Several investigators have suggested that two factors dictate the observation of these types of enhancement effects. The first is that the number of evaluations and their appropriateness are important in dictating whether such effects will be observed. Both Clark and Lawless (1994) and Frank *et al.* (1993) reported that multiple rating sets (i.e. rating sweetness and fruitiness in the above example of strawberry and sucrose) tend to diminish enhancement effects, whilst limited rating sets (i.e. just rating sweetness or just rating fruitiness) tend to produce enhancement. However, multiple- versus single-attribute ratings alone cannot explain all enhancement effects, as several studies have obtained them even when multiple and appropriate rating sets are employed (e.g. Labbe *et al.* 2006, von-Sydow *et al.* 1974). Moreover, one study has reported that odour–taste combinations may differ in their sensitivity to the effects of multiple, appropriate rating scales, with some still demonstrating enhancement effects even when such scale sets are employed (Valentin *et al.* 2006).

A second factor is that enhancement effects appear to depend upon the perceived similarity of the tastant and the odourant (e.g. van der Klaauw and Frank 1996, Schifferstein and Verlegh 1996). Accordingly, when an odourant (e.g. strawberry) and a tastant (e.g. sucrose) are perceptually similar (i.e. the strawberry is perceived to smell somewhat sweet—and sucrose, of course, is sweet too), then if a fruitiness rating is not present, participants will conflate the strawberry qualities (sweet/fruity) into a sweetness rating.

Two predictions can be derived from this two-factor account of odour–taste interaction effects. First, that where multiple 'inappropriate' response alternatives are provided (e.g. bitterness and sweetness, rather than fruitiness and sweetness), no loss of enhancement will occur. This has been confirmed (van der Klaauw and Frank 1996). Second, that where two stimuli are not perceptually similar, there will be little change in ratings between single and multiple rating sets. Some supportive evidence for this has been obtained in the taste domain, where mixtures of sucrose and quinine (highly dissimilar) are contrasted with citric acid and quinine (more similar). For these stimuli, varying the size of the rating set (using appropriate descriptors) significantly affects ratings for citric acid and quinine, but not for quinine and sucrose (Frank *et al.* 1993). Whilst these findings are supportive, they do not test odours and tastes and, given that suppression effects for sucrose and quinine are mediated to a significant degree (as described earlier) by peripheral interactions, one must wonder whether this is a good test of a process predicted to occur at a central level—a point the authors themselves make clear.

A more fitting test would employ odour–taste pairs. Frank *et al.* (1993) reported such a test, using lemon–quinine and almond–quinine mixtures, which are reported as differing in perceived similarity. However, they did not obtain any favourable evidence for their hypothesis, as the shift from single to multiple appropriate rating sets did not have a greater effect on the perceptually more similar pair. Perhaps this was not the most favourable test. Indeed, similarity ratings were not obtained from participants in the experiment, and the difference in similarity was by no means as large as that between sucrose and quinine and quinine and citric acid.

Finally, perceptual similarity is only one facet of any overall similarity judgement. Similarity judgements could equally rely upon either conceptual (i.e. 'knowing' that lemon is a pleasant accompaniment to (bitter) tonic water) or hedonic factors (i.e. if two things are disliked (or liked), then they may be judged similar on this characteristic). However, the latter at least may not be important. Schifferstein and Verlegh (1993) examined whether the pleasantness ratings of three types of odour–taste mixtures could account for the degree of sweetness enhancement. Pleasantness of the mixture could not account for the enhancement effect. In fact, the only variable that could significantly predict enhancement was the sweetness rating of the odourant.

Schifferstein and Verlegh's (1993) findings point again to the likely importance of perceptual similarity in generating enhancement effects over and above any effect produced by varying the rating scales employed. Indeed, Stevenson et al. (1999) found that participants' ratings of sweetness made orthonasally for a range of odourants, was the single best predictor of the degree to which these odours would enhance the sweetness of sucrose when presented retronasally in a mixture. This finding has recently been replicated. Valentin et al. (2006) obtained ratings of harmony, congruence, similarity, and smelled taste, of a set of odour–taste mixtures (or the orthonasal odour for smelled taste). The smelled taste and the similarity of the odour and the taste were the best predictors of odour-induced taste enhancement. To summarize, participants' ratings of odour sweetness likely reflect the perceptual similarity of the odour and the (sweet) taste, so that, under conditions where the rating set is held constant, enhancement is a function of perceptual similarity (i.e. greater similarity between odour and sweet taste = greater enhancement). A more compelling reason to suspect that perceptual similarity is important comes from findings outside of the domain of odour–taste interactions, namely data from learning and neuropsychological investigations, which are examined in the next chapter.

A further line of evidence for qualitative odour–taste interactions comes from employing an alternative approach reliant, instead, upon subthreshold additivity. If, e.g. an odour has a sweet smell, does the addition of a sweet taste make it easier to detect that smell? Of the five studies that have utilized this type of approach, all but one suggest that it does (the exception being Bingham et al. 1990). Dalton et al. (2000) tested participants' detection threshold for the sweet-smelling odourant benzaldehyde (almond/marzipan smell), both in saccharin and in water. Participants were able to detect benzaldehyde at a significantly lower concentration in saccharin. To test if this effect was taste specific, they repeated the experiment using monosodium glutamate (MSG) rather than saccharin, but MSG did not affect detection threshold for benzaldehyde (and see Delwiche and Heffelfinger (2005) for similar results). Finally, Pfeiffer et al. (2005) examined whether temporal synchrony was a necessary condition for taste-induced odour-threshold enhancement to occur.

They reported that the taste and smell have to be perceived simultaneously, for a detectable threshold-enhancement effect to occur, although individual differences between participants were clearly evident (see also Elgart and Marks (2006) who obtained favourable evidence for subthreshold integration of taste and smell, but with notable individual differences in performance).

A final type of interaction, which is related to those above, was reported by Davidson *et al.* (1999). Participants chewed gum flavoured with menthone and sucrose. Some participants served in trials in which saliva samples were obtained to estimate the amount of sucrose in the mouth. Other participants had the concentration of menthone reaching the nose recorded by *in vivo* measurement, and a trained sensory panel evaluated menthone sensations whilst chewing the gum. All three types of measure were obtained across time (see Figure 2.1). The results indicated that whilst menthone levels remained fairly constant over time, sucrose levels progressively declined. Most interestingly of all was the finding that menthone judgements (i.e. odour) tracked the decline in sucrose concentration—even though, as noted above, menthone concentrations did not change. There are at least two ways these data can be interpreted. One possibility is that participants conflate the odour and the taste. Davidson *et al.* (1999) suggest this is unlikely as they were a trained panel, but it is possible that, for certain odour–taste combinations, training

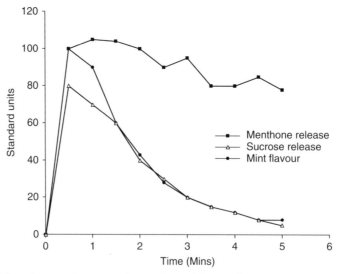

Fig. 2.1 Menthone and sucrose release, along with mint-flavour ratings across time using a chewing gum base. Adapted from Davidson *et al.* 1999.

may not improve the ability of participants to discriminate between the taste and olfactory components. A second possibility is that participants progressively adapt to the menthone, given the constant exposure to it over time.

In conclusion, qualitative perceptual interactions between taste and smell clearly occur, and they have a psychological basis. These interactions can be detected in several ways, notably by rating particular taste or olfactory qualities or by subthreshold additivity experiments. More specifically, these interactions may arise via perceptual similarity. Whilst the number and type of rating scales employed can clearly affect this form of interaction, it cannot explain subthreshold integration effects or the presence of enhancement effects when scale use is appropriately controlled (Valentin *et al.* 2006).

Taste and somatosensation

This section examines interactions between taste and irritant stimuli, taste and temperature, and taste and tactile stimuli.

Taste and irritant stimuli

Naive participants report that irritants, especially capsaicin, adversely affect their ability to 'taste' (Prescott and Stevenson 1995). Certain tastants could also affect perception of irritation. Indeed, sour and salty tastants are, especially at high concentrations, irritants as well as tastants, and so it would be surprising if they did not affect the perception of other irritants with fewer taste properties. In addition, sucrose has been found to have analgesic properties, and so this could act to reduce irritant (i.e. pain-like) sensations. This section starts by examining the effect of tastants on irritant perception, and then examines the effects of irritants on tastant perception.

Two irritants have been studied in depth—capsaicin and carbon dioxide. The latter produces irritation via the formation of carbonic acid on the tongue. For capsaicin, sucrose appears to exert a number of weak effects on participants' perception of irritation. Sizer and Harris (1985) found that threshold detection for capsaicin was elevated when the vehicle was sucrose. There was also a non-significant tendency for easier detection when the vehicle contained citric acid or salt. Both Nasrawi and Pangborn (1989) and Prescott *et al.* (1994) found that capsaicin irritation at suprathreshold levels could be reduced by the presence of sucrose, although this effect was neither large nor particularly consistent. Prescott *et al.* (1994) found that salt tended to enhance capsaicin irritation, but Nasrawi and Pangborn (1989) found no effect for either salt or citric acid. For carbonation, sucrose has been observed to suppress irritation, at high concentrations (Yau and McDaniel 1991b), but not at lower concentrations (Cometto-Muniz *et al.* 1987). Yau and McDaniel (1991b) also reported that citric acid enhanced irritation produced by carbonation, and

Cometto-Muniz *et al.* (1987) found a similar effect for the sour-tasting tartaric acid and for saline. They also noted that quinine tended to reduce irritation generated by carbonation at low carbon dioxide concentration and at high concentrations of quinine. A broad conclusion from these studies then (and one which may see some limited extension for other irritants such as zingerone (from ginger) and piperine) is that sucrose exerts a weakly suppressive effect on perceived irritation, which sour and salty tastants may enhance.

The basis for these effects is likely to be varied. For sucrose, viscosity is certainly a possibility, as Yau and McDaniel (1991b) found that aspartame, of equal sweetness, did not reduce irritation. This result would tend to argue against a central effect (e.g. analgesia) and, instead, suggest a peripheral effect based upon some impact that viscosity might have on the rate at which capsaicin reaches receptors. A further explanation might relate to dilution of the irritant by excess salivation, as sucrose is particularly effective at promoting salivation (Lyman and Green 1990). The enhancing effect of citric acid and salt may come from their ability to generate irritation, producing what in effect is a more concentrated irritant stimulus.

As described above, participants often report that irritants make it harder to perceive the 'taste' of food. Psychophysical studies of taste–irritant mixtures provide some support for this perspective, but *only* as it applies to true tastes, rather than odour–taste mixtures. Lawless and Stevens (1984) examined the effects of pre-rinses with capsaicin or piperine on perception of four tastants. Capsaicin reduced the perceived intensity of sucrose at high concentrations and citric acid and quinine at both high and low concentrations. It exerted no effect on salt. Piperine reduced the perceived intensity of all tastants at both high and low concentrations. Cowart (1987) found far less evidence of irritant–taste interactions, with no effects on sucrose or salt but some reduction for the bitter taste of quinine. Whilst Cowart (1987) used considerably weaker concentrations of capsaicin (2 vs. 60 ppm in the Lawless and Stevens (1984) study) which might have accounted for this difference in effect, her study also involved presenting the irritant and tastant simultaneously. Prescott *et al.* (1994) also used simultaneous presentation, but included higher capsaicin concentrations than Cowart (1987). They observed sweetness suppression, but no decrement in perception of saltiness. Prescott and Stevenson (1995) also observed a sweetness-suppressive effect of capsaicin, but no effect on the sour tastant citric acid.

A more recent study provides some closure to the varying effects described above. Simons *et al.* (2002) applied capsaicin (32 ppm) to one side of the tongue, and then applied tastants to the capsaicin-treated and non-treated sides. Participants had to judge on which side the tastant tasted stronger.

In their first experiment, they reported that sucrose and quinine were both judged to taste more intense on the non-treated side, with no effect for citric acid, salt, or monosodium glutamate (MSG). In further experiments, they observed that reducing the tastant concentration produced the same effect for quinine and sucrose, and also now for MSG. Reducing capsaicin concentration to 1.5 ppm yielded the same effects for sucrose and MSG, but not for quinine. These findings suggest, when considered with the others above, that sucrose is generally suppressed by capsaicin-induced irritation, with some evidence of the same effect for bitter-tasting quinine.

The effects of carbonation-induced irritation on taste perception are not so well explored. Cometto-Muniz et al. (1987) found no effect on the sweetness of sucrose, as with Yau and McDaniel (1991b). Both these groups reported that the sourness of tartaric and citric acid was enhanced by carbonation, and Cometto-Muniz et al. (1987) also found enhancement of saltiness, and that effects on bitterness were quinine-concentration dependent—with suppression at high concentrations and enhancement at low. Cowart (1998), however, found evidence for much more substantial effects of carbon dioxide on the perception of sucrose 'sweetness' (i.e. rating that quality, rather than the intensity, of the taste) with reductions in the order of 25%. Similar effects were observed for salt, with 33% reductions in saltiness relative to uncarbonated controls. Little effect was observed for citric acid or quinine, even though sucrose was judged as sourer tasting when carbonated. Apart from concluding that taste perception is affected by carbonation, the specifics of this effect have not been studied well enough to draw any general conclusions.

Several mechanisms have been suggested to account for capsicum's effects on taste, especially the sweet taste of sucrose. This matter was considered by Lawless and Stevens (1984, for all tastes), and they outlined several possible mechanisms. These included: (1) an attentional effect in which the most dominant aspect of the stimulus (i.e. the chilli burn) would detract from concentrating on the less dominant aspect, taste; (2) an effect of taste dilution produced by irritant-induced salivation; (3) neural inhibition of taste generated by concurrent irritation; (4) chemical interactions between the capsaicin and the tastant prior to receptor-tastant binding; (5) contractile response by the taste pore, reducing tastant entry to the receptors; and (6) recruitment of primarily taste-responsive neurons to carry trigeminal information. At least some of these possibilities can now be eliminated (Simons et al. 2002). Attention-based effects appear unlikely in the light of later findings in which capsaicin does not affect all tastes equally—a prediction that an attentional theory would make. Pore closure also appears unlikely, again because of the selective nature of the effect of capsaicin (i.e. not all tastes affected). Simons et al. (2002) favour a peripheral explanation, noting that the effects of capsaicin tend to be primarily upon tastants that rely upon G-protein coupled receptors (i.e. sweet and bitter) rather than on those relying upon ionic-based receptor channels.

Taste and temperature

Most research has concentrated on the effect of stimulus temperature on perception of various tastants. Sweet tastes have been extensively explored and there is a broad consistency across studies, with a modest increase in perceived sweetness above room temperature and decrease with cooler temperatures (e.g. Bartoshuk *et al.* 1982, Schiffman *et al.* 2000). Not all sweeteners appear susceptible to this temperature-related effect. Schiffman *et al.* (2000), although observing a small general trend for increased sweetness intensity with higher temperature (50°C), when compared to lower temperatures (6°C), did not find these effects for all sweeteners tested, and where these effects were observed, they tended to be for the high-potency sweeteners (e.g. aspartame).

Participants' ability to detect tastants, including sweeteners, has also been determined. The general conclusion here, irrespective of the tastant, is that detection sensitivity is best within the physiological range of temperatures (i.e. 20–40°C; McBurney *et al.* 1973, Paulus and Reich 1980, Pangborn *et al.* 1970).

Only two studies have examined the effect of actually heating or cooling the tongue to a specific temperature and then examining the effect of this on stimuli presented at the same temperature (Green and Frankmann 1987, Green and Frankmann 1988). Green and Frankmann (1987) found that tongue-temperature changes were the dominant factor in changed taste-intensity perception. Cold temperatures significantly reduced judgements of the sweetness of sucrose and the bitterness of caffeine, but had no effect on judgements of salty or sour tastants. Similarly, Green and Frankmann (1988) again observed that cooler temperatures led to reductions in sucrose sweetness, but this time they also observed an increase in sweetness following warming of the tongue. As with Schiffman *et al.*'s (2000) findings, the other sweeteners they tested did not always behave in the same way, e.g. saccharin was not affected by temperature, whilst aspartame was.

Whilst different methodologies must account for some of the observed discrepancies between studies, the effect of temperature on sucrose sweetness, albeit rather small, does appear to be a consistent observation. This may result from the fact that taste receptors themselves are thermally sensitive, especially perhaps sweetness receptors. To explore this, Cruz and Green (2000) examined whether changing the temperature of the tongue might actually generate sensations of taste. This was observed, with warming on the front of the tongue generating a sweet taste and cooling generating a sour/salty taste. These findings led

Green and colleagues to explore whether individual differences in the ability to perceive thermally induced tastes might relate to their ability to perceive tastes in general (i.e. as more or less intense) and this observation was borne out. Thermal tasters are more responsive to all basic tastants, i.e. they report them as more intense (e.g. Green *et al.* 2005). This finding suggests one possible explanation for the effect of temperature on taste perception, namely that warm temperatures can, in a proportion of participants, activate taste receptors, leading to detectable levels of taste sensation, which then add (or subtract) from the effect of an actual tastant in the mouth. So, e.g. with a warm sucrose solution, both the warmth and the sucrose will activate taste receptors, leading to a small increase in the perceived intensity of sweetness. This would suggest a likely peripheral basis for temperature–taste-based interactions.

Taste and tactile stimuli

Within the tactile domain, the principal areas of study have been between taste and viscosity, taste and 'hardness' (typically of gels and gums), with a few studies examining taste and astringency. Most of the work examining taste and viscosity has emphasized the effect of viscosity on taste perception, and there is far less literature on the effect of tastants on the perception of viscosity. Stone and Oliver (1966) used a range of hydrocolloid thickeners, which varied in viscosity. There was generally a good agreement between instrumental measure of viscosity and participants' perception of it. They found that whilst viscosity significantly impaired sucrose detection thresholds, it had a less clear effect on perception of suprathreshold sweetness. In fact, there was a tendency for the more viscous solutions to be ranked as sweeter. Vaisey *et al.* (1969), again using a range of hydrocolloid thickeners of varying viscosity, found that sweetness recognition was slower for the more viscous solutions. Whilst viscosity had no effect on sweetness matching, it tended to reduce perceived sweetness, as well as making rankings of different concentrations of sucrose— within a particular thickener—less accurate. Arabie and Moskowitz (1971), using the hydrocolloid carboxymethyl cellulose (CMC) at varying concentrations, found that sweetness of both, saccharin and sucrose, decreased monotonically with increasing viscosity.

The other type of parameter that has been extensively manipulated in textural studies is hardness. Using the artificial sweetener saccharin, Marshall and Vaisey (1972) used gels of varying hardness as the vehicle. They found that gels of increasing hardness were judged as significantly less sweet and that the judged textual properties of the gel accounted for a significant proportion of the variation in perceived sweetness. Texture could influence the gel at a psychological level (i.e. inhibition of taste) or at a non-psychological level via reducing the quantity of the tastant available to the receptors or by greater hydrogen bonding of the sweetener to the gel. These issues of cause (psychological vs. non-psychological) also loom large in more recent work.

Moskowitz and Arabie (1970) extended their examination of the effects of viscosity to the four basic taste qualities, sweet, sour, salty, and bitter, in a similar set of CMC solutions varying in viscosity. They reported that increasing viscosity decreased perceived taste intensity for all four basic tastes, to a similar degree. The commonality of this effect across tastants (of varying chemical structure) argues against bonding between tastant and CMC because of the varying chemical nature of the tastants. In contrast, Pangborn *et al.* (1973) did not find generalized effects. Using five different kinds of hydrocolloid, varying in viscosity, they found that only taste intensity for sucrose decreased with increasing viscosity. Whilst the perception of other basic tastants was affected by differing hydrocolloids, these effects were not obviously related to instrumental or perceptually derived measures of viscosity. For example, citric acid sourness was reduced in all of the hydrocolloids, but this was not related to differences in viscosity. Similarly, saccharin sweetness appeared to be increased by certain hydrocolloids, but not others, and again this effect was independent of variations in viscosity. These findings suggest that some of the effects were the product of specific non-psychological interactions between tastant and hydrocolloid (e.g. for citric acid), whilst the effects for sucrose were indeterminate. Christensen (1980a)—using different forms of CMC, but with matched levels of viscosity—found that the effect on tastants was thickener specific, i.e. general effects of viscosity were not observed for *any* taste. Christensen (1980a) suggested that the specific nature of these effects probably pointed to physiochemical interactions between specific hydrocolloids and specific tastants.

Two further experiments suggest that textural effects on tastants may be mediated by variation in the rate at which the tastant can reach the taste receptors. Lynch *et al.* (1993) had participants rinse their mouths with, coconut oil, sunflower oil, or water, after which a gel block containing one of four basic tastants was placed on the tongue. For sucrose, only coconut oil reduced perceived sweetness, whilst for the other tastants, both oils were equally effective in reducing salty, bitter, and sour tastes. As coconut oil was generally better at reducing perceived intensity of all the tastants (but especially sucrose), they suggested that it was its greater viscosity—and thus its better ability to physically prevent diffusion of the tastant on to the tongue—which accounted for the observed effects. Similarly, Calvino *et al.* (1993), found that the tastants caffeine and sucrose were judged significantly less intense in a gel base, but not in CMC. They suggested this resulted from the gel releasing the tastant at a slower rate than from CMC.

Whilst the preceding reports have found somewhat conflicting evidence for viscosity on taste perception, the general consensus has been that where these effects occur they result from a peripheral cause. A notable exception is a more recent study by Cook et al., (2002). They chose a number of hydrocolloid thickeners that were either above or below a particular threshold termed C*. C* refers to the point at which there is critical coil overlap and entangling in polysaccharide thickeners. This occurs at different concentrations for different thickeners. Using a forced choice paired-comparison procedure, participants were given two samples which, unbeknownst to them, contained the same concentration of sucrose, but differed in that the thickener in one solution was above the C* threshold and below it in the other. Four sweeteners, varying markedly in chemical composition were used, and these were all judged less sweet on trials in which one solution was below C* and the other above. Similar effects were observed for salt, but not for quinine or citric acid. At least two possible explanations can be advanced to account for these effects. Cook et al. (2002) suggest that their effect may have a psychological locus (for the sweeteners at least), on the basis that perceptual changes in viscosity are quite marked across the C* boundary, and that this change appears to affect 'all sweeteners' equally, even though they vary considerably in chemical composition. However, an older explanation—and one more in tune with those advanced to account for textural effects in the studies above, comes from work by Kokini (1987). Kokini (1987) reported that diffusion coefficients decrease with increasing viscosity, which would appear to offer a physical explanation—slower diffusion of tastants to receptors and hence reduced taste intensity (Kokini et al. 1982). It remains to be seen whether this also accounts for effects across the C* boundary.

Whilst hardness and viscosity may affect the perception of tastants, tastants can also affect the textural properties of the vehicle in which the tastant is dissolved. One effect, which has been widely noted, is that sucrose can influence both instrumental and perceptual measures of viscosity, with higher concentrations of sucrose increasing physical viscosity (e.g. Pangborn et al. 1973). Christensen (1980b) explored these effects in some detail, and also found that sucrose increased perceived viscosity (except for high levels of viscosity where the reverse effect was observed), whilst sour and salty tastants tended to decrease it. Christensen (1980b) suggested that sucrose might restore Newtonian properties to certain viscous solutions, so that their viscosity remained constant across changes in sheer rate. Christensen (1980b) also argued that citric acid and salt may increase sheer thinning, and she obtained some evidence favouring these hypotheses from instrumental measures of viscosity. More recently, Theunissen and Kroeze (1995) attempted to replicate

Christensen's (1980b) finding of increased viscosity with sucrose, when added to CMC. Surprisingly, they found that sucrose decreased perceived viscosity across a range of viscous solutions, whilst aspartame had no effect.

These data above do not make for clear conclusions, and some of this variability likely results from the complexity of the stimuli. Notwithstanding this, it is likely that sweetness is reduced by increasing viscosity (and that sucrose may also increase perceived and actual viscosity), but for other tastants the picture is inconclusive. Whilst most investigators have tended to favour non-psychological explanations, it may be that some form of central taste suppression, especially of sweet tastes, may occur. But this begs the rather difficult question as to why sweet tastes should be special, and it does look as if non-psychological causes (perhaps based on diffusion coefficients) are the dominant factor.

One further type of tactile–taste interaction, which has received some attention, is that between astringency and taste—astringency having a signifi-cant somatosensory component independent of any taste it may elicit (Breslin et al. 1993, Green 1993b). Using a timed intensity-scaling procedure of bitter-ness, sweetness, and dry mouth (astringency), Lyman and Green (1990) found that a mixture of tannic acid and sucrose was judged as significantly less sweet (than sucrose alone) and significantly less bitter (than tannic acid alone). In addition, the presence of sucrose reduced the reported degree of astringency of tannic acid. The effect on sweetness ratings—and indeed the finding by Brannan et al. (2001) that salt-, citric acid-, and caffeine-taste intensity can be suppressed by both, tannic acid and alum (but not sucrose, although there was a trend for this in their data)—may arise directly from the effect of these astringent agents on taste receptors. Schiffman et al. (1992) reported that, in Gerbils, all tastants evoked a smaller response in the presence of tannic acid, in terms of recordings made from the chorda tympani, suggesting a possible peripheral locus.

The reduction in astringency produced by sucrose may arise from a combi-nation of effects. Lyman and Green (1990) found that whilst tannic acid alone did not suppress salivation, sucrose (and sucrose and tannic acid combined) significantly increased salivation. This may reduce the sensations of friction between the surfaces of the mouth, produced by the astringent agent's ability to precipitate salivary mucoproteins—a process that is apparently more effective as the pH of the mouth becomes more acidic (Guinard et al. 1985). However, this is not the only mechanism by which sucrose may reduce sensations of astringency. Lyman and Green (1990) also found that whilst aspartame was able to reduce astringency, it was not as efficient at this as sucrose. Whilst the aspartame was somewhat less effective at generating saliva (more effective than tannic acid alone, but less effective than sucrose alone), sucrose solutions are more viscous than those of aspartame. Lyman and Green (1990) suggest that the somewhat viscous sucrose solution may act as a lubricant, and so reduce friction between the oral surfaces (and see Brannan *et al.*'s 2001 observation that carboxymethyl cellulose solutions are also effective at reducing astringent sensations). This lubricating effect may be in addition to any effects generated by excess saliva, which of course might be expected to dilute the sucrose solution and so reduce its viscosity. In sum, both the effects, of astringency on taste perception and of sucrose on perceptions of dry mouth and puckering (i.e. astringency), appear to be peripherally mediated effects.

Odour and somatosensation

This section reviews the interaction of odours with irritants, temperature, and tactile stimuli. Whilst there is a reasonable body of literature on irritant–odour and temperature–odour interactions, there are almost no papers that deal exclusively with odour–tactile relationships. Rather, they deal instead with odour–taste–tactile relationships, simply because many of these stimuli are very unpalatable without the addition of a sweetening agent and because, in some cases, the tactile agent may require the addition of a chemical agent to assist thickening—and this itself may have a taste. For this reason, odour–tactile relationships are *generally* examined in the context of odour–taste–tactile relationships later in this chapter.

Odour and irritant stimuli

The suppressive effect of irritation on odour perception has been well documented (see Brand 2006). Cain and Murphy (1980), e.g. had participants sniff mixtures of carbon dioxide and amyl butyrate, as well as presenting these stimuli individually (but simultaneously) to different nostrils. In both cases, the presence of carbon dioxide suppressed perception of amyl butyrate, with this effect becoming more pronounced with increasing carbon dioxide concentration. When a time lag was introduced, such that the carbon dioxide was presented first, participants reported a far smaller odour-suppression effect. Both of these findings suggest that the effects of this irritant were centrally mediated.

Whilst this finding suggests that the irritant carbon dioxide can suppress orthonasal odour perception, somewhat different effects may occur when the target odourants are perceived at levels closer to threshold. Jacquot *et al.* (2004) found that sniffing allyl isothiocyanate (the pungent principle of mustard), prior to engaging in detection trials for butanol and phenyl ethyl alcohol, had the effect of enhancing their detectability. These authors suggested a peripheral basis for this effect.

If it is assumed that carbon dioxide is a fairly representative irritant, then central suppression might also occur when an odour is presented retronasally along with an irritant in the mouth. This situation is, of course, very common during eating and drinking, and participants readily report that highly spiced food 'deadens' the flavour (Prescott and Stevenson 1995). To investigate this claim, Prescott and Stevenson (1995) undertook two experiments, both employing various concentrations of capsaicin. In Experiment 1, participants were presented with a vanilla or orange odourant, sucrose and citric acid, along with varying levels of capsaicin. Participants swilled and expectorated these samples and judged, alongside other qualities, flavour intensity. Ratings of flavour were suppressed on the strongest capsaicin trials, but were not affected by weaker concentrations. Whilst these results ostensibly show that an oral irritant may affect retronasal perception of an odourant, these results could have occurred as a consequence of participants conflating sweetness and flavour ratings, especially as sweetness too was suppressed by capsaicin. Thus, in Experiment 2, capsaicin, at the same concentrations, was presented in a mixture with just strawberry odourant, and only strawberry flavour and burn intensity were assessed. This time, no evidence of odour suppression was obtained. These results would suggest that oral irritants, whilst affecting taste perception (see above), might have relatively little effect on retronasal odour perception.

Odour and temperature

Increasing temperature is associated with increasing volatility of aromatic agents (e.g. see Gray 1972), thus the increase in concentration should lead to increase in judgements of odour intensity. Whilst this may be observed when participants sniff a sample presented at differing temperatures (e.g. Voirol and Daget 1989), the situation in the mouth is more complicated. This is because the mouth will actively resist changes in temperature. Of course, this will depend upon the magnitude of the difference between oral temperature and stimulus temperature, and larger differences are easier to achieve when the stimulus is cooled rather than warmed. For cooled stimuli, such as tomato and orange juice (served at either 0 or 22°C), Pangborn et al. (1978) found that the cooler temperature was associated with reduced flavour intensity. However, where the temperature variation is somewhat less extreme, the effects (although in the expected direction— i.e. cooler, less flavour; warmer, more flavour) are either small (e.g. Olson et al. 1980, Engelen et al. 2003) or not detectable (e.g. Cliff and Noble 1990).

Interactions within the somatosensory domain

Somatosensory stimuli are diverse, and there is clearly considerable overlap in the receptors that detect different stimuli (e.g. thermal–irritant) within this domain (see Chapter 1). For this reason, peripheral causes for any observed interaction effects might be expected, and this does appear to be the case.

Irritants and tactile stimuli

Several types of interaction have been explored between chemaesthetic agents, mainly capsaicin, and then fat, viscosity, oral movement, and astringency. The literature on viscosity and fat is the most extensive. For physiochemical reasons—the lipophillicity of capsaicin—presenting capsaicin in a more fatty stimulus reduces judgements of burn intensity (Baron and Penfield 1996, Lawless *et al*. 2000). In the most detailed exploration, Lawless *et al*. (2000) found that presenting capsaicin in an oil base increased thresholds 30-fold, and that approximately 50 times the amount of capsaicin in oil was required to match the perceived intensity of capsaicin in water.

Whilst these oil-based effects probably reflect the way in which capsaicin partitions between the base and saliva, and saliva and the receptors, investigators have also examined whether viscosity might influence burn intensity. Nasrawi and Pangborn (1989) found that xanthan gum acted to reduce burn intensity, suggesting that increased viscosity has an effect, but Baron and Penfield (1996) found no correlation between instrumental measures of viscosity for a range of capsaicin-impregnated foodstuffs and burn intensity. Similarly, Forde and Delahunty (2002) found that viscosity had no effect on judgements of the irritant menthol, but they did find that menthol made it harder to judge viscosity.

Casual observation suggests that mechanical action of food in the mouth may reduce burn intensity. Several studies suggest this—in that whilst eating foods as varied as rice, butter, pineapple juice, and milk burn intensity may be reduced, only for it to rebound once the mechanical stimulation ends (e.g. Hutchinson *et al*. 1990, Nasrawi and Pangborn 1990). Part of this effect may be food dependent, note that butter and milk are fatty, and as Lawless *et al*. (2000) note, these foods were slightly more successful in reducing the burn. The effect of mouth movements on oral burn intensity with capsaicin has not been directly explored. However, Green (1990) applied capsaicin to the border of participants' lips and masked the burn until the vibratory stimulus could be applied. He found a small but significant reduction in burn intensity with vibration at 60 Hz. For another irritant, ethanol, Green (1990) observed that static pressure on the tongue tip following ethanol application produced a significant increase in perceived irritation, suggesting that the effects of mechanical stimulation may be dependent both on frequency and the irritant as well. Finally, a further type of tactile stimulus—astringency produced by citric acid and quinine—is reduced by prior capsaicin desensitization (Karrer and Bartoshuk 1995), suggesting, as with the Green (1990) data above, that tactile and chemaesthetic agents interact.

Irritants and temperature

Sensory descriptions of irritant chemicals borrow terms both from the thermal and pain lexicons. Burning and hot, and cooling, are typically used by participants to describe their experience of capsaicin and menthol, respectively. It is not, therefore, surprising that there has been some interest in how perception of these chemical irritants is affected by temperature and vice versa.

Capsaicin was the first chemical irritant to be explored, although the early investigations did little more than note an apparent synergy between capsaicin and the vehicle temperature. The first systematic examination, by Sizer and Harris (1985), found that detection thresholds for capsaicin were lowered when the stimuli were presented at higher temperatures. A suprathreshold study by Green (1986b) found evidence consistent with this, in that solutions of 2-ppm capsaicin were found to increase perceived warmth between 38–45°C and to reduce perceptions of coolness as cooler stimuli (i.e. lower than body temperature) were presented. Temperature of the stimuli also produced a parallel effect on perception of irritation, with temperature increasing irritation and cooling reducing it. Thermal modulation of capsaicin irritation was the more powerful effect. Similar effects of warmer temperatures on irritant perception were observed by Prescott et al. (1994), although these were inconsistent across experiments.

A more recent study by Albin et al. (2008) provides evidence not only of a clear interaction between temperature and chemical irritation, but also information on its cause. In a particularly elegant design, they simultaneously applied capsaicin (and other irritants too, which will be dealt with below) to one side of the fore-tip of the tongue and the vehicle to the other. The tongue was then pressed against a thermode at either 9.5 or 49°C. The participants' task was to judge which side of their tongue felt hotter or cooler. Participants also rated perceived heat or cold pain. Not only did capsaicin increase heat pain, participants chose the capsaicin-treated side as hotter at a level significantly above chance. Capsaicin, then, does appear to affect perception of painfully hot thermal sensations. No effect on cold perception was noted. In a further experiment, they tested whether desensitizing the tongue with capsaicin would produce a similar effect. This is an important question because, if the participant is unable to experience any sensation from capsaicin, but there is still an effect on noxious heat perception, this would strongly suggest a peripheral basis for the enhancement effect obtained in their first experiment. This is exactly what they found. In fact, the potentiation of thermal pain and detection of the 'hotter' side were almost identical to those obtained when the capsaicin was producing a perceptible burning sensation on the tongue. This suggests a significant overlap between irritant and thermal receptors (see Chapter 1), and a clear peripheral cause.

Another study by Green (2005) observed effects, which at first sight are in direct conflict with those described above. Following capsaicin pre-treatment of the fore-tongue, perception of thermal and nociceptive sensations—when a warm or hot thermode was applied to the tongue—revealed *reduced* perceptions of warmth and irritation. However, the temperature manipulation was taken some 15 min following capsaicin pre-treatment, compared to within 5 min for the Albin *et al.* (2008) study. In fact, Albin *et al.* (2008) noted that at 10 min following pre-treatment, the enhancing effect of capsaicin had dissipated; so it may be that even further out (i.e. as with the Green (2005) study), this renders thermal receptors insensitive.

The effects of menthol have also been explored. Green (1985a) examined the effects of menthol on temperature perception in three experiments. Experiment 1 produced quite surprising results, in that mixtures of menthol in a cool vehicle (10–28°C) had only a small effect on thermal perception of cold (i.e. menthol made the fluid feel cooler). However, it had a much larger effect in warm fluids (38–46 C), making them appear warmer, relative to the vehicle control. This may have resulted from the fact that menthol may take a while to reach its peak perceptual effect. So, in Experiment 2, 5-min pre-treatment with menthol was followed by samples of cold and hot fluids. This time menthol produced significant cooling, as well as reducing of the perceived warmth of the hotter solutions. In Experiment 3, a longer interval was used (10 min); this generated an even more marked cooling effect with colder fluids, but no effect on warmth perception. The reduction in perceived warmth following menthol pre-treatment has also been observed in another study reported by Green (2005), but this time with no effect on cooling. In this study, irritant sensations generated by menthol were also examined and these were not affected by temperature—a quite different pattern to that of capsaicin, and again a pointer to the likely peripheral basis of this effect. Finally, Albin *et al.* (2008), using the split-tongue technique described above, found that participants reported increased cold pain and reduced heat pain when stimulated with menthol. However, menthol only affected judgements of which side of the tongue was perceived as cooler—namely the menthol side.

The other irritant, which has been explored in relation to temperature, is carbon dioxide. These studies have all examined interactions with colder temperatures. In these studies, there is clear evidence that the level of carbon dioxide in the fluid is not physically affected by manipulating temperature (at least in the experimental range), so any observed effects are not the result of a change in this parameter. Yau and McDaniel (1991a) examined participants' judgement of carbonation at varying volumes of carbon dioxide, with temperatures between 3 and 22°C. Perceived carbonation was increased with cooler temperatures, especially for higher levels of carbonation. Similarly, Harper and McDaniel (1993) observed that irritant sensations generated by carbonation were also significantly more acute at colder temperatures. Green (1992) also manipulated temperature (2–24°C) and level of carbonation, and obtained both thermal and irritative intensity ratings. Irritation was significantly higher for colder stimuli with higher levels of carbonation. Moreover, with higher levels of carbon dioxide and cold temperature, participants reported greater oral pain and irritation for the coldest and most carbonated stimuli. Whilst there is no psychophysical data indicating the basis for this interaction, it is likely that this too is a peripheral effect, dominated by the shared sensitivity of certain receptors to chemical and thermal stimuli.

Albin *et al.* (2008) also examined two other chemical irritants, mustard oil and cinnamaldehyde (an irritant derived from cinnamon). Both were found to interact with stimulus temperature. Mustard oil increased heat-pain ratings and participants were also more likely to choose the mustard oil-treated side of their tongue as hotter. Mustard oil also enhanced cold pain and participants' choice of which side of their tongue was cooler, but only immediately after treatment. Cinnamaldehyde also produced effects on warmth and cold, with enhanced heat-pain ratings and choice of the cinnamaldehyde-treated side with hot stimuli, and enhanced cold-pain ratings. The same conclusion probably applies here, too, in respect to a likely peripheral locus.

Temperature and tactile stimuli

Two types of effect have been noted for temperature–tactile interactions. First, the temperature of the mouth may affect sensitivity to vibratory stimuli. Green (1987) observed that cooling the tongue to 20°C produced a reduction in sensitivity to high-frequency vibratory stimuli, but not to low-frequency stimuli. Whilst this effect suggests reduced sensitivity, Green (1987) noted that more transient exposure to cold stimuli in the mouth may have the opposite effect, in that it may increase the perceived intensity of tactile stimuli and improve detection of its spatial location. This has not as yet been confirmed in the mouth, nor for that matter have the effects of warming the mouth on tactile sensitivity. More generally, whether any temperature effect on tactile perception would reliably influence the way in which we experience the texture of food has yet to be determined.

A second type of effect is that produced physically on the structure of the food (or experimental stimulus) by warming or cooling. Both, Baron and Penfield (1996) and Engelen *et al.* (2003), reported quite large changes in instrumental measures of viscosity with temperature—namely reduced viscosity with increasing temperature. Such effects are clearly of importance when eating foods such as ice cream, where the food itself undergoes major textural change as it warms in the mouth. Temperature transitions are routine for most foods and will be accompanied by varying degrees of textural change, and thus changes on perception of the food. However, these interactions, whilst of great significance for our enjoyment of food, do not appear (at this stage) to reflect interesting psychological interactions.

Interactions between odour, tactile, and taste stimuli

This section is split into two subsections, the first dealing with the effect of tactile stimuli on the perception of odour and to a lesser extent, taste. This subsection starts with a quick look at the more basic studies, followed by a more in-depth examination of those which employed either *in vivo* measurements of odourants in the nose or controlled odourant delivery—i.e. studies with excellent stimulus control. This is followed by an evaluation of the relative contribution of psychological and physical causes of the observed tactile–taste–odour interactions. The second part deals with the effect that odours and tastants have on tactile perception and the physical characteristics of the tactile stimulus.

Tactile effects on odour and taste perception

Tactile–odour interaction studies, which do not measure or manipulate the quantity of odourants reaching the nose are hard to interpret, because it is not possible to say whether any effect on odour perception is a consequence of changes in odourant release (i.e. more or less of the respective chemicals are present in the nose) or a result of some central process. These less controlled studies present a mixed picture in respect to the effect of tactile stimuli on odour perception. Pangborn and Koyasko (1981) found that, for the same food presented as either a liquid or a solid, the solid was judged sweeter and slightly more chocolaty. Using a set of odourous stimuli, where viscosity was manipulated by varying the hydrocolloid used, Pangborn and Szczesniak (1974) concluded that the effect of thickeners on retronasal odour perception was likely to be a consequence of specific interactions between the thickening 'agent' and the odourant.

Ferry *et al.* (2006) employed a range of hydrocolloid thickeners, but flavoured with salt and basil. They found no consistent relationship between instrumental measures of viscosity and retronasal odour perception. The one physical correlate they did observe was the mixing behaviour of the dyed hydrocolloid with water. Those that mixed poorly (i.e. the dye took longer to reach equilibrium with the water above) were also the thickening agents that were most able to suppress perception of the basil odour. Poor mixing may also occur in the mouth, reducing the rate at which the 'tastant' can access taste receptors. This, in turn (i.e. reduced taste intensity), might affect odour perception, especially under conditions of perceptual similarity between the odour and taste (see odour–taste interactions above).

The effect of hardness and softness, using gels, on odour and taste perception has also been explored quite extensively, and harder gels appear to reduce perceived flavour intensity of sweetened and odourized samples (Guinard and Marty 1995, Jaime *et al.* 1993, Lundgren *et al.* 1986, Wilson and Brown 1997). In all of these cases, orthonasal *and* retronasal judgements of intensity were similarly affected, suggesting a non-psychological basis for the effect. However, Juteau *et al.* (2004) examined orthonasal and retronasal discrimination of intensity between the same odour presented in either a soft or hard gel. For the retronasal comparisons, of the eight odourants used, five were judged to be less intense in the harder gel, but few differences were observed for orthonasal comparisons. For some of these odourants, their physiochemical parameters appeared to predict their behaviour in the gels, but for others this could not account for the reduced intensity, leading the authors to suggest a psychological cause.

A significant advance in understanding the influence of tactile stimuli on retronasal odour perception comes from being able to measure the volatile components *in vivo*. Typically, this involves sampling air that has been expelled from the nose (or mouth) and then feeding samples of this expired air into a measurement device, usually a mass spectrometer. Not only does this allow identification of certain volatiles, but also allows quantification of the amount. If this technique is then combined with perceptual time–intensity measurements, a more complete picture can be developed of the relationship between the stimulus and the percept, and how the tactile stimulus is modulating either or both. Two caveats need to be considered before examining this literature. The first is that the *in vivo* measurements, whilst accurate in terms of quantification, may not always be able to measure all possible volatiles in a complex mixture. Thus, in some cases, concluding that there was a reduction in the stimulus concentration could, in actuality, reflect a reduction in *just* the components measured—the remaining unmeasured ones may not have changed or could even have increased (see Saint-Eve *et al.* 2006). Needless to say, this is not a problem when the stimulus is composed of just one or a limited number of odourants.

The second problem—and it is a far more pressing one as will become apparent—is that, in most of the studies described next, an odour and a taste are used, yet no comparable *in vivo* measures of the tastant are made. To illustrate why this may be a problem, recall the findings reviewed earlier in this chapter about the interaction of taste and smell (and indeed the salt and basil study above). If a tastant's ability to reach the receptors on the tongue is reduced by the medium in which it is delivered, then *even if there is no physical change in in vivo measures of odourant concentration and type* participants may still report a less intense smell—a consequence of the absence of taste, rather than a direct effect of the tactile stimulus on retronasal odour perception.

Of the several studies, which have included perceptual measures and *in vivo* instrumental measures of odourants, most have suggested a perceptual impact of texture (gel hardness or viscosity) on odour perception. One interesting exception is Linforth *et al.* (1999). Here participants ate gels of varying hardness, which had been flavoured with sucrose or glucose, with added dimethyl pyrazine or menthol (in gelatine gels) or ethyl butyrate (in pectin/gelatine gels). Perceptual and instrumental measures were closely correlated for dimethyl pyrazine and menthol, with the harder gels producing a longer persistence of the odourant. Thus the effects of texture here are likely to be driven by changes in volatile concentrations. Interestingly, the ethyl butyrate and pectin/gelatine gels behaved rather differently. There was a much poorer correspondence between the instrumental and perceptual measures, with retronasal odour perception accurately tracking the rise of odourant concentration, but not its decline—i.e. there was a persistence of the percept even when the stimulus had vastly diminished, and this was especially so for the softer gels. This could be explained by reference to the perceptual similarity between ethyl butyrate (sweet and fruity) and the sweetener, with the sweetener release driving ethyl butyrate ratings (see Davidson *et al.* 1999, and see Figure 2.1 for analogous findings).

A much larger group of studies have found textural effects on odour perception. Baek *et al.* (1999) employed gels of varying hardness flavoured with the sweet and fruity odourant furfuryl acetate and sucrose. Perceptual measures of flavour and *in vivo* measures of odourant concentration were obtained. Whilst there was no significant variation in odourant release between gels, ratings of flavour (retronasal odour) were considerably lower for the hardest gels. A similar taste-based explanation to the one above could also be used here to account for this effect, if the harder gels released the sweetener at a slower rate (this type of explanation could also account for several other findings of this general sort; see Bayarri *et al.* 2006, Cook *et al.* 2003, Hollowood *et al.* 2002).

Boland *et al.* (2006) also utilized odourized sweetened gels. Sweetness ratings declined with gel hardness as did strawberry-flavour ratings. The interesting finding here, pertinent to a non-taste-driven explanation—i.e. a direct effect of texture on odour perception—was the observation that *in vivo* measurements of the odourant indicated that the highest concentration (between and within stimuli) occurred when swallowing the harder gels (see Figure 2.2) even though

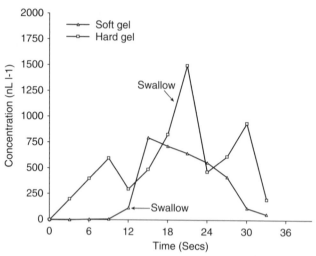

Fig. 2.2 *In vivo* measure of ethyl butyrate concentration for a hard and soft gelatine gel before and after swallowing. Adapted from Boland *et al.* 2006.

flavour-intensity ratings were lower. A contrast effect might explain the
perceptual findings here, in that changes in odourant concentration from pre-
to post-swallow were considerably *larger* for the softer gels, than for the harder
gels. This contrast may have dictated the overall weaker judgements of
strawberry-odour intensity in the harder gels. Whilst a contrast effect is clearly
a psychological explanation, a further possibility is that participants adapted to
the odourant released prior to swallowing the harder gels, thus the spike in
concentration (far exceeding that produced by the softer gel) may have been
perceived as less intense.

The key concern so far is that variations in sweetness resulting from the
physical properties of the stimulus (e.g. diffusion rates) could drive differences
in odour perception, rather than from some direct psychological effect of
texture on odour perception. A very important study in this regard is Weel
et al. (2002) where gels of varying hardness were flavoured with either ethyl
butyrate or diacetyl (cream odour). No sweetener or other tastant was added
to the gels, yet both odourants were perceived as less intense in the harder gels.
There were no changes in the volatiles recorded *in vivo*, i.e. the gels did not
affect odourant release. This strongly suggests that the olfactory component of
flavour is suppressed by changes in texture perception (hardness in this case).
Figure 2.3a and b illustrate these effects for the intensity and concentration
data, respectively.

Two further papers have adopted a rather different approach to measuring the impact of texture on odour perception. In both cases, catheters were positioned under endoscopic control, either into the nasopharynx or a few centimetres into the anterior nares. The odourant, under precise control, was then delivered at some point in the eating cycle. In one study using this technique, it is again not possible to tell whether the effect of texture on odour

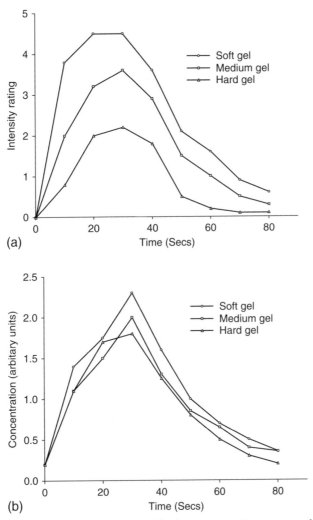

Fig. 2.3a and b Time-intensity ratings and *in vivo* concentration measures for ethyl butyrate in soft, medium, and hard gels. Adapted from Weel *et al.* 2002.

perception is driven by the effect of texture on taste or by the effect of texture on odour (Visscher *et al.* 2006). However, a second study using this technique suggests more definitively that texture affects odour perception via a psychological mechanism. Bult *et al.* (2007) presented participants with plain or thickened milk. Whilst milk contains a small amount of lactose, it is not appreciably sweet, and so these samples can be regarded as effectively unsweetened. Cream odourant was piped either to the anterior nares or to the nasopharynx. Rated flavour intensity was reduced in the thickened milk, irrespective of whether the flavour was presented ortho- or retronasally, or whether it occurred with the milk, with mouth movements, or on swallowing. These findings, taken together with the Weel *et al.* (2002) study, suggest very strongly that tactile perception, be it increasing hardness or viscosity, can act to suppress odour perception in the *absence* of any effect on the physical quantity of odourant available to the receptor. Thus, increasing oral tactile stimulation appears to suppress odour perception. This phenomenon may be exaggerated further by the direct physical effect that viscous (or hard) agents have on tastant release, reducing taste intensity and, thus (via interaction between taste and smell), further reducing perceived odour intensity.

Effect of odour and taste on tactile perception

Whilst the quantity of odourant within a food is typically small, the odourant can physically modify texture, although the effect may not be large. Pangborn and Szczesniak (1974) measured the viscosity of a variety of hydrocolloids (each at five different levels of instrumentally determined viscosity), with and without particular odourants—namely acetaldehyde, acetophenone, butyric acid, and dimethyl sulphide. Butyric acid significantly reduced instrumentally measured viscosity as well as perceived viscosity, but the other odourants did not have any systematic effect. Although these results suggest that the physical effect of an odourant may be small, they highlight the need to be aware that any observed effect of an odorant on tactile perception could 'potentially' result from an actual physiochemical cause.

Studies into the effect of odour stimuli (and taste) on tactile perception can be grouped into three methodological classes: (1) those in which the effects are just presumed to be based on psychological effects; (2) those which confirm a probable psychological influence of the odour on texture perception by using a nose-clip; and (3) studies in which odour delivery is independently controlled by the experimenter allowing a more definitive conclusion about psychological cause.

Jaime *et al.* (1993) examined the effect of adding raspberry and butterscotch odourants to gels of varying hardness. The odourants had no effect on perception of gel texture. With stimuli where the main variable is viscosity rather than hardness, odourants that are typically associated with the thickened stimulus (or a thinned stimulus) do appear to exert an effect. Tepper and Kuang (1996) found that the addition of cream flavour to a dairy stimulus did affect participants' evaluation of its texture. Physical parameters were (not surprisingly) identified as the most important factor in determining texture perception (i.e. fat globule size, number, and viscosity), with flavour second in importance (in terms of variance accounted for). De Wijk *et al.* (2003) added different quantities of either, the creamy-smelling odourant diacetyl or vanilla, to custard desserts. Vanilla exerted no appreciable effect, but diacetyl in fact *decreased* perceived fattiness, an effect the authors speculated might have resulted from a physical effect of this agent on the custard. Finally, Saint-Eve *et al.* (2004) produced yoghurts with differing viscosity by mechanically extruding it through different nozzles. All were sweetened, and then different odourants were added singly or in combination to each of the yoghurts. Green-smelling odourants tended to have a thinning effect on participants textural judgements, whilst buttery- and coconut-smelling odourants had a thickening effect. Single odourants led to yoghurts being perceived as thicker than those containing odour mixtures—an effect that was presumed to be related to variations in perceived intensity (i.e. stronger odour being associated with lower viscosity).

More specific odourant-based effects can be gauged from studies which have examined these interactions with and without a nose-clip. Thus, in one of the experimental conditions, judgements of texture are made with no retronasal olfaction. Mela (1988) reported that fattiness judgements of a range of milks varying in fat content were unaffected by the presence or absence of retronasal olfaction. However, other more recent studies present a rather different picture. Yackinous and Guinard (2000) found not only that the addition of a fat-related odourant enhanced judgements of fatty intensity in certain foods (mashed potatoes and chips), but also that the presence of a nose-clip significantly reduced rated fattiness for nearly all of the foods. Weenen *et al.* (2005) had participants evaluate a range of foodstuffs which varied in creaminess. These samples (which were naturalistically flavoured—i.e. the products usual odourants were in place) were evaluated as less fatty and creamy when wearing a nose-clip, indicating that retronasal olfaction significantly enhanced these textural judgements. Kora *et al.* (2003) reported a conceptually similar finding in that the addition of odourants to yoghurts of varying viscosity affected textural judgements. Odourants with a 'green' smell significantly reduced rated thickness (i.e. perceived viscosity), and this effect was eliminated when wearing a nose-clip. These more recent studies suggest that odourants can both enhance and suppress textural attributes such as fattiness and thickness, and the loss of these effects when the nose is occluded indicate a likely central cause.

When considering the effect of texture on odourant perception, the paper by Bult *et al.* (2007) was of particular interest, because of its method of controlling odourant delivery. Not only did they assess the impact of texture on odour perception, they also had participants evaluate textural parameters, notably thickness. For retronasally delivered odourants, that were delivered either whilst mouth movements were taking place or after swallowing, they found that participants judged the stimulus to be thicker. This effect was reduced when air was delivered rather than the odourant, suggesting an odour-specific effect. This again implies that odourants can affect judgements of texture—in this case enhancing them—and this effect must have a central locus. In sum, odourants can affect texture perception and, in the main, the evidence favours a centrally based cause.

Interactions with vision

Pretty much, all of the interactions reviewed so far involved the simultaneous effect of one stimulus upon another in the mouth. A substantial literature suggests this is not the only type of interaction that can affect the way in which we perceive flavour. Appearance variables, notably food colour, precede the perception of flavour, and also clearly affect it. Such effects are very likely to have a psychological basis. Of course, this assumes that the physical basis of the appearance variable, such as colour, does not itself have a taste or a smell (e.g. unlike say paprika, turmeric, etc.). In the following section, the effects of colour on taste and odour perception, and on the perception of odour–taste mixtures, are examined. Whilst there are clearly other important visual variables, notably texture-related features (e.g. wilting, turbidity, and glossiness; Lawless and Heymann 1998), as well as the shape of food (e.g. a chocolate brownie shaped as a dog faeces might influence ones desire to eat that food; Simpson *et al.* 2007), the effect of these on flavour perception has not been examined systematically.

Vision and taste

Studies in which only colour and taste are examined are few in number. Maga (1974) examined taste identification at threshold, to see whether the colour of the solution influenced the concentration at which participants would correctly identify a taste. Identification thresholds for sucrose were lower (i.e. 'better') in green solutions, than in colourless solutions, and highest in red or yellow. For citric acid, this was lowest in a colourless solution, and higher in all coloured fluids. Bitter, too, was detected better in a colourless solution. Yellow and green fluids followed, with the highest thresholds in red. Colour had no effect on salty identification thresholds.

Whilst these results indicate that colour can affect identification thresholds, colour does not appear to affect taste intensity when just a tastant and a tasteless colourant are present. Alley and Alley (1998), using 12-year olds, found no effect of colour (red, green, yellow, and blue) on judgements of sweetness intensity. Similarly, Frank et al. (1989) observed no effect of red colour on judgements of sweetness intensity in adults. Finally, Pangborn conducted two discrimination studies to examine whether colour affected participants' ability to tell apart sucrose solutions of similar concentration. She found that colour impaired discrimination in one study (Pangborn and Hansen 1963), but not in another (Pangborn 1960).

Vision and olfaction

Engen (1972) reported a psychophysical study using three participants where they had to judge which out of two stimuli had a smell. The target odourant was close to threshold, and on some trials the odourant was coloured while on others the blank was coloured. Even though participants were instructed to disregard any cue other than smell, colour increased false alarm rates in all three participants, even when a payoff was introduced to shift participants to a more conservative decision criterion. These results suggest that colour may inadvertently bias participants to judge a smell as being present, even when it is not. After all, coloured fluids often smell and colourless ones, notably water, do not.

Engen's (1972) observation has been consistently supported. Coloured fluids that contain suprathreshold odours are found to smell more intense than their uncoloured counterparts and these effects occur even when the demand characteristics of the situation are carefully controlled (Blackwell 1995, Zellner and Kautz 1990, Zellner and Whitten 1999). Colour enhancement of odour intensity appears to be generic, in that there is no robust evidence that particular colours differentially affect intensity judgements of odours with which they are commonly associated (e.g. strawberry-odour intensity is enhanced irrespective of the colourant; Zellner and Kautz 1990). However, particular colour–odour associations (rather than generic ones) do appear to matter for certain tasks. Inappropriate colours (e.g. green orange odour) can impair identification (Blackwell 1995) and discrimination (Stevenson and Oaten 2008), whilst appropriate colour–odour combinations facilitate identification (Davis 1981, Zellner et al. 1991). In the study by Zellner et al. (1991), this facilitatory effect was only observed for appropriate colour–odour pairs that were 'typical'—in other words, those colour–odour associations that were very well established. This gels with work using a different paradigm, the implicit association test, which has been used to demonstrate the automatic nature of the links between high-strength odour–colour pairs (Dematte, Sanabria, and Spence 2006).

Where the odour is experienced orthonasally, there appear to be two psychological effects in operation: a generic colour–odour association, in which the mere presence of colour inflates judgements of intensity and the likelihood of judging an odour as being present (even if it is not), and particular colour–odour associations that affect identification and discrimination judgements. But what about when the odourant is experienced retronasally? Only one study has explored this. Koza *et al.* (2005) found that whilst red-coloured water enhanced intensity ratings of a fruity odour when sniffed, this effect disappeared when the judgement was made retronasally. This interesting observation clearly needs following up, as its cause is not understood.

Vision, taste, and smell (and somatosensation)

A good place to start reviewing this literature is to look at the one study that has attempted to use an objective index of colour–flavour interactions. In the earlier section on taste–smell interactions, four studies were described which examined whether appropriate (vs. inappropriate) tastants could affect the detection threshold for an odour. Johnson and Clydesdale (1982) pioneered a similar approach. They obtained participants' detection thresholds for sucrose under a variety of conditions—with a sweet-smelling odour, with a red colour, and with both together. The results are somewhat complicated to interpret because there were no significant main effects of either colour or odour, although, as one might predict, thresholds for sucrose were indeed lower in the presence of a sweet odour and in the presence of a colour (red) that is frequently associated with this taste (and smell). The presence of significant interactions between subject and odour, and subject and colour, may suggest that some participants were more susceptible than others to these sub-additive effects.

A large body of published work exists on the effect of colour on intensity judgements of odour–taste mixture components. Of the studies reviewed, at least four did not obtain any systematic effect on judgements of intensity in student-age participants (of either taste and odour, or flavour) using real foods (Chan and Kane-Martnelli 1997, Christensen 1985) or coloured, flavoured solutions (Philipsen *et al.* 1995, Zampini *et al.* 2007). In three of these studies, however, elderly people were also tested, and in two cases enhanced flavour-intensity judgements—when the food or solution was more darkly coloured (i.e. the lightness dimension)—were observed in the elderly (Philipsen *et al.* 1995, Chan and Kane-Martinelli 1985), but not in Christensen's (1985) experiment.

Several other studies have obtained significant effects of colour on flavour intensity. However, these studies have two problems that hinder interpretation.

First, because in many cases they employ tastes and smells that are both perceptually similar, any effect on ratings of one variable (e.g. judgements of sweetness) cannot be readily distinguished from the other (e.g. judgements of strawberry flavour). Drawing upon the literature reviewed above for colour and odour, and colour and taste, it would seem likely that smell is more strongly influenced by colour than taste. Still, this remains a supposition, especially given the findings of Koza *et al.* (2005) who found that colour exerted no effect on odour perception when the judgements were made retronasally. A second problem relates to colour appropriateness. The studies finding an intensity-enhancement effect typically do not employ colour-appropriate and -inappropriate conditions, so it is not possible to tell whether colour effects on flavour judgements are generic or whether they rely on specific associations between a flavour and a colour.

At least six studies demonstrate that colour influences judgements of flavour intensity. Lavin and Lawless (1998), testing children and adults, obtained flavour-intensity enhancement by use of colour in adults. Effects for children were mixed, suggesting that they had, perhaps, not yet acquired such strong colour–odour–taste associations as adults. In a series of similar experiments using cherry odour, with varying concentrations of sucrose and red colour (Johnson and Clydesdale 1982, Johnson *et al.* 1983, Johnson *et al.* 1982) and sweetened lemon and lime odours and colours (Roth *et al.* 1988), increasing sweetness ratings tended to accompany decreasing colour lightness. It is not clear whether this arose from the impact of colour on odour, then its effect on taste, or from colour directly affecting taste. A similar interpretative problem surrounds findings from Bayarri *et al.* (2001) and Calvo *et al.* (2001). They used a range of appropriately coloured sweetened fruity-flavoured solutions and found effects of colour on odour-related judgements, but not on sweetness.

The effects of colour on odour-quality judgements and identification have been explored far more systematically. DuBose *et al.* (1980) observed that colour could exert quite profound effects on the qualitative characteristics that participants perceive in sweetened, fruit-flavoured drinks (at least to the extent that their chosen label for each flavour reflects its quality). Some data illustrative of this experiment are presented in Table 2.1. As can be seen here, colour had a significant impact in three ways. It facilitated identification when the colour was appropriate (relative to uncoloured). It inflated ratings of flavours that were not present, when the coloured solution was flavoured (e.g. 19% of participants misidentified lime as cherry when lime was presented in red fluid). Finally, it appeared to induce the illusion of flavour in solutions that had, in fact, no flavour.

Table 2.1 Proportion identifying the target odourant or blank (retronasally) in various coloured solutions and in uncoloured fluid. Data from DuBose *et al.* 1980

Odourant Proportion identifying as:	In red	In orange	In green	Colourless
Cherry				
Cherry (%)	70	41	33	37
Lime (%)	0	0	26	7
Orange				
Orange (%)	33	82	30	30
Lemon (%)	4	0	22	15
Lime				
Lime (%)	15	19	48	44
Cherry (%)	19	0	0	0
No odour				
Cherry (%)	9	0	0	0
Orange (%)	0	22	0	0
Lime (%)	0	0	26	0
Flavourless (%)	41	44	41	48

Whilst the facilitatory effect of colour on flavour identification has been more difficult to obtain across studies (but see Stillman (1993)), the finding that inappropriate colour impairs identification (and often results in quite dramatic misidentification) is well established (e.g. Hyman 1983, Stillman 1993, Zampini *et al.* 2007). Teerling (1992) found, using wine gums, that inappropriate colours impaired flavour recognition and that departures from the usual colour of yoghurt changed their flavour profiles. Presumably these are related effects, and this has been most forcefully demonstrated by Morot *et al.* (2001) who observed that merely changing the colour of a white wine to red, using a flavourless red colourant, shifted participants' flavour profiles, so that they now more closely matched red-wine, not white.

These types of effects presumably depend upon participants acquiring associations between flavours and colours. As noted above, Lavin and Lawless (1998) and Allen and Allen (1998) both found that colour effects were attenuated or absent in children. However, in contrast, Oram *et al.* (1995) reported that colour exerted a far more profound effect on children's identification of flavours than it did on adults, especially when the colour was inappropriate for the flavour (i.e. orange chocolate flavour). This finding suggests that children (aged 2–7) may already have acquired flavour–colour associations, and that these are more likely to influence their identification judgements, perhaps because their odour identification and discrimination abilities are typically poorer than adults (Stevenson *et al.* 2007).

Three studies have extended research on visual characteristics beyond smell and taste, to texture. One such study, reported by Christensen (1983) found no effect of colour on texture perception. In contrast, De Wijk *et al.* (2004) had participants suck custard up through a straw from a hidden lower compartment. Although colour and odour of the custard in the upper compartment had no impact on judgements of the ingested custard (Experiment 2), its appearance did. Visual-texture cues (thinner vs. thicker) of the custard in the upper compartment affected participants' judgements of the custard in the hidden lower compartment in a lawful manner.

Kappes *et al.* (2006) used six carbonated drinks to which they added a caramel colour. The added caramel colour decreased participants' judgements of carbonation, reducing bite, burn, and numbing ratings. For ratings connected with the drinks' viscosity, colour increased ratings of body and mouth-feel, even though it is very unlikely (as with irritation) that the 'physical' characteristics of the stimulus were in anyway altered by the addition of caramel colour. For both chemaesthetic and tactile effects, some of these intensity enhancements were still maintained under conditions in which multiple, appropriate rating scales were included. Finally, the colour also affected olfactory and taste ratings. It tended to reduce citrus ratings and increase caramel and vanilla flavours, as well as boosting bitter taste. There was no effect on sweetness.

The impact of colour on flavour probably has at least two components. The first is relatively straightforward, and, as with colour and odour, may reflect the simple observation that uncoloured fluids are generally flavourless whilst coloured fluids are generally flavourful. The second impact probably relates to participants' expectations that flow from their previous experience with certain colour–flavour combinations. This can lead to misidentification and qualitative shifts or, indeed, the apparent perception of qualities that are not physically present. A major question is whether these latter effects result from a change in the way that participants perceive the stimulus or from the way in which they report it. Put more bluntly, are these effects genuinely perceptual or are they a consequence of semantic knowledge? This question is addressed in the latter part of Chapter 3.

Interactions with audition

Certain foods produce particular patterns of sound when they are eaten. Crispness is by far the best example, and it has even been suggested that crispness is primarily an acoustic percept (Vickers and Bourne 1976a). The archetypal crispy food is the potato crisp (or chip). If participants make judgements of crispness by listening to tape-recorded sounds of other people eating them, after which they eat samples from the same set of crisps and judge crispness, there is a substantial correlation between these ratings—around 0.85 (Vickers 1987). Vickers and Bourne's (1976b) strong claim that crispness is *primarily* an acoustic percept is not supported by the finding that the presence of an auditory block (white noise) whilst making crispness judgements has no effect on participants' ratings relative to a no-block condition. This would suggest that texture and sound both carry similar information on crispness—an example of information redundancy.

Zampini and Spence (2004) examined whether manipulating particular aspects of the sound of biting a crisp would affect participants' perception of the crisp's crispness and freshness. They obtained the bite sound whilst the participant was biting the crisp and immediately played this back via headphones. Two aspects of the sound were manipulated whilst the crisps remained (unbeknownst to the participant) identical. First they manipulated loudness, by having a standard condition (no change in loudness) and two conditions where it was attenuated by 10 and 20 dB, respectively. Second, the high-frequency component of the crisp sound was amplified, left as it was, or attenuated. Based upon Vickers' (1984) work, in which crispness was found to be associated with high-frequency sounds, and with louder sounds too (Vickers and Christensen 1980), they suggested that crispness (and freshness) should be enhanced with high-frequency amplified sounds, and that crispness should be reduced (as well as freshness) where loudness was reduced, and especially with attenuation of the high-frequency component. Data from this experiment is illustrated in Figure 2.4, where it can be seen that these predictions were borne out. Crispness ratings increased with high-frequency amplification, and decreased with high-frequency attenuation. Similarly, reducing loudness reduced crispness. These factors interacted, in that the sound-frequency manipulation had little effect at the highest levels of loudness attenuation. Clearly, sound can influence texture perception, and this is an unambiguous example of a psychological interaction.

Crispness is, of course, not the only flavour quality that has a significant acoustic component. A further example is carbonation, with the fizzing and popping of the bubbles providing a cue as to whether the drink is carbonated, and the degree of carbonation. Zampini and Spence (2005) explored whether participants could judge carbonation from auditory cues alone, and in addition, manipulated the sounds by having participants hold the carbonated drink under a microphone whilst the sound was again subjected to the same pattern of modification that they used for their crisp study. As with crisps, they found that manipulating the sound of the drink did indeed affect participants' judgements of carbonation level. However, unlike the crisps

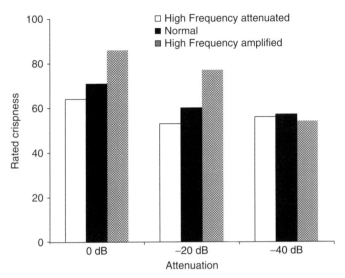

Fig. 2.4 Effect of manipulating loudness (attenuation) and high-frequency sounds (amplified or attenuated) on perception of the crispness of crisps. Data adapted from Zampini and Spence 2004.

study, when this was attempted 'in the mouth', no effect of sound manipulation could be obtained, suggesting in this case that carbonation perception is driven primarily by somatosensory cues. As Spence and Zampini (2006) note, auditory influences on perception in other modalities are pervasive, and it is highly likely that other examples of interaction with flavour will be identified.

Conclusion

This chapter aimed to identify psychological (or centrally based) interactions between the various modalities and sub-modalities that comprise the flavour system. The interactions reviewed above can be categorized into three groups: (1) unambiguous examples of psychological/centrally driven interactions; (2) ambiguous cases; and (3) unambiguous examples of peripherally driven interactions. This section will briefly summarize category (1) because these interactions will form the material that is examined in the next chapter, where the issue of cause will be more directly addressed. That some psychological interactions may have been missed (or indeed that the standard of evidence is too harsh) may be fair criticisms to level at this approach, but it does seem preferable to concentrate on interactions that have a well-established psychological basis.

Table 2.2 Clear-cut cases of psychological or centrally driven interactions within the flavour system

Interaction	Nature of psychological/ central interaction effect(s)
1. Taste–taste	Component quality suppression (only certain tastes)
2. Odour–odour	Component quality suppression (most odours)
3. Taste–smell	Qualitative enhancement, sub-additive detection
4. Smell–chemaesthesis	Suppression (orthonasal only)
5. Odour–(taste)–tactile	Odour suppression, tactile enhancement by odour
6. Colour–orthonasal smell	Generic effect of colour on detection/intensity
	Specific effect on identification/quality
7. Colour–(taste)–retronasal smell	Generic effect of colour on detection/intensity
	Specific effect on identification/quality
8. Auditory–tactile	Enhancement and suppression of crispness

Table 2.2 presents the interactions that appear to have a demonstrable psychological basis. Items one and two are important and have been well documented in the literature. The effects here are rather straightforward to describe, namely that suppression appears to characterize these interactions. Item three clearly has a psychological basis and is a very central component to nearly all foods and drinks. The same comment can be extended to item five. Item four, although clearly psychological, is of less interest as it is a purely ortho-nasal phenomenon that may not occur when the irritant is in the mouth. Consequently, item four will not be discussed in the next chapter. Item six, whilst also being an orthonasal phenomena, is worth considering, as it appears to extend into retronasal perception and thus flavour (item seven). Item eight is also important, even though it rests upon relatively little experimental work.

Before turning to the issue of cause in Chapter 3, notice how central olfac-tion and vision are to most of these psychological interactions. Apart, of course, from the obvious fact that these are anatomically discrete (thereby reducing the likelihood of peripheral or stimulus-based interactions) it likely reflects functional concerns of the sort discussed in Chapter 1. That is, the eyes and the nose evaluate food, *before* it is placed in the mouth. As argued throughout this book, this reflects the brain's capacity to learn about flavour and to use this knowledge via the exteroceptive senses of vision and orthonasal olfaction, in deciding what to eat or drink. This may offer one explanation for certain interaction effects, but this is to anticipate the next chapter.

Chapter 3

Causes of flavour interaction

Introduction

The purpose of this chapter is to examine the distal and proximal causes of the central/psychological interactions identified in Chapter 2. Four different types of interactions are featured in Chapter 2. The first type, which is not considered here, were those interactions occurring within the stimulus during its transit through the mouth (e.g. variations in diffusion rates, chemical reactions, etc.) and interactions directly involving the receptors (e.g. competition for the same receptor type, thermal tastes, etc.). These types of interactions do, however, feature in the discussion of how flavour components are bound in Chapter 6.

A second type of interaction reflects processes which depend upon low-level activity in the brain. The term 'low-level' here refers to forms of information processing and their content that are not available to consciousness. Two types of interactions described in Chapter 2 *may* be examples of this, namely interactions between different tastants, and interactions between different odourants. Whilst they are not cross-modal interactions, these represent such crucial components of flavour that they warrant attention. This is especially so for olfaction, where complex mixtures of chemicals typify what is routinely encountered in food and drink (e.g. Maarse (1991) and see Chapter 1). If these complex mixtures produce a percept which is cognitively impenetrable, then a major component of flavour *may* be permanently beyond anyone's ability to 'dissect' into its parts. The same may not be true for taste. Consequently, for these two forms of interaction, it is necessary not only to consider how this occurs, but also to address the issue of whether the components are identifiable.

A third type of interaction may occur via information redundancy, in which two or more sensory channels carry similar information and this, in combination, may be used to enhance stimulus detection, location, or identification—the classic functional benefits of multisensory processing. A clear example of this is the interaction between audition and tactile stimulation. Here two independent channels of information are complimentary and one may—under appropriate circumstances—impact upon the other. An important issue in this case is whether the interaction is symmetrical or asymmetrical. This type of question draws upon a wider psychological literature, because it is necessary to identify the factors which are used to resolve potential conflicts between redundant channels—i.e. does one channel always 'win out' generating an asymmetry? Whilst auditory–tactile interactions are one example, creaminess appears to be another. This was not discussed in Chapter 2 for reasons that will become apparent later on. Creaminess seems to draw upon multiple, redundant channels of information, especially as it appears possible to alter various aspects of the physical stimulus and produce an appreciably similar level of creaminess. A further example involves certain forms of colour–flavour interaction. The most compelling is that of white wine coloured red, which results in flavour judgements akin to those obtained for real red wine. In this case there are two channels of information, the wine's flavour, and its colour, with colour winning out.

Colour–flavour interactions are notably different from both creaminess and auditory–tactile interactions and so are considered separately from them. This is because colour is an attribute of food or drink that is perceived prior to ingestion, not simultaneously as with tactile–auditory stimulation or creamy percepts. This is an important distinction as it also applies, in a different but functionally related way, to interactions between taste and smell, and certain tactile/taste and smell interactions too. Humans, and of course other organisms too, need to detect, locate, and identify food and then decide whether to place it in the mouth. To do so, they must keep a record—memories—of what is and what is not food. To detect, locate, and identify food, humans must rely primarily upon the exteroceptive (distance) senses, notably vision and orthonasal olfaction. This will also apply when the food is up close and a decision is made about whether or not to ingest. It may then be misleading to believe that all interactions observed 'in the mouth', are reflections of 'functional' multimodal processing (as with auditory/tactile interactions or creaminess). Rather, the effects of colour on flavour perception or the interactions between taste and smell, and certain smell–tactile–taste interactions, could be inadvertent consequences—i.e. side effects—of learning about flavour; learning that is focussed on providing information that is later deployed 'outside of the mouth' by the exteroceptive visual and orthonasal olfactory systems.

It is for this reason that a fourth type of interaction is defined here. This is one where the functional benefits occur primarily outside of the mouth (the term 'primarily' is used deliberately here because there is a further delayed functional benefit relating to flavour memory that operates within the mouth discussed in Chapter 5 and 6). These types of interactions all result from learning about flavour, but there is a further distinction that has to be made. Some learning processes appear to result in a change in the way a stimulus is perceived, whilst others are expressed as a change in what is known about a stimulus. Sometimes, these forms of learning occur together, and at other times they may occur independently. Especially for odours and tastes, and arguably for certain odour–taste–tactile interactions, it is a change in perception, which appears to be important. For learning involving colour, this may manifest as a change in what is known about a stimulus and what it is expected to taste like. By far the bulk of scientific knowledge, both psychological and neuroscientific, has been collected about this fourth type of interaction and so inevitably this forms a central part of the chapter.

Impenetrable interactions

The focus of this section is to examine interactions that occur within taste and smell. For taste, the literature is more limited and so inevitably a greater part of the discussion below deals with olfaction.

Taste

The split-tongue experiments (e.g. Kroeze and Bartoshuk 1985) demonstrate that the suppression of individual taste qualities in mixtures has both peripheral and central components. Electrophysiological data is consistent with these behavioural observations. Recordings from both, single nerve cells in the chorda tympani nerve (Frank 1989) and from the parabrachial nucleus in the pons of the hamster (Smith 1989), indicate that neurons are less responsive to mixtures of tastants (matched for intensity) than one would predict from their responsiveness to individual tastants. This reduced neuronal responsiveness to mixtures versus single tastants also extends to single-unit recordings made in the primary taste cortex of monkeys (Miyaoka and Pritchard 1996, Plata-Salaman *et al.* 1996). Needless to say, one can only infer that the same pattern would be observed in humans, but these animals have broadly similar taste responsiveness, so this is not an unreasonable inference.

These animal data indicate that suppression may be the dominant feature of neural responding to taste mixtures at all levels of the nervous system, suggesting, as in humans, that taste-mixture components are perceived (generally, and dependent upon concentration) as less intense. Three questions emerge: How does this occur? Why should this be so? and what of individual taste qualities? In respect to the first question, as far as one can tell from animal neurophysiology, neither the suppression mechanism(s), nor its locus (loci), have been fully identified. However, Bartoshuk (1975) suggests one possibility drawing upon single-cell recordings from frogs, namely peripheral antidromic inhibition of taste receptors. Here, it is suggested, increasing stimulation of receptors leads to progressively greater antidromic feedback, suppressing receptor activity, and thus requiring much greater increases in stimulus concentration to achieve a further noticeable increase in intensity.

An answer to the second question (suggested earlier) may reside in the form of an individual tastants' psychophysical function (e.g. Bartoshuk 1975, Keast and Breslin 2002). The nervous system has to deal with a large range of stimulus values (chemical concentration here), and this is achieved, in part, by compressing the psychophysical function as concentration increases (and, of course, the mechanism suggested by Bartoshuk above is one way to achieve this at the neural level). A mixture of two tastes effectively represents an increase in concentration, and so the neural response is then less than the sum of its parts (from a linear additive model) because of this response compression.

The third question concerns the perception of individual tastants in mixtures. As noted in Chapter 2, participants 'appear' to have no difficulty in identifying individual tastants (as far as judging their intensity goes) in four-component mixes (i.e. salt, sucrose, quinine, and hydrochloric acid; Bartoshuk 1975). So whilst mixture suppression may reduce the apparent intensity of the components, it does not 'appear' to affect their identifiability. Judgements of individual taste intensities are based, of course, on the assumption that the components can be identified, and several studies have addressed this assumption directly.

Laing et al. (2002) presented trained participants with both, single tastants and mixtures of tastants (up to five—sucrose, salt, citric acid, caffeine, and inositol monophosphate (umami)). The participants' task was to identify one particular target taste within single, or mixtures of, tastants. Sucrose and bitter were identified above chance in all but the five component mixtures, whilst salt was identified even in this stimulus. Sour and umami tastes were not identified in mixtures with three or more components. These results provide some answers and, as always, some further questions. At least for bitter, sweet, and salty tastes, participants are generally able to identify these qualities even in complex mixtures. This, of course, may depend upon the tastant used by the experimenter, as Laing et al.'s (2002) results for sour taste suggest. Bartoshuk (1975) observed that, for the sour taste of hydrochloric acid, this was the most distinctive stimulus in terms of perceived intensity ratings of components in ternary and quaternary mixtures (see her Table 3.1, op. cit.).

An interesting question Laing et al.'s (2002) data raise is whether the failure to identify certain tastants in more complex mixtures reflects the emergence of some new taste quality or qualities. This possibility cuts to the heart of an old and very live debate as to whether taste should be considered as an analytic or synthetic sense (see e.g. McBurney and Gent 1979). Evidence favourable to the emergence of new taste qualities has been obtained (e.g. Kuznicki and Ashbaugh 1982), but perhaps here the most important point is that, in general, mixing tastes does not preclude identification of the components. Functionally, this would make sense, especially if taste serves to rapidly identify bitter (i.e. potential poisons), sweet (i.e. potential energy), umami (i.e. protein), sour (i.e. tissue damage, ripeness, etc.), or salty (i.e. mineral balance) tastants in food, so as to decide rapidly whether to ingest or eject. In this case a significant analytic capability, especially for bitter tastes, would be highly advantageous.

Smell

A common finding when odourants are mixed together is that the combination is perceived as less intense than the sum of its components—hypoadditivity. As described in Chapter 2, this effect in humans appears to have both peripheral and central components, as indicated by presenting one odourant to one nostril and the other odourant to the other nostril simultaneously (e.g. Laing and Wilcox 1987). The observation of hypoadditivity with odourants raises a similar set of questions to those that were addressed for taste. What is its underlying neural cause, what is its function, and are the contents of component processing cognitively impenetrable? Each of these questions is addressed below.

The neural basis of mixture suppression has been found, perhaps not surprisingly given the psychophysical data, to also have peripheral and central components. Duchamp-Viret *et al.* (2003) recorded the activity of rat olfactory receptor neurons (ORN) when stimulated with single odourants and binary mixtures of these odourants. Hypoadditivity, as measured by the predicted discharge spike frequency of the particular ORN in response to single odourants, was the most common finding when a binary mixture was presented. Hypoadditivity has also been observed within the olfactory bulb, from single-cell recordings of mitral cells (Giraudet *et al.* 2001). In this case, 'dominance' was the most frequently observed pattern in that a mitral cell's response more closely resembled its output pattern to just one of the two odourants in the mixture (i.e. the output was less than the input might lead one to expect).

The question of function, neural basis, and cognitive impenetrability are all entwined. For tastes, it was argued above that suppression arose primarily as a consequence of the way in which the brain has to deal with a broad range of stimulus concentrations—from low to high. This results in compression, especially for mid- to high-range stimuli. To an extent, this will also be true for odour mixtures. However, there is very likely to be a problem in judging the intensity of components, which may be unique to olfaction and derives from the different way in which the brain processes odours, relative to the way it processes tastes. For tastes, there are good functional reasons for an analytical strategy, as noted above, thus potentially allowing a participant to assess the intensity of individual components. For olfaction, where the stimulus is often a mixture with 10's or 100's of elements (e.g. see Maarse 1991), processing is different, because the function is different, namely to recognize and identify the 'smell' (i.e. the mixture). In this case, judgements of intensity for mixture components, beyond binary or ternary mixtures, may be very difficult or impossible, because there may no longer be conscious access to each component.

A series of studies by Laing and colleagues demonstrates convincingly that there is an absolute limit to the detection of components in odour mixtures. In his early studies, participants were presented with olfactory stimuli that were single, binary, or contained three, four, five, six, or more component odourants. Participants were trained beforehand to identify each of the components individually, before being presented with the test stimuli. Participants identified single odourants on 82% of trials, and the components of binary ones on 35% of trials, ternary ones on 14% of trials, four-component ones on 4% of trials, but they were never able to identify all of the components in a five-odourant mixture (Laing and Francis 1989). Needless to say, this is a hard task, and poorer performance with the more complex mixtures might reflect cognitive load (i.e. demands on executive processes) rather than reflecting limits of the perceptual system. However, Laing and Glenmarec (1987) asked participants to just identify a single, target component in each test stimulus. Results from this experiment revealed the same finding that a limit on detecting components occurs when three or more odourants are presented together as a mixture. Similar results have also been obtained with poor and good blending odours (Livermore and Laing 1998a) and when using complex odourants, rather than single, pure chemicals as the stimuli (e.g. a mixture of chocolate and rose; Livermore and Laing 1998b). This latter finding is especially interesting, as it suggests again that complex mixtures and single chemicals are both treated as 'units'—i.e. as temporally discrete patterns of neural activity.

The data reviewed above suggest that odour perception is a synthetic sense. The use of the term 'synthetic' is not absolute, and clearly we have some limited capacity to identify components, but it is heavily constrained. The neural processing that underpins this type of synthetic olfactory perception has been reviewed extensively (e.g. Wilson and Stevenson 2006, Stevenson and Wilson 2007), and it is reassuringly consistent with the synthetic account that emerges from the psychological data.

A final and important issue here concerns the way in which people communicate information about odour quality. This is normally in the form of 'it smells like X'.

The fact that odours can be profiled by comparing then either directly to a range of other odours (Schultz 1964) or to odour names (e.g. Dravnieks 1986) might suggest an ability to decompose odours into their component features. Indeed, precisely this claim was made above for rating the intensity of component tastes in complex taste mixtures. However, this is probably not the case, because what participants may be doing when profiling an odour is making similarity judgements between the target and an either real or imagined quality (i.e. the odour is evaluated on a semantic profile or against a set of real odours that reflect the qualities of each component of the semantic profile). In fact, there may be a deeper analogy here between semantic profiling and what the brain does when it processes the complex neural activity pattern that is generated by an odourant. The neural output pattern may be compared to all available stored patterns (i.e. previously experienced smells), and the degree of computed similarity between the patterns may reflect the reported degree of similarity that is obtained in semantic profiling studies (see Stevenson and Boakes 2003). Indeed, some empirical support for this analogy has been obtained (Mingo and Stevenson 2007). In sum, whilst taste perception may maintain a generally analytical stance, odour perception appears to be generally synthetic. Part of the cost of synthetic processing may be the loss of information about the component parts—unlike taste.

Information redundancy in the mouth

A general property of animal sensory systems is that information about an event in the external world is usually carried via multiple sensory channels (Stein, Wallace, and Stanford 2001). This is highly adaptive, as it allows for substitution (e.g. touch and sound for finding things in the dark), and enhanced detection and identification of events in the external world (De Gelder and Bertelson 2003). In addition, whilst different sensory modalities may carry overlapping (redundant) information, they may also carry different features of the same stimulus. This ability to capitalize on information redundancy makes it a ubiquitous feature of human and animal perception, and so it should not be surprising that it operates within the context of flavour. Because information redundancy can generate a number of different effects (i.e. substitution, detection, identification, etc.), one task here is to determine what type of effect is being demonstrated for each flavour-related example and the function this might serve.

Auditory–tactile interactions

As described in Chapter 2, presenting participants with an altered sound of their crisp bite can have a significant impact on their judgements of how crispy or fresh the crisp is (Zampini and Spence 2004). In this case, there are two channels of information. The auditory channel can clearly carry information that is informative about the rheological properties of foods, as participants can judge a food's likely textural qualities quite accurately from simply hearing the sound of someone else eating it (Christensen and Vickers 1981). The somaesthetic channel can also carry information (not surprisingly) about the tactile properties of food, and this can also be used to make judgements of crispness, again quite accurately, even when the sound of eating is eliminated by a white-noise mask (Christensen and Vickers 1981).

Zampini and Spence (2004) used a classic intersensory discrepancy approach to examine the interaction between these channels of information (Welch and Warren 1980). Here, one channel is held constant whilst the other is distorted. In this case, Zampini and Spence (2004) obtained data suggesting that ratings of crispness were lawfully distorted by the adjustment of loudness (more crispy) and attenuation of high-frequency sounds (less crispy) or amplification of these sounds (more crispy). Three general classes of explanation have been advanced for how these intersensory distortions may arise (see Welch and Warren 1980): (1) The more precise modality wins out, i.e. the channel that carries the more accurate information. (2) The modality that attracts greater attentional resources wins out. (3) The modality that is better suited to carry information relative to the task at hand wins out. Neither explanation (1) nor (3) appear likely, as there are no grounds to suspect that either the tactile or auditory modality is any better than the other at determining crispness, nor in fact any better suited for the particular task at hand. Explanation (2) appears the most probable, as participants were wearing headphones and so were likely to be attending more to this channel of information than they might otherwise have been.

The type of interaction here appears to be most similar to an enhancement of identification. Normally, stale crisps would be associated with softer bite and a quieter, less high-pitched sound (and vice versa for fresh crisps) and so the auditory channel provides information that is normally complimentary to the tactile channel for making this form of identification judgement (stale or fresh). Notice how this interpretation assumes that participants have learnt to associate the output of the tactile and auditory channel—if this were not so, then one channel could not affect the other in this lawful manner. A similar point is made by Welch and Warren (1980) in their review of intersensory discrepancies.

A second point concerns the psychological locus of this effect. Clearly, Zampini and Spence's (2004) experiment does not preclude a decision (or semantic) explanation. Participants could have reasoned that sound was being manipulated or alternatively drawn upon conscious knowledge of what such sounds mean in the context of this type of food. Alternatively, the effect could have a perceptual locus, in that the auditory information actually altered participants' tactile perceptions of crispness. Their experiment cannot determine the answer to this common problem in intersensory discrepancy research (see De Gelder and Bertelson 2003), but Zampini and Spence (2004) noted that 75% of their participants thought that the crisps were coming from different bags—i.e. they believed that the samples were different, not the same as in fact they were. This would suggest a perceptual locus.

The neural basis of this type of interaction probably draws upon the same sort of basic mechanisms that have been suggested for other examples of information redundancy, where that information converges on multimodal neurons (Calvert *et al.* 1998). These multimodal neurons that are presumably responsive to combinations of sound and texture might be expected to be located in the orbitofrontal cortex—a structure of high significance in flavour processing, as it appears to contain cells that are responsive to multiple flavour-related inputs (e.g. Rolls and Baylis 1994). This is conjecture, but a reasonable one. A further conjecture is how such multimodal neurons influence perception. Drawing upon Mesulam (2000), multimodal neurons may function as the node that links information stored in cortical areas that deal with the unimodal percepts—tactile and auditory here. Thus, an auditory input may activate a multimodal node, which in turn activates the unimodal tactile cortex, resulting in a percept that is distorted (more or less crispy).

Whilst auditory–tactile interactions are clearly demonstrated with crisp texture, this is not the case for carbonation. In this case, the channel information argument holds, in that participants can appropriately detect variations in carbonation, with carbonation sound alone (see Experiment 2, Zampini and Spence 2005), and similarly can detect variations in carbonation dependent on chemaesthesis (recall this is also a somatosensory modality). However, in this case no interaction was obtained under the conditions, which did obtain an effect for crispness. Two explanations suggest themselves. First, in this case attention may have been potently directed to the mouth by the irritant nature of the stimulus. Second, judgements of carbonation—in the mouth—may not normally rely upon auditory cues, but instead on chemaesthetic ones.

Creaminess

Discussion of creaminess was largely absent from Chapter 2. This is interesting because of what it tells us about this phenomenon. Most interactions can be adequately specified by examining the senses that contribute to them and, indeed, this is why Chapter 2 was organized in this way. Creaminess is a case where the perceptual dimension is quite specific (as detailed below), but where both, the relative contribution of the senses and the relevant stimulus parameters, are unclear (see de Wijk *et al.* 2006, Frost and Janhoj 2007). Thus, creaminess was very difficult to capture within the framework of Chapter 2, because it may result from different contributions from each sense, which vary on a food-by-food basis. Whilst it may be an orphan in terms of Chapter 2, it is an excellent example of multisensory integration and of information redundancy.

Two characteristics of creaminess are important. The first is that the use of this quality in describing foods does not appear to change markedly from naive participants to trained sensory panellists (de Wijk *et al.* 2006). This suggests that the concept is a fairly basic one in respect to the perception of flavour (e.g. more like sweetness). The second is that the use of the creaminess descriptor appears to describe broadly the same percept across a range of foods, although there clearly is some variation here (Tournier *et al.* 2007). This would also seem to indicate that it is a fairly basic flavour-related percept (e.g. again consider sweetness across foods).

Whilst creaminess may be a fairly stable percept across foods and between participants, the stimuli that contribute to it are not. Take two examples. The first is drawn from milk products. Richardson *et al.* (1993) varied three parameters: fat-globule size (via homogenizing or not homogenizing the milk), fat content (3.5 vs. 4.8%), and thickness (addition or not of carboxymethyl cellulose). Homogenized high-fat milk was perceived to be approximately as creamy as non-homogenized low-fat milk. Similarly, the creaminess of low-fat homogenized and thickened milk was almost identical to that of high-fat non-homogenized unthickened milk. The point here is that varying single or multiple physical features of the stimulus can result in broadly the same percept of creaminess, suggesting that multiple, redundant channels of information underpin this.

The second example draws more broadly from the literature and looks across food groupings for factors that influence creaminess (see de Wijk *et al.* 2006). These include: (1) the odour (ortho and retronasal) of yoghurts and cheeses, and the colour of cheese (Frost and Janhoj 2007); (2) the visual textural appearance (de Wijk *et al.* 2004) and sweet taste of custards (de Wijk *et al.* 2003); (3) the viscosity and flow behaviour of soups (Daget and Joerg 1991) and desert creams (Daget *et al.* 1987); and (4) the fat content of ice creams (Frost *et al.* 2001) and the oil-droplet size and fat content of emulsion gels (Clegg *et al.* 2003). In addition, the list would not be complete without inclusion of the role of viscosity and frictional forces, acting between the tongue and hard palate, which may be common to many (but not all) judgements of creaminess (Kokini and Cussler 1983). Thus, together, these include physical parameters that affect the visual, olfactory, taste, and especially the somatosensory systems, as well as a range of other variables, including time course, bolus size, and the effect of saliva, which were not included above. Presumably, information from these disparate sources, varying between foods, is combined to produce the percept of creaminess.

Creaminess is an important variable for the food industry because it is predictive of whether people will like a particular food product, especially if their expectations of creaminess are violated—say in low-fat products (de Wijk *et al.* 2006). In terms of biological function, it is likely that it is one way (others might include crispiness and appearance; Drewnowski 1992) in which the fat content of food, and thus more broadly, its caloric content is evaluated. Whilst correlations with fat content are generally moderate to poor, creaminess does appear to relate to participants' perception of fat content (e.g. Tournier *et al.* 2007, de Wijk and Prinz 2005). This may reflect, perhaps, that in less processed foods (e.g. dairy products), creaminess may be a reasonable predictor of fat content, even if it is not always so in more processed foods. This is essentially an evolutionary argument for creaminess perception as one means of sensing fat. The close relationship between hedonics and creaminess, as with hedonics and sweetness, also points to this conclusion.

With this possible functional basis in mind (fat/calories), it is necessary to consider the form that this information redundancy takes and its locus. In terms of form it would appear, as with the auditory–tactile interaction above, to represent an example of identification enhancement. Rather than relying on one channel to identify fat (or calories), information from several channels is combined (see Chale-Rush *et al.* 2007) to produce a more reliable percept (creamy here) and thus increase appropriate identification of calorie-rich food. An additional consideration is that creaminess is also an example of substitution, analogous to the use of different channels of redundant information under different circumstances (i.e. different foods here). This is nicely illustrated by the range of textural parameters that can generate creaminess in dairy products (e.g. Richardson, Booth, and Stanley 1993) and in other food groups too.

In terms of locus, this must involve multiple levels. Odour and colour effects suggest high-level (cortical) interactions, whilst fat-globule size, viscosity, and friction represent both, complex interactions with tactile receptors in the mouth as well as between the output of different types of tactile receptors at a more central level. As for the auditory–tactile case, a similar explanatory approach to central integration of these multiple redundant inputs can be adopted here. The difference in this case is that there is more supporting evidence.

Single-cell recordings in the primate orbitofrontal cortex provide clear evidence for cells that are responsive to differing concentrations of carboxymethyl cellulose (CMC). Some of these cells respond in a graded fashion, becoming more responsive as CMC concentration increases (i.e. increasing viscosity) whilst others respond preferentially to certain viscosity ranges (Rolls *et al.* 2003). Other cells demonstrate responsiveness only to oils (i.e. to fats) and also to pure hydrocarbons such as mineral oil. Importantly, some of these cells are not responsive to viscosity, suggesting that it is some other characteristic of the stimulus that is being detected—a tactile quality—which is viscosity independent (Verhagen *et al.* 2003). In this latter study, cells were also found that responded to changes in viscosity, independently of fat or oil content, suggesting that the orbitofrontal cortex has at least three channels of information that are relevant: (1) fat/oil-sensitive cells that must draw from tactile source because they are responsive to fats *and* oils (i.e. similar textural quality); (2) fat/oil- and viscosity-sensitive cells (which were detected by Verhagen *et al.* 2003); and (3) viscosity-sensitive cells that are not sensitive to fats/oils. In addition to this, Rolls *et al.* (1999) also found evidence of cells that were responsive to fat and to its associated odour (cream). All three of these studies (above) also obtained evidence of cells that were sensitive to viscosity/taste and taste/fat and taste/fat/viscosity combinations. It is also likely that cells will be found that are sensitive to the visual appearance of fat, although none were noted in these studies. Finally, whilst these data were obtained in primates, it is very likely that the human orbitofrontal cortex is also central for encoding similar properties. In a neuroimaging study using chocolate milk and tomato juice as stimuli, activity was detected in the orbitofrontal cortex suggesting that this is a likely locus for convergence of perceptual information relating to the textural (and other) qualities of food (Kringelbach *et al.* 2003). In sum, the orbitofrontal cortex offers a likely point of convergence for the formation of a creaminess percept, drawing upon viscosity, fat content (perhaps friction, globule size, oral coating, etc.), taste, and odour.

Interactions as side effects of learning

In Chapter 2, two olfactory-related interactions were particularly apparent—those between odours and tastes and those between odours and tactile stimuli (along with tastes). A further interaction, with a clear psychological basis, was also identified there, namely that between colour, odour, and taste (i.e. colour–flavour). The aim of this section is to examine the distal and proximal causes of these various interactions, especially their distal cause as this has important functional implications. The following sections deal, first, with odour–taste interactions; then with odour, taste, and tactile interactions; and finally with colour–flavour interactions.

Odour–taste interactions—Functional issues

The basic argument advanced here is that interactions between odours and tastes in 'flavour' are a side effect of learning. Arguably the main purpose of odour–taste learning is to assist the organism, via orthonasal olfaction, to decide whether or not to place a food in the mouth, and more broadly to assist in the detection and location of food in the environment. To this end, learning associations between taste and smell in the mouth have a number of functional benefits that are expressed outside of the mouth. First, when a taste–smell combination is encountered in the mouth, this combination is learnt. When the food is encountered again, the smell of the food is able to redintegrate (recover as a whole) the memory of the food's flavour. A key component of this flavour memory is, of course, its taste. If the food smells sweet, then this is very likely to indicate calories, and so a sweet-smelling odour is signalling, even before its source is tasted, the likely presence of an energy source. Similarly, if the food were to smell salty, sour, or bitter, these too would have functional significance, in just the same way that the signal of the tastes themselves do; salty for mineral balance, sour for potential irritants/ripeness, and bitter for potential poisons, etc.

A second benefit is that this signalling system appears to be complementary to, but independent of, odour hedonics. For example, sucrose-paired odours are liked more than bitter-paired odours, (see De Houwer et al. 2001) making an odour-based flavour signal (i.e. smelling sweet or bitter) a complimentary cue. However, the affective value of foods can change as a consequence of ingestion and so whilst the smell of a food is indicative of its likely pleasant (or unpleasant) consequences (see Chapter 5), identification of future food sources when sated would be problematic. The advantage then of perceiving foods as smelling, say, sweet or bitter is that it gives important information irrespective of the organism's state as well as providing information redundancy.

A key point then from the functional argument above is that it is the signal value of an odourant's orthonasal smell (i.e. smelling sweet) that is important. This would suggest that interaction effects in the mouth between certain tastes and smells are an incidental consequence of the redintegration process (e.g. retronasally perceived strawberry odour in the mouth redintegrates a sweet-strawberry flavour memory and it is this that generates the interaction). Two asymmetries are suggested by this account. First, tastes should *not* trigger odour percepts (i.e. the signal value is all in the odour-triggering taste).

Second, the effect of odours on taste perception and taste on odour perception (i.e. orally based interaction effects) should be more inconsistent than observations pertaining to odour-induced tastes (i.e. orthonasally perceived tastes). This is because the former are incidental effects and the latter are functional effects. Is there any evidence for these claims?

Starting with the first claim, that tastes should not induce odour percepts, this would appear to be true, but with some caveats. As noted in Chapter 2, tastants can smell (Mojet *et al.* 2005). The question is why? One possibility is that even purified tastants contain trace volatiles that have either escaped purification or that are a consequence of chemical processes occurring after purification. A further possibility is that tastants themselves can trigger an odour percept, but this is unlikely. In Mojet *et al.*'s (2005) experiment in at least one condition, participants could identify the likely taste of a sample by orthonasal olfaction alone. This suggests that volatiles were being released by the sample and that these volatiles were predictive of the tastant, suggesting a common and prior history of co-occurrence. A final possibility is that small quantities of the tastant were swept up via the nose and detected in the nasopharynx where there are taste receptors. This is a possibility, but it does not appear to be a very likely one.

A second finding is that the addition of sweet tastes can sometimes enhance certain olfactory attributes (e.g. fruity, berry-like, etc.) and depress others (e.g. pungent, green, etc.; see Von Sydow *et al.* 1974). These findings could be interpreted as suggesting that taste 'generates' an olfactory percept, which is then added to that generated directly by the odourant. This possibility appears unlikely given that subtractive effects can also occur (i.e. depression of green and pungent notes). It appears more likely that taste-induced odour-enhancement effects occur as a consequence of the association of particular odour qualities with particular taste qualities. In the example above, fruity and berry notes were enhanced by the addition of sucrose and, indeed, these type of odourants commonly co-occur with sweet tastes. Similarly, pungent and green notes may be associated with sour tastes, and sour tastes are suppressed by sweet.

This is a good point to examine the proximal cause of these types of interactions (see van der Klaauw and Frank (1996) for a similar account to the one here). First, these interactions depend upon a history of co-occurrence between the odour and a taste, which results in an association forming between them (the distal cause). This association can then act to blur the perceptual boundary between the odour and its associated taste percept in the mouth (i.e. they start to act as integral dimensions in Garner's (1974) terminology). For example, if a participant with a history of such co-occurrence is then asked to rate strawberryness in a strawberry–sucrose mixture, then it will be difficult for them to judge where 'strawberryness' stops and 'sweetness' starts. Put another way, attending to the feature 'strawberry' in the example here automatically invokes attention to sweetness; the two can no longer be attended to in isolation because of the association between them. This boundary blurring can also account for why this type of interaction effect may be susceptible to manipulation of rating scale type and number (see Chapter 2). This is because it is more likely that, e.g. strawberryness will be conflated into sweetness ratings, if *only* a sweetness rating is available (and vice versa). This represents one way in which odour–taste interactions can occur, but it is not the only way. Valentin *et al.* (2006) have suggested that certain odour–taste interactions may result from other processes that are independent of prior learning. These may reflect more general effects of flavour binding—in particular, the default tendency to process flavour in the mouth as a unitary percept (this the focus of the next Chapter and a significant part of Chapter 6). However, as Valentin *et al.* (2006) also note, odour–taste interactions that do result from prior learning reflect an additional interactive component.

There is, though, another proximal mechanism that is complimentary to boundary blurring, which also depends upon learning. As discussed more extensively below, certain odours can induce taste-like percepts (e.g. sweetness). This extra (psychological) 'taste' can impact perception when an odour with a history of co-occurrence with a particular taste (e.g. sweet) is placed in the mouth with that associated taste being physically present (e.g. drawing on the example above, strawberry odour and sucrose). The extra redintegrated (psychological) taste may then add to the perceived sweetness of the mixture, or possibly even exert a suppressive effect if a different taste is physically present (e.g. a sweet-smelling odour with a sour taste). These two learning-based effects, boundary blurring and redintegrated taste, may combine to produce suppressive effects. For example, a bitter-smelling odour with a physically present sweet taste may result in a reduction in the perceived intensity of particular odour qualities. The sweet taste may mask both the bitter redintegrated taste and, by virtue of the latter's association to the odour, the odour too. Finally, subthreshold integration, where a taste can facilitate detection of a subthreshold odour also likely relies upon both of these processes. The association between taste and smell allows the combination to be perceived as a unitary stimulus, with redintegrated taste and the odour adding to the physically present associated taste, thereby enhancing intensity, and so aiding detection.

Returning to the issue of asymmetry, a final point here concerns contingency. Tastes occur with hundreds or thousands of odourants, yet particular combinations of odourants typically occur with a limited (or very limited) number of tastants. Consequently, one taste might predict many odours, but a particular odour is likely to predict just one taste. In addition to this predictive (i.e. contingency-based) argument, sampling a taste brings with it the risk of poisoning; a risk that is almost wholly absent if a food is sniffed. Indeed, even if a food is novel it may have a similar olfactory profile to one that is familiar, and so would generate a similar odour-induced taste. Consider rose odour, for example. This may be described as sweet-smelling even though sweetened rose odours are not commonly encountered. The volatiles that make up rose odour overlap considerably with those generated by other members of the *Rosoideae* subfamily. These include, raspberries, blackberries, and strawberries, all of which smell sweet.

The second asymmetry predicted by the functional account above concerns the reliability of the effect of odours on tastes and vice versa in the mouth, versus the reliability of an odour's ability to induce a taste sensation when sniffed. Valentin *et al.* (2006) present a very handy table listing the effects of odours on sweet-taste perception (see their Table 4.1, *op. cit.*). Excluding the 23 cases where the odour *may* not smell sweet, i.e. when a sweetness-enhancement effect might not be reasonably demonstrated (e.g. wintergreen, oolong tea, etc.), the table details reports on a further 48 cases. Of these 48, 28 used single-scale methodology (i.e. just ratings of sweetness) and sweetness enhancement was demonstrated in 24 of the 28 cases. A further 20 used a multiple-scale approach, and here only 7 of the 20 demonstrated a sweetness-enhancement effect. At least as far as sweetness enhancement goes, the effect is clearly there, especially under the single-scale condition, but the effect is considerably less evident under the multiple-scale condition. Thus, one could conclude that sweetness enhancement is a reliable effect—but one that is apparently sensitive to the way in which the judgement is made.

What about judgements of odour-induced taste, when the odourant is simply sniffed? For starters, it is hard to find evidence that such judgements (sweetness) are affected by the number of ratings that participants are asked to make in the same way that odour-induced sweetness-enhancement effects clearly are. The Dravnieks (1986) *Atlas of odor profiles* requires participants to make 146 judgements of each odourant, yet many typically sweet-smelling odours are still regarded as smelling sweet (e.g. Strawberry (Table 6, *op. cit.*), Pineapple (Table 8, *op. cit.*), Banana (Table 9, *op. cit.*), etc.). In fact in these three examples, 'sweet' was selected as the most applicable descriptor over and above their nominal quality (i.e. strawberry, pineapple, and banana, respectively). Assuming that these odourants would be judged sweet smelling under single-rating conditions, and there appears little reason to doubt that they would, then multiple ratings do not appear to affect these judgements in the way that multiple ratings impact on sweetness enhancement. The reason offered for this observation is that sweetness is a highly salient feature of certain odours.

If odour-induced tastes are especially salient, then participants should use taste-based terms to spontaneously describe odours. The only experiment that comes close to addressing this was reported by Harper *et al.* (1968) who had participants sniff and spontaneously evaluate the qualities of 53 odourants. A list of 31 descriptive qualities were available on request if the participant could not readily bring to mind the name of the quality they perceived. Sweet was the most frequently used descriptive term and was employed to describe a range of sweetness from weak to sickly sweet. Whilst there is not the data yet to directly compare the robustness of orthonasal sweetness judgements (single vs. multiple scales) in comparison to retronasal sweetness-enhancement judgements (single vs. multiple scales), it would appear reasonable to conclude that orthonasal ratings of sweetness are the more robust.

If the functional argument is correct that odours come to smell sweet (or whatever taste they have been paired with) because this is a useful signal for calories (in the case of sweet), then this ability should also be present in animals, especially those that obtain food from multiple sources, such as omnivores like the rat. However, it is not easy to demonstrate that rats come to find certain odours as smelling sweet or sour, because unlike humans they obviously cannot be asked to directly report upon their subjective experience. Nonetheless, several studies suggest that rats can come to perceive these types of taste-like qualities for odours.

In one study, Sakai and Imada (2003) had rats consume odour A paired with saline and odour B with water. During this training period, odour B in water was consistently preferred to odour A in saline, by a large margin. During a subsequent test phase, half of the rats received injections of furosemide to induce a salt imbalance and thus a hunger for salt. All of the animals were then tested for their preference for odour A in water versus odour B in water. The salt-hungry animals demonstrated a preference for odour A in water over odour B, a preference not observed in the animals that were not salt hungry—i.e. the salt-hungry animals preferred the odour that had originally been paired with saline. Because all of the animals *initially* preferred odour B in water, the shift in preference observed during salt hunger is likely to reflect an association formed between the perceptual quality of the taste (i.e. its saltiness) and the odour. Thus when the animals become salt deprived, it is this taste information derived from smell that forms the basis for their choice of 'salty' odour A over 'non-salty' odour B, when both these odours are presented in plain water.

If, as Pearce (2002) suggests, rats treat a flavour, that is an odour–taste mixture as a compound, then later when the odour component is presented alone this will have the capacity to activate the associated compound, and thus the taste. One implication of this is that there should be summation between the associative taste and a physically present tastant, if the two are the same (notice here the broad parallel between this and odour-induced sweetness-taste enhancement). To test this idea, Harris and Thein (2005) explored the effects of sucrose- and salt-paired odours on rats' unconditioned preference for sweet and salty tastes.

In the non-thirsty rat, preference for sucrose peaks at about 15% and then flattens out with further increases in concentration. For the thirsty rat, preference peaks at around 20% before dropping dramatically as concentration increases further. For non-thirsty rats that had received odour A paired with 5% sucrose and B paired with 30% sucrose, they preferred a 5% sucrose solution mixed with odour B (over a 5% solution with odour A). However, when offered a 30% solution flavoured with odour A or B, there was now no difference in preference. For thirsty animals, trained in the same manner, whilst they showed the same preference for B in 5% sucrose, they preferred odour A in 30% sucrose. These findings suggest that the odours added extra sweetness, an extra sweetness that made little difference to non-thirsty animals tested with 30% sucrose where additional increases in sucrose concentration have no effect on preference, but a big difference for thirsty animals, where increased sucrose concentration is progressively more aversive. That these animals chose odour A over B under this condition suggests that odour A added less sweetness than odour B, a conclusion consistent with that of the authors. Finally, similar results were also obtained with salt-paired odours, suggesting that these too could add extra saltiness to saline solutions.

A third study also points to the same conclusion. Again using rats, Dwyer (2005) presented rats with pairings of odour A-sucrose, odour B-maltodextrin, and odour C-water. The rats were then made sick either to sucrose or maltodextrin and the effect on their consumption of odour A and B in water was then assessed. A similar approach was adopted in a second experiment, except here the rats had their preference for either sucrose or maltodextrin reduced by pre-feeding with one or the other stimulus (sucrose or maltodextrin) just before the choice test between odour A and B in water. Both studies revealed the same outcome, namely that devaluing one reinforcer 'selectively' reduced preference for the odour that had been associated with that reinforcer. These findings suggest that the animals preferences for these odours was underpinned by an association to the perceptual properties of that *particular* tastant. If the tastant was devalued, then so was the odour. These findings, along with those above, suggest that rats, like humans, can access information about the taste that an odour was originally presented with. This suggests a common functional role in assisting the omnivore (and possibly the herbivore in cases where the animal eats a variety of different plant-based foods) to identify foods rich in calories, and to identify novel foods that may be similarly calorie-rich.

Odour–taste interactions—Nature

Two related questions are addressed in this section. The first is whether reports of orthonasal (and retronasal) odour sweetness—and sweetness will mainly concern us because the bulk of work is on this parameter—represent a percept that is the same as that generated by a sweet taste. The second is whether other taste qualities, notably salty, bitter, sour, and umami, can also be induced by odours.

In addressing whether tasted and odour-induced sweetness is the same psychological (and possibly neural) entity, one starting point is to consider the two most obvious alternative explanations. The first one is that the use of the term sweet might be metaphoric. In colloquial use, people may refer to certain other people as 'sweet', 'bitter', or 'sour' (but not, generally, as salty), however they clearly do not mean that they taste sweet, sour, or bitter, but rather that they like or dislike them. In this sense, the metaphoric usage of sweet (or sour, etc.) is conveying a hedonic message. There are several grounds for suggesting that hedonic usage is not what participants mean when they say strawberry smells sweet. One powerful line of evidence comes from learning-based explanations of odour-induced tastes, which will be discussed in more detail below. Suffice it to say here, that it is possible to alter an odour-induced taste (sweetness) independently of its hedonic attributes (Stevenson and Boakes 2004, Yeomans et al. 2006) and that by varying motivational state (hunger/satiety), odour-hedonic and odour-induced tastes can also be independently manipulated (Yeomans and Mobini 2006).

A further reason to suspect that odour-induced sweetness and hedonics are independent comes from a study to be considered below, in which a pleasant sweet-smelling odour affected a behavioural parameter (pain tolerance) known to be affected by sweet taste, but an 'equally pleasant', but non-sweet odour did not (Prescott and Wilkie 2007). More generally, and as the Prescott and Wilkie (2007) study makes clear, odours can be liked even if they are not reported as sweet smelling, although the reverse is not true, as most sweet-smelling odours are liked. In this sense, sweetness is a poor metaphor for liking, because it clearly does not capture liking for non-sweet-smelling perfumes and fragrances, and especially for savoury foods. It would appear that whilst sweet-smelling odours are liked, odour liking and odour sweetness are independent entities.

The second possibility is that odour sweetness is perceptually identical (or at least very close to being so) to tasted sweetness. In effect, some evidence pertinent to this possibility was discussed in Chapter 2 and relatedly in the animal data above. A starting point for Harris and Thein's (2005) experiment was that the conditioned sensory property of the odour that been paired with sucrose would combine additively, when this odour was later combined with that taste. They confirmed this prediction, essentially one that assumes that such additive combinations arise from perceptual similarity. This same assumption has underpinned much of the human odour-induced taste-enhancement literature, and the evidence for this is generally favourable. That is, participants do appear to be able to conflate odour-induced sweetness with tasted sweetness in such a manner that the combination is generally perceived as sweeter than the taste alone. The reverse of this principle also seems to hold, although there is far less evidence for it—namely, that odours that smell sour may act to reduce perceived sweetness in the same manner that sour tastes do (e.g. Pelletier *et al.* 2004). When combined with the finding that the magnitude of sweetness-enhancement effects is predicted by the degree to which the odour smells sweet when sniffed (Stevenson *et al.* 1999, Valentin *et al.* 2006) and by the degree of perceived similarity between the odour and a sweet taste—the latter and the former being highly correlated (Valentin *et al.* 2006)—then the odour-induced taste-enhancement literature is consistent with odour-induced sweetness and tasted sweetness being perceptually alike.

Whilst the number of rating scales used in evaluating odour–taste mixtures may complicate this issue, several studies, and again as noted in Chapter 2, suggest that perceptual similarity is a key consideration in explaining sweetness-taste enhancement. Similarly, the finding of subthreshold additivity, whereby low concentrations of tastant and odourant can improve detection thresholds for sweet-smelling odours, also points to substantial perceptual similarity. Another is that detection of non-sweet-smelling odourants can be adversely affected when the detection task takes place in a weakly sweet-tasting solution (Djordjevic *et al.* 2004). Again, all of these findings are consistent with the observation of perceptual similarity (or dissimilarity) between certain odours and tastes.

These various lines of evidence, notably interactions between taste and smell, were covered in more depth in Chapter 2, but there are several more recent studies that have attempted to demonstrate that the similarity between taste and odour-induced taste runs very deep (i.e. suggesting a processing and/ or neural commonality). The first is a report by Prescott and Wilkie (2007), who examined whether sweet-smelling odours may affect pain tolerance in the same manner that sweet tastes do in adults and children (Blass and Shah 1995, Lewkowsko *et al.* 2003). The logic here is straightforward. If odours induce taste percepts that are really like sweet tastes, then the neural processes engaged by smelling a sweet odour should also be similar as well. Consequently, if sweet tastes can increase pain tolerance, then so should sweet smells. To test this, participants completed a cold pressor task twice (immersing the forearm and hand in 5°C water). Latency to withdraw the arm (tolerance) and pain ratings were the two dependent variables. The cold pressor task was conducted once with an odour present and once without. Three groups of participants were formed, one received a sweet-smelling and pleasant odour, another received a pleasant but non-sweet-smelling odour, and a third received a non-sweet and unpleasant smell. Whilst the odours had no effect on pain intensity, the sweet-smelling odour selectively increased latency to withdraw (see Figure 3.1). These findings mirror those obtained with sweet tastes and suggest, first, that sweet smells appear to activate the same neural processes that are present when a sweet tastant is tasted and, second, that it is the taste quality, not hedonics, that is important.

The second study, conducted by White and Prescott (2007), investigated whether a sweet smell could facilitate identification of a sweet taste and retard that of a sour taste, and whether a sour smell could do the reverse. Using two-chamber

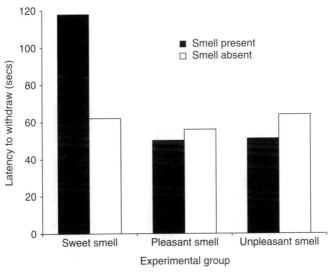

Fig. 3.1 Mean latency to withdraw the forearm and hand on the cold pressor task as a function of the odour that participants were exposed to, and whether or not this odour was present (adapted from Prescott & Wilkie (2007)).

suck/smell bottles, in which a straw connects to the lower chamber containing the tastant and the participant sniffs at an open upper chamber (the two chambers being separate and invisible to the participant), participants were presented with six combinations of stimuli. These were sweet smell–sweet taste, sweet smell–sour taste, no smell–sweet taste, no smell–sour taste, sour smell–sweet taste, and sour smell–sour taste. If sweet smells really do smell like sweet tastes, and sour smells smell like sour tastes taste, then there should be a facilitatory effect on taste identification on what are effectively congruent trials, and an inhibitory effect on incongruent trials (i.e. where the odour-induced taste does not match the real taste). As can be seen in Figure 3.2, this type of outcome was observed, with congruent trials having faster reaction times than incongruent trials, and with incongruent trials being somewhat slower than the water control. In sum, these findings again suggest perceptual similarity between odour-induced tastes and real tastes.

The third set of findings comes from a rather different direction. The premise that Stevenson *et al.* (2008) adopted was to assume that if odour-induced tastes and real tastes depend upon the same (or similar) neural substrate, then (1) patients with a brain injury who demonstrate impaired taste should also demonstrate impaired perception of odour-induced tastes and (2) those who demonstrate impairments in perception of odour-induced tastes should also have impaired taste perception. To test this, patients were recruited in two ways. The first was to screen neurology out-patients to find people who appeared to be unable to appreciate odour-induced tastes (e.g. not finding

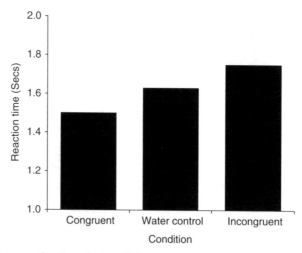

Fig. 3.2 Mean reaction times for identifying a target taste, under congruent, control, and incongruent odour–taste conditions (adapted from White & Prescott (2007)).

strawberry sweet smelling) or who could not recognize or judge appropriately the intensity/quality of certain tastants, including sucrose. The second was to identify patients with relatively selective damage to the insular cortex. Damage to this structure has been linked to impaired taste perception in several studies (e.g. Mak *et al.* 2005, Pritchard *et al.* 1999), and neuroimaging indicates that it is responsive to both unimodal tastes and smell stimuli, and to their combination—flavour (e.g. Small *et al.* 2004).

Whilst identifying potential participants was relatively easy to specify, a more difficult task was to determine how, exactly, an impairment in odour-induced tastes might manifest. Three predictions were derived. The first was the simplest, namely that when sniffing odourants that are commonly reported as having a sweet (or sour, etc.) smell, patients with impaired odour-induced taste perception would report these characteristics as being less salient (i.e. as less intense) than matched controls. However, they would still need to be able to smell, so they would need to report the overall intensity of the odour as similar to that of controls, even if they reported that they could perceive little or no odour-induced taste. The second prediction followed from the first. Whilst a set of sweet-smelling odours may differ in their other qualities (e.g. chocolate and strawberry both smell sweet, but strawberry is not chocolate-like and vice versa), the fact that they share a common perceptual quality (i.e. sweetness) should render a set of sweet odours as *more similar to each other* than a set of non-sweet odours, that is a set which does not share a common element. Thus, control participants should judge the sweet set as more similar to each other than the non-sweet set, whilst this should not be the case for patients who may not be able to smell the common element—sweetness—anymore. The third prediction followed from the second—if a sweet set of odours no longer smelled sweet to the patients, then they should be better able to discriminate between them than control participants.

An obvious problem in any neuropsychological study is that the pattern of performance in the patient group could reflect some more general set of impairments that are not specific to the actual tasks the experimenter is interested in. To tackle this, measures of visual discrimination and visual similarity were obtained using procedures that placed similar cognitive demands on participants to those obtaining in the olfactory and taste tasks. In addition, it was obviously also important to obtain measures of taste functioning, namely taste discrimination, taste intensity, and recognition judgements, as well as taste and odour hedonic ratings—as these would be crucial in establishing the relationship between real taste perception and odour-induced taste perception. Finally, more general neuropsychological measures were also included to assess cognitive function.

Three separate approaches were taken to analyse the data generated in the study. The first approach was to examine the patients' performance on the three measures of odour-induced taste perception and to identify patients who were impaired on these tests, relative to the matched controls. Four patients were identified who were impaired in their perception of odour-induced tastes. The first key question was whether these four patients, relative to the controls, would also be impaired on the measures of taste perception. Figure 3.3a–e illustrates the mean performance of these four patients and the controls on

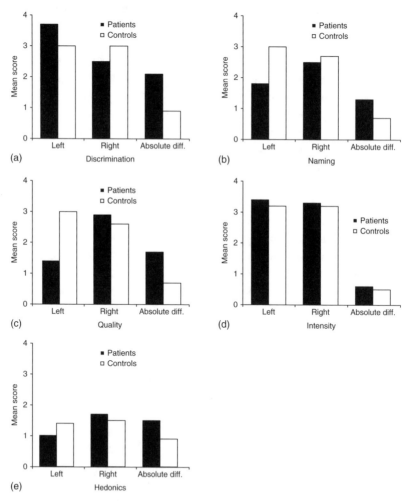

Fig. 3.3a–e From top left to bottom left, (a) taste discrimination, (b) naming, (c) quality, (d) intensity, and (e) hedonics, for the selected patients and controls (adapted from Stevenson, Miller, and Thayer (2008)).

each measure of taste perception. Significant impairments were evident in the four patients for taste discrimination, naming, and quality perception, but not on taste intensity or hedonics. For taste discrimination, impairment was especially marked in terms of the absolute difference between the left and right hemitongues, as with taste-quality perception. Performance on taste naming and quality perception was also notably worse on the left hemitongue. Whilst these differences suggest that taste perception is impaired in these same patients who were also impaired in the perception of odour-induced tastes, one outstanding question remains—were these patients also impaired on the control tasks? The patients did not significantly differ from the controls in age or education, nor in their scores of pre-morbid intelligence (National Adult Reading Test), nor on the mini-mental state exam (a measure of overall cognitive function). However, they were somewhat worse on the Boston Naming Test, a measure of ability to name pictures. No significant differences were observed in visual discrimination or visual similarity performance, relative to controls, nor in measures of odour intensity or naming. Thus these patients were, by and large, as cognitively able as controls, and were not anosmic. It, therefore, appears that taste impairments accompany impairment in the perception of odour-induced tastes. If you cannot perceive sweet tastes appropriately, you cannot perceive sweet smells appropriately either.

As all of the patients (excepting those with lesions of the insular cortex) were inducted into the study because the screening test identified either poor taste or odour-induced taste perception (relative to screening control data), Stevenson *et al.* (2008) also explored the whole data set using regression to determine the variables that best predicted impairment in odour-induced taste perception. The results from this analysis, using both controls and patients, revealed four key predictors that together explained 54% of the variability in odour-induced taste performance. These were: level of education, the Boston Naming Test, pooled performance on taste tasks presented to the left hemitongue, and absolute difference in taste-quality perception. Significant individual contributions (i.e. squared semi-partial correlation coefficients) were made by education, the Boston Naming Test, and absolute difference in taste-quality scores. When the same regression analysis (i.e. using the same variables) was employed on just the patient group, this accounted for 61% of the variability in odour induced taste performance, and there was only one significant individual contribution, namely absolute difference in taste-quality perception. These results suggest that taste impairment, especially in the perception of taste quality (i.e. sweetness, sourness, etc.), is related independently to odour-induced taste performance, even when potentially confounding variables are taken into account.

A further set of analyses were also reported on the patients with insular lesions, but discussion of these findings, and of the anatomical data linked to impaired odour-induced taste perception, is postponed till later, as it appears more sensible to discuss this material in the context of neuroimaging data, pertinent to the neural basis of these effects. The key point from the study by Stevenson *et al.* (2008), and indeed from that of White and Prescott (2007) and Prescott and Wilkie (2007) too, is that the similarity between tasted sweetness and odour-induced sweetness extends far beyond participants' self-report. It would appear, as the evidence stands at the moment, that odour-induced tastes draw upon overlapping neural networks that also underpin taste perception and so result in both, similar qualia and effects on behaviour.

The only study, which appears to contradict this conclusion, was reported by Rankin and Marks (2000). Whilst this study confirmed the general impression that participants judge certain odours as sweet-smelling, this perceptual similarity between sweet tastes and sweet smells had no effect on the impact of stimulus context on intensity judgements. If sweetness and odour-induced sweetness draw upon the same underlying neural processes, then they should form a common judgemental context for sweetness, all other things being equal. This was not observed, and so suggests a contrary conclusion to the findings above. There are two possible explanations as to why this discrepancy might arise. First, increasing odour concentration may not result in a linear increase in sweetness intensity, in which case the only way to manipulate variations in odour-induced sweetness would be to vary the *odour* and not the concentration. Whilst there is some evidence that sweetness intensity is not directly yoked to odour concentration (see Stevenson *et al.* 1999), this relationship is not well explored; but if odour intensity was increasing whilst sweetness changed at a slower rate, this could account for their experimental results. A second possibility concerns the neural locus of differential context effects. Whilst Rankin and Marks (2000) suggest that taste-based differential context effects have a central neural basis, they have no evidence one way or the other to rule out a peripheral basis for the effect, as they themselves acknowledge. If, in the case of taste, there were a peripheral basis, then these results would have little relevance to whether tastes and odour-induced tastes are processed by similar brain structures. Without doubt, Rankin and Marks (2000) findings are interesting, but their full implications for the way in which taste and odour-induced tastes are processed are unclear.

So far, the discussion has focussed mainly on odour-induced sweet tastes. However, during eating and drinking, people are exposed to other combinations—notably to sour, salty, bitter, and umami tastes—all with relatively specific (but culturally dependent) odourants. These might include vinegar or citrus fruits (sour tastes), savoury foods (salty and umami tastes), and the relatively few instances of acceptable bitter-tasting foods (many being sweetened), such as certain almond products, coffee, certain spices, bitter lemon, Indian tonic water, and tamarind. On the basis of the frequency with which different tastes appear in our diet, one might expect that after sweet, savoury and sour would predominate, with bitter a distant third. On this basis, odours should be able to induce tastes other than sweet, especially savoury and sour and possibly bitter. Is there any evidence that certain odours can induce these other tastes?

Three strands of evidence suggest that they can. The first is simply to look at sets of odour descriptors, such as Dravniek's (1986) *Atlas of odour profiles*. Sour-smelling odours are certainly quite frequent here (descriptors 106—sour, vinegar, and 105—sharp, pungent, and acid). However, many are clearly acids and these will almost certainly have affects on nasal trigeminal receptors, just as in the mouth their irritant qualities would contribute to a sour (acid) taste. For savoury-smelling odours, there is no unique category, but examples can be readily found for conceptually similar categories, such as fried chicken (descriptor 123), cooked meat (124), and cooked vegetables (126). For bitter, there is a unique descriptor (104—bitter) and several odourants are rated as possessing this quality. However, with the exception of sour (106), none of these descriptors are used with anything like the frequency that sweetness is deployed. Pretty much the same conclusions can be drawn from looking at the more spontaneous descriptors generated in the study by Harper *et al.* (1968).

A second approach is to examine the limited perceptual similarity data—i.e. taste-enhancement studies—that have used tastants other than those that generate a sweet taste. These are remarkably few in number, and only four are of direct interest here. The first, Bonnans and Noble (1993), added varying amounts of citric acid and sucrose to a constant level of orange odourant. Orange odour might reasonably be proposed as inducing both sour and sweet tastes, and consistent with this Bonnans and Noble (1993) observed that both sucrose and citric acid, independently (and together) could increase perceived orange fruity flavour. Recalling the discussion above regarding whether tastes can generate olfactory sensations, it was suggested there that tastes might affect judgements of purely olfactory notes via their associated taste properties. That both citric acid and sucrose were able to increase orange fruity flavour would then imply that both of these taste qualities were generated by the orange odourant.

A second study by Stevenson *et al.* (1999) examined whether certain odourants could enhance the sourness of citric acid. Whilst no sourness-enhancement effects were detected, it is noteworthy here that the odourants used in this study would not be ones that frequently co-occurred with sour tastes, so this may not have been a very adequate test. A better approach was reported in a third study. Pelletier *et al.* (2004) found that mixing a sour-smelling lemon odorant with a solution of citric acid and sucrose resulted in an additional increase in perceived sourness and a reduction in sweetness when citric acid concentration increased.

A fourth study examined interactions within an oil–water emulsion base between cis-3-hexanol (a 'green' smell) and the bitter tastant quinine (Caporale *et al.* 2004). Here, the bitter taste of quinine was enhanced by the presence of cis-3-hexanol, and this effect was eliminated by the presence of a nose-clip during tasting, indicating its olfactory basis. This suggests that odourants with green notes may induce bitter tastes.

Although there is general agreement that sweet, sour, salty, bitter, and umami constitute the primary gustatory sensations; others have suggested that the number of possible taste qualities is much broader (see Schiffman 2002). One of the 'additional' qualities that have been reported is that of 'metallic taste'—a property peculiar to certain divalent salts (Lawless *et al.* 2005). Interestingly, these salts, especially $FeSO_4$, are odourless outside of the mouth, but in the mouth they react with fats, creating a range of volatile chemicals that have a distinct metallic smell when sniffed. Lawless *et al.* (2005) suggest that the metallic note that these volatile chemicals generate may arise via associative learning between the taste of these divalent salts (i.e. metallic) and concomitant retronasal olfactory stimulation—a topic discussed in the next section.

From the data above, it appears plausible that odours may induce sour and bitter tastes although the data is rather limited. A more substantial data set comes from a rather different direction, namely studies which have examined whether odour-induced tastes arise via associative learning. Not only do these studies provide support for the observation that odours can come to induce other tastes apart from sucrose (e.g. see above for metallic-smelling odourants), they provide strong evidence that these effects are the product of experience—learning. This would be expected if the function of odour-induced tastes were to provide important information about a potential food (e.g. calories, salt content, bitter poisons, etc.) *prior* to consumption.

Odour–taste interactions—Learning

This section has three aims. The first is to examine the evidence that experiencing an odour and a taste together in the mouth, as a mixture, can subsequently affect how that odour alone will later smell (i.e. orthonasally)—i.e. will the odour acquire taste-like properties? And can this occur for any taste? The second aim is to determine the characteristics of this learning. This can be broken down into two related issues: (1) considerations of particular relevance to the learning literature, notably awareness, extinction, and latent inhibition (note that these factors have considerable bearing upon the nature of the learning, i.e. whether it is semantic or perceptual) and (2) the practical application of these considerations to train participants to more accurately discriminate/identify the taste and olfactory components of flavour, and the impact such training may have on odour–taste learning. Issue (1) is covered here and issue (2) is considered in Chapter 4. The third aim is to identify whether odour–taste learning is independent from hedonic changes that are known to occur when pleasant (or unpleasant) tastes are paired with odours (Zellner et al. 1983).

Stevenson et al. (1995) examined whether an unfamiliar odour paired with sucrose would get to smell sweeter and an unfamiliar odour paired with citric acid would get to smell sourer. Using a rather laborious 5-day design, participants sniffed the two target odours on day 1 and rated them for sweetness, sourness, overall intensity, and liking. They then experienced each of the target odours in sucrose and citric acid, and sucrose and citric acid alone, again making the same evaluations. Over the next 3 days, participants tasted a total of nine mixtures of one odour in sucrose solution and a further nine mixtures of the second odour in citric acid solution. On day 5 they returned for the post-test, which was identical to the pre-test described above. The odour paired with sucrose was judged to smell sweeter, relative to the citric acid paired odour on post-test, than it had on pre-test. Similarly, the citric acid paired odour was judged to smell sourer, relative to the sucrose paired odour on post-test, than it had on pre-test. However, when the odours were evaluated with each tastant, as flavours, the only odour-related effect from pre- to post-test was for the citric acid-paired odourant. This reduced the sweetness of sucrose more at post-test than it had at pre-test. In common with all other studies reported below, participants reported little, if any, explicit knowledge about the nature of the pairings they had received, suggesting that they had acquired this information implicitly. To acquire the odour–taste association apparently without awareness is consistent with an underlying perceptual change, in contrast to a change in semantic knowledge (i.e. 'I know that smell has been mixed with a sweet taste').

A second experiment (Stevenson et al. 1995) replicated this effect for changes in odour-induced sweetness and sourness. Again, effects on taste enhancement were varied, with an effect this time for the sucrose-paired odour, which was found to enhance sweetness more on post-test than it had on pre-test, yet when tested in citric acid, it surprisingly enhanced sourness. Whilst these experiments clearly indicate that odours paired with sucrose get to smell sweeter, and those paired with citric acid, sourer, they do not show convincingly that these effects lead to reliable changes in taste enhancement (i.e. interaction effects). However, the enhancement tests in both experiments were conducted in quite concentrated taste solutions and this may have worked against a successful demonstration. Enhancement (interaction) effects appear more consistently in weaker solutions (see Frank *et al.* 1989).

In a follow-up study, Stevenson *et al.* (1998) examined whether odour–sucrose pairings, when contrasted to a second odour presented in water, would still evidence a change in sweetness—i.e. the original experiment described above, whilst sensitive to a differential conditioning effect, could not demonstrate whether the effect occurred for sucrose alone or for citric acid alone. Experiment One here clearly indicated a significant learning effect using a design similar to the studies above (i.e. pre-test, training, and post-test), with the sucrose-paired odour smelling sweeter, but with no change in odour-sweetness ratings for the odour paired with water.

Experiment Two in this series examined whether the effect could be obtained under conditions where the participant did not have the opportunity to smell the odourant prior to ingestion. Following a pre-test, where both odours were sniffed and rated, participants received pairings of one odour and sucrose consistently sucked through a straw, and a second odour in sucrose, sipped from a cup. The latter afforded the opportunity to sniff the odour beforehand whilst the former did not. The magnitude of the change in perceived sweetness for both odours was identical. Both came to smell sweeter, indicating that it is the simultaneous perception of the odour and the taste in the mouth, which is responsible for the effect, not sequential associations between the orthonasal odour and the taste of sucrose in the mouth.

As noted for Stevenson *et al.* (1995) little evidence of contingency knowledge was demonstrated, i.e. participants appeared to acquire the odour–taste associations with minimal conscious awareness. This is a contentious claim, as it is difficult to establish conclusively whether or not it is correct. However, no study to date has reported evidence that odour–taste learning effects 'depend' upon explicitly knowing that one odour has been paired with a particular taste. For example, when participants have been grouped into those that do demonstrate some awareness (i.e. they recognize that odour A was paired with sucrose and B with citric acid), they demonstrate no significant benefit in learning relative to those not classified as aware. It is important to note here that the odour-induced taste appears to be used as a cue by some participants when they try to answer these types of 'contingency awareness' questions (i.e. 'what taste was this smell presented with earlier today?'). Whilst the claim of implicit learning has its detractors (e.g. Lovibond and Shanks 2002) and supporters (e.g. Brunstrom 2004), the evidence so far is consistent with the claim that 'explicit' awareness of the odour–taste relationship is not necessary for learning to take place (see Stevenson and Boakes (2004) for further discussion).

Once odour–taste associations are acquired, they appear to be relatively robust. Re-testing participants either 24 h after learning ceased or immediately reveals, if anything, a tendency for improved performance after the delay (Stevenson et al. 1998). Over a longer interval of 1 month, a similar finding was obtained, with no evident loss of information—citric acid-paired odours still smelled sour, and sucrose-paired odours still smelled sweet (Stevenson et al. 2000a). A more exacting test was also reported from this study, in which one odour was paired with citric acid, a second also with citric acid, and a third with sucrose. One of the citric acid-paired odours was then presented several times in water—more times in fact than it had been in citric acid (i.e. an extinction procedure). This had no effect on participants' judgements of the odour, i.e. it was still reported to smell sour—as sour as the non-extinguished citric acid-paired odour and significantly more sour than the sucrose-paired odour. A control condition using equivalent pairings of colours and tastes demonstrated that the procedure was sensitive enough to detect extinction of colour–taste pairings.

A further study (Stevenson et al. 2000b) adopted a similar design, but rather than presenting the citric acid-paired odour in water (i.e. extinction), the odour was now presented several times in sucrose (i.e. counter-conditioning). This too, whilst affecting equivalent colour–odour pairings, had no effect on odour pairings. These findings suggest that once odour–taste associations are acquired, they are highly resistant to interference.

A related question is whether pre-exposure to an odour alone, prior to pairing with a taste, will then prevent odour–taste learning occurring—i.e. latent inhibition. Results here are less straightforward. In an unpublished study (see Stevenson and Boakes (2004) for description), we obtained evidence favouring a latent inhibition effect. Indeed, a general premise in all of our work, and other groups too who have used the odour–taste learning procedure, is to choose odours that most participants are unfamiliar with. Notwithstanding this, Stevenson et al. (2000a) did not obtain a latent inhibition effect where this was tested for (arguably using less than ideal controls), but in a further study, Stevenson and Case (2003) did (again using arguably less than ideal controls). Part of the ambiguity here arises from the fact that, apart from our unpublished study, no experiment has set out to examine latent inhibition effects alone. Indeed, they were part of Stevenson and Case's (2003) study in the context of exploring the effects of training on odour–taste learning (more in Chapter 4) and in Stevenson et al. (2000a) for the purpose of keeping exposure to odours and tastes constant across training and extinction. Whilst this may sound of little interest to any but to the most committed learning theorists, this is far from the case because pre-exposure to a stimulus, especially an odour, may have marked effects on a participant's ability to discriminate it (e.g. Rabin 1988). Further discussion of this important topic is deferred to Chapter 4.

More recent studies of odour–taste learning have found that the effect can be obtained with as little as a single exposure to an odour–taste pair (Prescott, Johnstone, and Francis 2004), and more recent studies have tended to reduce both, the number of pairings and testing sessions. Apart from demonstrating that odours can acquire sweet-taste properties from pairings with sucrose, and sour-taste properties from pairings with citric acid, a number of other types of pairing have also been explored. The most consistently positive findings have been obtained with pairings of an odour and bitter-tasting quinine. Not only can this lead to an odour acquiring a bitter-like quality, it also appears to reduce the degree to which the odour is judged as sweet smelling (as with sour-taste pairings; Yeomans and Mobini 2006, Yeomans *et al.* 2007, Yeomans *et al.* 2006).

Pairings with salty/savoury tastes have not been so well explored. Yeomans *et al.* (2006) attempted to test this, and found some suggestive evidence. Pairing an unfamiliar odour with a mixture of salt and monosodium glutamate led to a reliable reduction in the degree to which the odour smelled sweet (relative to a water-paired control). Whilst there was a small change in the expected direction for ratings of odour meatiness and savouriness, no significant effects were obtained. It remains to be seen whether savoury taste–odour pairings can generate conditioned effects similar to those obtained for sweet, sour, and bitter tastes, but the fact that plenty of foods do smell meaty/savoury, etc., would suggest this possibility.

A final and especially important consideration, is whether changes in odour sweetness (and by implication, odour sourness and bitterness) depend upon concurrent changes in the hedonic reaction evoked by the target odour. Stevenson and Boakes (2004) were clearly troubled by this possibility, especially that participants might conflate judgements of liking and sweetness and disliking and sour/bitterness (see above). However, recent experimental evidence strongly suggests that for odour sweetness at least, this cannot be the case.

Yeomans *et al.* (2006) pre-tested participants liking for sucrose and, on this basis, formed two groups of participants: sucrose likers and dislikers. After evaluating the two target odours, participants received pairings of one odour with sucrose and a second with water. Whilst odour-sweetness ratings for the sucrose-paired odour significantly increased for both groups—and did not significantly differ—liking ratings for the sucrose-paired odour *only* increased for participants who liked sucrose (see Figure 3.4). This suggests

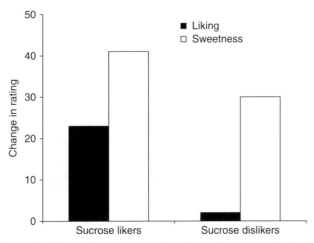

Fig. 3.4 Change in liking and sweetness ratings (post minus pre-test) relative to the water-paired control, for sucrose-taste likers and dislikers (adapted from Yeomans, Mobini, Elliman, Walker, and Stevenson (2006)).

quite strongly that changes in the perceived sweet quality of the odour are independent of changes in the hedonic aspect. Clearly, hedonic changes could not account for changes in odour sweetness in the participants who disliked sucrose sweetness.

A further experiment provided even more conclusive findings (Yeomans and Mobini 2006). First, the experimenters selected only participants who liked sucrose. These participants were then trained when hungry, by pairing one odour with sucrose, another with quinine, and a further odour with water. Participants were then tested after being given water (i.e. hungry), after a low-calorie preload (i.e. hungry), or after a high-calorie preload (i.e. sated). These differences in hunger were all confirmed by self-report ratings. Crucially, on test, changes in liking for the sucrose-paired odour were only observed for participants who were hungry, not for those sated by the high-calorie preload (see Figure 3.5), whilst changes in odour sweetness were observed in all three groups to the same degree (see Figure 3.5). This form of testing, whilst affecting the sucrose-paired odour for liking, had no effect on the quinine-paired odour which was disliked equally by participants in all three groups, and was also reported as smelling significantly bitterer post-conditioning.

In summary, convincing evidence exists that experience with odour–taste mixtures can result in changes in the way that the odourous component is later perceived. These changes are robust, require minimal conscious awareness, and are independent—definitively so for sucrose paired odours—of concomitant

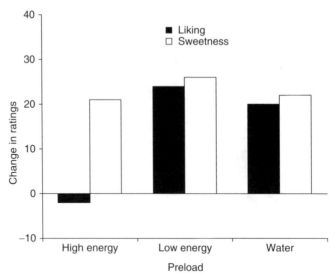

Fig. 3.5 Change in liking and sweetness ratings (post minus pre-test) relative to the water-paired control odour, for participants given a high-energy, low-energy, or water preload (adapted from Yeomans and Mobini (2006)).

changes in liking. Finally, these changes in taste-like properties can be readily demonstrated for sweet, sour, and bitter tastes, but the evidence for such changes with salty and savoury tastes has not yet been convincingly established. What is currently lacking is good evidence that these laboratory-based changes in orthonasal odour-induced tastes can result in the type of interaction effects described in Chapter 2.

Odour–taste interactions—Neural basis

A reasonable question to ask at this point is, the neural basis of what? The material above establishes that odours can come to acquire taste-like properties, and that these taste-like properties, notably sweetness, appear to be very similar indeed to the sensation generated by tastants, especially sugars. A further finding is that when a familiar odour–taste combination is experienced in the mouth, participants often behave as if the perceptual boundaries between these two dimensions are blurred. Relatedly, subthreshold integration may occur in which low concentrations of a taste may boost detectability of an odour, but again only when the combination is a familiar one. It seems then that there are at least three processes at work here. First, that certain odours can induce sensations that appear to be appreciably similar to sensations generated by real tastants (odour-induced tastes). Second, that a combination of odour and taste has to be learned (odour–taste learning). Third, that for learned combinations these can interact when both are presented together as a flavour (odour–taste interaction).

Arguably, these three processes may have separate, but related, neural underpinnings, because they clearly have separate, but related, histories and functions. A brief example is illustrative: (1) A novel flavour is encountered (e.g. sour-fish). (2) The flavour is implicitly learnt (i.e. sour-fish) and this results in two consequences. (3) Smelling the flavour's volatiles (i.e. fish) orthonasally results in a re-experiencing of something very much like the original flavour (i.e. sour-fish). (4) Eating the food results in direct experience of its taste, *plus* the flavour memory that is generated by the smell. Points (1) and (2) refer to odour–taste learning, point (3) to an odour-induced taste and point (4) to an odour–taste interaction.

The neuroscience literature offers some insights into these three processes. There is not much on odour-induced tastes, more on odour–taste learning, and most on odour–taste interaction. Verhagen and Engelen (2006) provide a detailed and thoughtful theoretical examination of the three processes described above, and certainly share a similar view to the one articulated here as to how they interrelate. They suggest that the brain utilizes an auto-association network that both, rapidly acquires odour–taste associations and recovers them when only the odour component is present. There are at least three neural systems that appear to operate such auto-association networks—the hippocampus, the olfactory system (notably the piriform cortex), and a more distributed network involving the piriform, the insular, and orbitofrontal cortices. The likely involvement of all of these structures was supported by their meta-analysis of a set of unimodal neuroimaging studies of taste and of smell (Verhagen and Engelen 2006). This revealed that certain structures, notably the insula, orbitofrontal cortex, and the hippocampus, could all be activated by *either* taste or smell.

A limited number of neuroimaging studies have now begun to look at combinations of odour and taste in the mouth, and, in particular, at combinations that are 'jointly' familiar or unfamiliar. From these studies, at least two specific types of contrast emerge as conceptually important. To reveal the neural substrates that may be involved in acquiring unfamiliar flavours (i.e. where the components *together* are unfamiliar) needs a contrast of 'jointly' unfamiliar minus 'jointly' familiar, or 'jointly' unfamiliar minus the single components. The former is required, because this will reveal whether the substrate for learning is different (or the same) from the substrate that generates an interaction effect. The latter is needed, because this will reveal whether specific structures are involved in acquiring the combinations that are not active when either component is presented alone. The second form of contrast is that between 'jointly' familiar combinations minus the familiar components that make these up. This will reveal the structures that are involved in the interactions that presumably result in taste enhancement and sub-threshold integration.

Two studies have examined the second form of contrast, 'jointly' familiar combination minus the familiar components. De Araujo *et al.* (2003) examined this for strawberry and sucrose versus strawberry alone and sucrose alone. Activation was observed solely in the anterior region of the orbitofrontal cortex. Small *et al.* (2004) conducted a much more extensive set of contrasts, building upon the basic familiar combination versus its components' approach outlined above. This revealed activation in several areas for vanilla and sucrose, relative to vanilla alone and sucrose alone. These activations occurred most notably in the insula and adjacent areas of the orbitofrontal cortex, frontal operculum, anterior cingulate cortex, ventrolateral prefrontal cortex, and posterior parietal cortex. Whilst there is, clearly, divergence in the outcomes of these two studies, both indicate involvement of the orbitofrontal cortex, albeit in different regions. In addition, identification of the insular and the orbitofrontal cortices is consistent with the structures revealed by analysis of the convergence of activation of unimodal taste and smell stimuli. As Verhagen and Engelen (2006) note, the failure to observe any activity from the piriform cortex is surprising, but probably a consequence of the difficulties involved in imaging this structure. It may turn out to be more crucial than these two studies would appear to suggest (see Marciani *et al.* (2006) for some suggestive evidence in this regard).

The first form of contrast, i.e. identifying the area/s that might be involved in processing (and thus learning) unfamiliar combinations, has only been examined by Small *et al.* (2004). She reported that the contrast of vanilla in saline versus vanilla alone and saline alone, revealed activation at the temporal/parietal junction, the ventral striatum, and the anterior ventral insular and adjacent orbitofrontal cortex. Whilst activity within the ventral striatum may relate to the identification of novel combinations, it may be that activity within the insular/ orbitofrontal cortex is important for acquisition of new combinations. This would be consistent with the role of these structures in interactions (albeit in a different locus), and with the observation that cells of the orbitofrontal cortex respond selectively to familiar combinations of taste and odour (Rolls and Baylis 1994). However, vanilla is a familiar odour, and this may represent a rather poor test of the likely neural substrates of odour–taste learning. A better test would be an unfamiliar odour and a sweet taste—as typically deployed in odour–taste-learning studies—to avoid possible latent inhibition. In sum, these data would suggest that insular/orbitofrontal structures may be involved in both, acquiring odour–taste combinations and expressing their interaction—but with the caveat noted above concerning the piriform cortex.

Odours can induce tastes when sniffed orthonasally. The brain regions responsible for these types of activations are not well understood, but some evidence is available. First, unimodal olfactory stimulation can result in activation of brain areas that are undoubtedly involved in taste processing, especially the insula, operculum, and orbitofrontal cortex (e.g. de Araujo *et al.* 2003, Savic *et al.* 2000). Second, at least one study suggests that food-related odours might activate the primary taste cortex to a greater extent than non-food-related odours (Leger *et al.* 2003). This may imply that food-related odours (i.e. those which induce a taste) might activate taste-based processing areas, which would be consistent with conscious experience of a taste percept. Third, Stevenson, Miller, and Thayer (2008) obtained a small group ($n = 6$) of insular-lesioned patients, and tested them for taste and odour-induced taste deficits. This group clearly evidenced taste-based deficits. These deficits were present for discrimination, naming, intensity, quality, and hedonics. In addition, they showed impairment on an overall measure of odour-induced taste performance. These impairments could not be readily accounted for by more generalized deficits in other cognitive abilities. However, what is perhaps more interesting, is that only one of these six patients had a highly discrete lesion, in this case in the posterior right insular. This patient, FC, demonstrated normal olfactory (naming and intensity judgements) and visual (discrimination and similarity) abilities, but had notable impairments on the Boston Naming Test. This is not surprising, as others have noted that insular lesions can produce language-related deficits (e.g. Manes *et al.* 1999). FC had a clear impairment in the perception of taste quality, hedonics, and naming, but not of taste intensity or discrimination, with these deficits most apparent in the absolute difference in performance between the left and right hemitongue (i.e. for taste quality, FC was better than controls on the right and worse on the left, as with hedonics and, to a lesser extent, naming). FC also had very marked impairments in odour-induced taste perception, with better discrimination of sweet-smelling odours than controls, more marked dissimilarity for the sweet-smelling odours, and poorer appreciation of their taste-like qualities. These findings point to two conclusions. First, that the right insular may be active in generating taste-like sensations for certain odours. Second, and again, that taste deficits and odour-induced taste deficits co-occur in a meaningful way.

Whilst the insula may be important, it may not be the whole story, because a further patient, GW, had no detectable insular damage, but displayed a broadly similar pattern of odour-induced taste deficits to that of FC. GW had had a right temporal lobe resection, which included most of the amygdala.

Small *et al.* (1997a) have suggested, amongst others, that a circuit involving the right insula and the amygdala may be important for taste recognition. In this case, FC's and GW's pattern of impairment may be similar—even though the ostensible lesion is different—because both lesions disrupt a common circuit that is required for the perception of taste quality. It may be then that the right insular–amygdala circuit requires activation for an odour to induce a taste.

If an odour induces a taste, why is this sensation attributed to the olfactory modality and not to the mouth as it is during the perception of flavour? Stevenson and Tomiczek (2007) have suggested that this may be a consequence of the unusual neural architecture of olfaction. Unlike other senses, olfactory information can reach the neocortex both directly (piriform/bulb to orbitofrontal cortex) and indirectly via the mediodorsal thalamic nucleus (piriform to thalamus to orbitofrontal cortex). Stevenson and Tomiczek (2007) suggest that, under conditions where an odour is sniffed, direct cortical activation recovers flavour memory by activating the type of structures detailed above (i.e. insular/amygdala, orbitofrontal cortex, etc.), but also the piriform cortex, i.e. primary olfactory cortex. Crucially, this pattern of activation is attributed to the olfactory modality because of sole and concurrent activation of the mediothalamic cortical pathway, which may assign modality identity to the experience (i.e. 'smell in the outside world'). Under conditions of retronasal olfaction, where somatosensory and taste stimulation can occur concurrently, the presence of these other forms of activity may act to anchor the experience as emanating from the mouth, rather than the 'nose'. This would at least explain why tastes or oral somatosensory experience do not routinely induce olfactory or other experiences (excepting those generated by receptor co-activation, such as thermal tastes) because they do not have direct cortical access like olfaction. It is important to stress that there is little empirical evdence to favour this hypothesis, although several lines of argument suggest it (see Stevenson and Tomiczek (2007) for more discussion). This possibility, and others, are discussed more extensively in Chapter 6.

Odour–taste interactions—Conclusion

When a familiar odour–taste combination is experienced, the taste, or sometimes the smell, may be enhanced and the taste may facilitate identification of smell at threshold. These interactions arise, so it is argued here, as a side effect of learning the odour–taste combination. More importantly, this allows olfaction alone—when a food is smelled prior to ingestion—to recover an impression of its flavour, including components from other senses, notably taste. As the identification of a foodstuff will fall heavily upon the visual system—indeed, it has been argued that colour vision arose in primates to facilitate identification of fruit and vegetation—the olfactory system can appreciably add to this process by providing further information about the likely flavour of the food. As described below, odours may also acquire other information via learning that adds further value to its importance in deciding whether or not to ingest a particular food.

Odour–tactile/taste interactions

Two types of tactile interaction were identified in Chapter 2. The first was that the more viscous or hard the vehicle, the lower the perceived intensity of the retronasal odour. The second—and the primary focus here—was that certain odourants appear to exert an effect on participants' judgement of textural attributes, notably those for fattiness and creaminess. Whilst these data are not as extensive as for odour–taste interactions, the general consensus in the literature is that odours, which commonly co-occur with fatty/creamy/viscous foods, may enhance perception of these tactile properties (de Wijk *et al.* (2006) and Frost and Janhoj (2007), but see Mela and Marshall (1992) for a dissenting view). Essentially then, there are two problems here: the need to explain tactile-based suppression of retronasal olfaction and the need to explain odour–tactile interactions.

Tactile suppression of retronasal olfactory perception is not well accounted for in the literature, probably because it is only fairly recently that it has been convincingly demonstrated (i.e. Weel *et al.* 2002, Bult *et al.* 2007). One obvious possibility is that any intense stimulus in the mouth, irrespective of modality, may attract more attentional resources than other competing, but weaker, stimuli. Whilst this is not unreasonable, it does not appear to hold true for chemaesthetic oral irritants. One can recall from Chapter 2 that Prescott and Stevenson (1995) found no evidence for suppression of strawberry flavour (odour only) when the irritant capsaicin was present. On the other hand, the simple presence of a tactile stimulus in the mouth has been demonstrated to result in suppression of orthonasally presented odours (Hornung and Enns 1986), and an analogous effect has also been found using neuroimaging (Small *et al.* 1997b). Setting aside the orthonasal versus retronasal distinction, it is possible that oral tactile stimulation leads to a diminution of olfaction, a diminution that increases with increasing tactile stimulation. This could arguably reflect an automatic process, so that even when participants are directed to attend to the olfactory domain such as to make olfactory-intensity ratings, this suppression is still evident. Whilst directing attention to what must be the most salient aspect of the stimulus offers an explanation of sorts, it is not readily apparent what function it might serve. One possibility is that it might be a side effect of binding (i.e. concurrent oral somatosensory stimulation is needed to bind retronasal odour to 'the mouth'; see Chapter 6). Speculation aside, there is at present is no well-established explanation for tactile-based suppression of olfaction.

Interactions where odours enhance tactile perception can be explained within the same framework adopted for odours and tastes. Apart from a desire for parsimony, there are good empirical grounds for suggesting this. First, certain odours clearly smell fatty and, indeed, this term (along with other related concepts) can be found in both Dravniek's (1986) and in Harper *et al.*'s, (1968) list of odour descriptors. Relatedly, Aldrich's *Flavors and Fragrances* catalogue also identifies numerous compounds that have fat-related qualities, including 'Butter-like', 'Creamy', 'Cheese', and 'Oily'. Taken with the evidence reviewed in Chapter 2 for odour–tactile interactions—especially those that might serve to predict the fat-content of food (or drink)—allowing an odour to retrieve this aspect of flavour would be functionally advantageous, as it would provide a further indicator of the possible caloric value of the food. Thus, it would serve a similar identification function to that of odour-induced taste, with any oral-interaction effects again being viewed as a secondary consequence of learning odour–tactile relationships.

Only one study appears to have explored whether fat-related information can be acquired via the olfactory system. In this study, no attempt was made to determine whether the information acquired arose primarily via tactile means or via a combination of olfactory cues associated with the fatty stimulus and tactile cues (Sundqvist *et al.* 2006). Participants here were exposed to four different types of stimulus: Unsweetened low-fat milk with odour A, sweetened low-fat milk with odour B, unsweetened high-fat milk with odour C, and sweetened high-fat milk with odour D. Prior to the training, phase participants evaluated the four sucrose–milk mixtures for sweetness and fattiness. Participants could readily discern that the high-fat milks (3.6% fat) were fattier than the low-fat milks (0.1% fat). The difference in sweetness between sweetened and unsweetened milks was also significant, but was a much weaker effect. Interestingly, sucrose and fat interacted, with the presence of sucrose increasing fattiness judgements for the low-fat milk, but not for the high-fat milks. This *may* have been a consequence of sucrose increasing the viscosity of the milk. As noted above, more viscous solutions tend to lead to reduced retronasal olfactory-intensity judgements, and this was confirmed in a pilot experiment. Consequently, the odour concentrations of the high-fat milks were increased to a level that produced similar intensity ratings to those obtained for the low-fat milks.

Following judgements of the milks alone and the odours alone, partici-pants were given exposures to four pairings (and various distracters) of each odour–milk combination. They then returned a week later to complete a second session, which started with a further two pairings (and distracters) of each odour–milk combination. Participants again evaluated the milks alone, the odours alone, and were then given an enhancement test, where each odour was added to a slightly sweetened and slightly fatty milk to determine whether or not the odour would enhance perceptions of fattiness. The odour pre-/post-test revealed a significant change in odour-fattiness ratings, but only for odours that had been paired with either the high-fat milks, or the low-fat sweetened milk. On the enhancement test, odours that had been paired with high-fat milks only, enhanced the rated fattiness of the test milk significantly more than odours paired with the low-fat milks—demonstrating, this time, that learning can be a distal cause of interaction effects akin to those examined in Chapter 2. As with the odour–taste-learning experiments, there was no detectable relationship between what participants knew about the odour–milk relationships and their performance on the task. Whilst these findings (albeit preliminary) suggest that odours can come to acquire fat-like attributes, the results here do present a puzzle, i.e. why should the enhancement test have obtained an effect for only the high-fat-milk-paired odours, whilst the odour pre-/post-test detected an effect for the high-fat and low-fat sweetened milk? One possibility is that participants may have acquired two types of information; one that related to viscosity and another to the fat-like attributes (e.g. fatty odours present in milk). The odour pre-/post-test may have detected all of these sources of information, whilst the enhancement test may have detected the effects of a more specific subset pertaining to milk-related fatty odours. Whatever the explanation, these findings certainly suggest that odours may act to induce somaesthetic-like sensations, which can then generate interaction effects of the sort observed in Chapter 2 (with presumably the same proximal basis as for odour–taste interactions discussed above).

Colour and flavour interactions

Colour is one of many visual features of a food (or drink) that helps to identify it *prior* to ingestion. The use of italics for prior is intended to stress the likely functional role of the visual signal here, namely that it allows (along with orthonasal olfaction) a ready means of eliminating what is and what is not food, without the risk of ingestion. The colour and visual appearance of food in the 'real world' are likely to be an accurate signal of identity and quality; the ripening of fruits, the colour/appearance of fungal or bacterial contamination, or the sheen and colour of fat on meat. But in the laboratory, this can of course be manipulated with quite marked effects on the ability to identify odours either via an ortho- or retronasal route. Relatedly, manipulating colour can also affect the quality of the experience, both hedonically and in terms of what the participant believes the food/drink 'tastes' like. Thus, where colour is manipulated, and the resultant colour does not normally predict the odour (and taste) combination present in the food/drink, participants' performance is usually biased towards reliance on the more veridical visual cue over that of taste and smell. This can be clearly seen in several of the experiments discussed in Chapter 2, but perhaps most clearly in Morrot *et al.*'s (2001) experiment with white wine coloured red, which was reported as tasting like red wine.

Identification of an odour in the absence of other cues is not particularly good (Desor and Beauchamp 1974), unless participants receive training to improve the strength of the odour–name association (see Cain 1979, Dempsey and Stevenson 2002). As Cain *et al.* (1998) noted, ' . . . unstable access to semantic information presumably largely governs performance at identification.' (p.320 *op.cit.*). This is very *unlikely* to be the case with visual cues, as in adults at least, most people have very little difficult in naming visually perceived objects. Similarly, in the case of colours their likely flavour associates can also be readily identified (see Zampini *et al.* 2007). Thus colour (and other visual variables that assist identification of a food/drink) may afford more precise identification (because of better semantic access) than smell. It is not, therefore, surprising that when conflicting visual/olfactory (taste) information is present, vision wins out.

A further and important question is whether the impact of this visual information simply affects identification and thus biases what participants report about a flavour stimulus (i.e. a semantic effect) or whether it actually alters, via some top-down means, what the participant perceives. Could, e.g. the red-coloured white wine *actually* taste like red wine? At present there is no definitive evidence, but it would appear as if a semantic explanation was the more likely. Three lines of evidence suggest this.

The first is the finding that when participants are asked to discriminate odours presented in inappropriate colours (e.g. green strawberry vs. green cherry), they perform more poorly than when presented in appropriate colours (e.g. red strawberry vs. red cherry) or in no colour at all. However, this effect is eliminated if participants are forced to engage in an articulatory suppression task—i.e. their discriminative performance *improves* under this condition (Stevenson and Oaten 2008). This would suggest that participants use colour to assist them in identifying the odours, and that incorrect colour disrupts this process, impairing discrimination—a semantic effect.

The second piece of evidence follows on from this. Let us assume that a misleading colour results in an incorrect odour identification and it is this incorrect identification which then results in top-down changes in perception (e.g. orange-coloured strawberry odour is misidentified as orange odour which then activates an orange-odour memory). In this case, the incorrect name could activate an olfactory percept more in line with the name than with the smell. In some sense, this is analogous to an odour-imagery task in which participants are asked to generate an image when provided with a name (e.g. imagine the smell of lemon). However, odour imagery under these sort of conditions is pretty difficult for most participants (see Stevenson and Case 2003) and so even this might not be able to generate a percept capable of overwriting the bottom-up-driven one.

A third piece of evidence comes from an experiment that examined whether pictorial visual information (e.g. picture of chocolate, cake, ice-cream, or biscuits) would facilitate the speed and detection of a 'semantically' congruent odour (e.g. vanilla),over an incongruent odour (e.g. rancid fish). The olfactory component of visual–odour congruent pairs was detected faster and more accurately than that of visual–odour incongruent pairs, an effect that is arguably semantic in nature, because the congruent odour and picture share only a common meaning (Gottfried and Dolan 2003). Whilst this does not directly inform us as to what may be happening with colour and odours, it would be reasonable to assume some similarity in process, namely that colours assist with (in this case) access to semantic information about the stimulus (i.e. the coloured fluid) which then facilitates or retards participants' olfactory/flavour identifications. This does not require any alteration in the olfactory percept, but it does require access to semantic information.

If visual cues then facilitate access to semantic information about smells, tastes, and also flavours, how does this come about? Several investigators have noted the consistency between certain colours and certain odours, both in respect to colour and odour identity (Gilbert et al. 1996) and between odour intensity and colour lightness (Kemp and Gilbert 1997). Dematte et al. (2006) have suggested that these consistencies, especially for colour and odour identity—and presumably for colour and flavour identity as well—may develop by their regular co-occurrence in the environment. Whilst some cross-modal correspondences *may* have deeper roots, such as those between intensive dimensions (in this case, odour intensity and colour lightness), it would appear that colour–odour (flavour) associations may be learnt. One reason for suggesting this is the rather obvious observation that the colour that is typically found to 'belong' to a particular odour logically relates to the colour of the physical object that emits the odour (i.e. a strawberry is red, and so red is associated with strawberry odour).

As Dematte et al. (2006) note, one problem with this assertion is the difficulty that some investigators have had in demonstrating paired-associate learning between visual and olfactory stimuli in humans (e.g. Davis 1977). However, Bowers *et al.* (1994) found that when a colour preceded an odour (i.e. yellow—then a smell), learning the association was as efficient as learning the association between two colours. This was not the case when the odour preceded the colour, or when two odours served as cues. Interestingly, Bower *et al.*'s (1994) participants described the widespread use of verbal strategies in acquiring colour–odour associations (e.g. this is blue vodka). These verbal strategies were far less common when the odour preceded the colour. This concurs with the conclusion above that colour effects on odour quality may result from semantic rather than perceptual processes.

The neural basis for colour–flavour associations has been examined directly in one study (Osterbauer *et al.* 2005) and indirectly in another (Gottfried and Dolan 2003). Turning first to the Gottfried and Dolan (2003) study (see above), they also obtained fMRI images during their behavioural task. Whilst it would be revealing to know the structures and systems that support learning colour–flavour associations, and which support their expression, Gottfried and Dolan's (2003) study only provides direct insights into the latter, although this has some interesting implications for the former. Recall that participants received either congruent or incongruent odour–picture pairs, odour alone, or pictures alone, as well as a baseline condition. The study's neuroimaging results revealed two interesting findings. First, that presenting odours and pictures together, irrespective of their congruency, revealed activation in brain areas shown previously to be involved in integrating information from different senses, especially with respect to location and identification, i.e. the intraparietal sulcus and the superior temporal sulcus (see Calvert 2001). Second, a further analysis, focussed on identifying activation particular to congruent odour–picture pairs, indicated activity in the hippocampus and rostromedial orbitofrontal cortex, suggesting that these areas are likely to be important in processing semantically congruent stimuli. The activity noted in the hippocampus is of particular interest, because it supports the notion that associations between visual features of an object and its odour are a consequence of explicit learning processes that are known to be mediated by this structure.

The Osterbauer *et al.* (2005) study presented participants simultaneously with colours and odours that varied in congruency, colours alone, and odours alone. By examining the correlation between congruency judgements and brain activation (as with Gottfried and Dolan (2003)), they observed significant associations with activity in the caudal orbitofrontal cortex and anterior insular, amongst other areas. Osterbauer *et al.* (2005) suggest that it is the hedonic aspect of the stimulus combination which arise from processing in the orbitofrontal cortex. Unfortunately, the study could not obtain any data relevant to hippocampal activity, and so it is not possible to tell here whether or not this structure was active.

In conclusion, the findings above suggest that participants learn colour–flavour associations, and that colour along with other associated visual features are used to assist identification, probably just as under naturalistic conditions when a potential food is encountered. This colour-assisted identification may then lead to expectations about the stimulus's flavour, potentially biasing olfactory judgements because the visual channel is; (1) likely to be more veridical (except in the laboratory) than the olfactory channel and (2) has better access to semantic information about the potential food. The exception to this account may be the effect of colour on perception of odour intensity. Whilst this too may be a product of learning (i.e. darker colours associated with stronger smells), its effects may occur at a lower level. Zellner and Kautz's (1990) finding that colour-intensity effects survived a manipulation that avoided experimental demand would also suggest this.

Interactions as side effects of learning—Conclusions

The dominant theme of this section is the role of experience—learning—as a distal cause for interactions between retronasal odours and tastes, retronasal odours and tactile stimuli (odour *affecting* tactile perception), and colour–flavour interactions. The essential premise is that a person acquires both, perceptual and semantic, memories of flavours they encounter. Perceptual flavour memories may be principally retrieved by smell (orthonasal or retronasal), and semantic flavour memories principally by vision. Together, this visual and olfactory information provide a very valuable source of information in judging whether or not to ingest a food or drink and this—along with finding food in the first place—is arguably the principal function in acquiring these perceptual and semantic flavour memories. However, it is *not* the only function because, as discussed in Chapter 5 and 6, flavour in the mouth is also contrasted to flavour memory, so as to detect inconsistencies—but more on this later.

A side effect of the flavour-learning process, is that these associations can come to affect the way in which a familiar food or drink is perceived (odour–taste or certain odour–tactile/taste interactions) or described (colour–odour/ taste/flavour interactions). Whilst these interactions are of major interest to how we *perceive* food, they may be of relatively little functional value. Indeed, detecting food and avoiding being poisoned are more important from the perspective of evolutionary fitness than our capacity to utilize knowledge of perceptual interactions in the culinary arts. From a purely scientific perspective, it may be that odour–taste interactions in the mouth are a rather poor example of multisensory processing, because what point does multisensory processing achieve here? Whilst it may be crucial to encode this multisensory information (providing a clear functional benefit for binding or multisensory integration), the flavour interaction itself does not lead to a useful or immediate benefit in terms of identification, detection, or localization, as does multisensory processing in other domains (see Chapter 6 and 7 for further discussion of this point). Rather, the benefits of multisensory processing of flavour are mainly delayed— i.e. they appear when the exteroceptive senses of vision and orthonasal olfaction are engaged in detecting, locating, and identifying food prior to ingestion.

Whilst learning may be a distal cause of odour–taste interactions and of odour–tactile interactions too, a proximal explanation draws upon the effect that learning has on the way the components are perceived in the mouth. Learning may result in blurred perceptual boundaries between a taste and a smell. This then makes it hard to judge one component independently of the other. In addition, where the odour induces a taste-like percept (and possibly a somaesthetic-like one, too), this may add to the taste (or somaesthetic) percept generated by the physically present stimulus. For colour-based interaction effects, these too have a distal basis in learning. The proximal cause for interaction effects here seems to depend upon the formation of expectancies that may then bias what the participant reports experiencing. Here, vision dictates the outcome because it is usually the more veridical channel.

Conclusion

This chapter examined the distal and proximal basis of the interactions between and within the flavour senses that were identified in Chapter 2 as having a psychological basis. For unimodal interactions within taste, and within smell, these revealed rather different outcomes in each case. Taste components remain largely identifiable and component suppression (i.e. the principal type of interaction) may arise from the way in which the nervous system deals with stimulus range (response compression). For smell, whilst response compression may occur, synthetic processing restricts conscious access to the component odourants that make up a mixture.

For auditory–tactile interactions and the perception of creaminess, both serve to identify particular salient features of flavour. In both these cases, a functional benefit of multisensory processing was apparent 'in the mouth'— for the former case, determining the freshness of food and, in the latter case, its probable fat content. The other examples, colour–flavour, odour–taste, and certain odour–taste–tactile interactions are arguably side effects of learning about flavour that principally manifest their functional benefit 'outside of the mouth'—i.e. outside the mouth, colour and odour draw upon perceptual and semantic flavour memory to identify, detect, and locate food and assess its likely edibility (i.e. one *knows* that peaches taste sweet, and peaches *smell* sweet too). The effects that are observed in the mouth are then a side effect of this process, arising from the interaction between perceptual flavour memory and stimulus-based information (for odour–taste and certain odour–taste–tactile interactions) or from semantically based expectations of what a particular food's appearance predicts about its likely flavour (colour–flavour interactions).

The interactions examined in this, and the last, chapter often depend upon the ability of the participant to detect particular components of flavour for evaluation. However, this chapter suggests that there may be limits to this process. Whilst taste components may generally be detectable, some olfactory ones may not. Similarly, a side effect of odour–taste or odour–taste/tactile learning may be that participants find it hard to identify the perceptual boundary between a taste and a smell or a smell and a fatty sensation. Indeed, what can we know about the components of flavour? and can this knowledge be improved with practice? More generally, whilst an analytic approach to flavour may be the standard by which scientists of all hues (neuroscience to sensory evaluation) approach flavour, is this anything like the way flavour is routinely perceived outside of the laboratory? It is to these questions that we turn next in Chapter 4.

Chapter 4

Wholes and parts

Introduction

Kubovy and Van Valkenburg (2001) suggest that a musical tune is a good example of a preservative emergent property. Flavour might count as a further example too. Many authors claim that flavour can be perceived as a unitary experience and as a series of parts (e.g. Auvray and Spence 2008, Lawless 1995, Small and Prescott 2000). The aim of this chapter is to explore this claim by addressing three specific questions: (1) Is flavour a unitary experience? (2) Can it be broken down into component parts? (3) If it can (or cannot) be, how does the mind/brain achieve this? In answering these questions, the starting point is to consider what is meant by unitary experience and what is meant by parts. A unitary perceptual experience is one in which: (1) the component parts are not *currently* available to consciousness; (2) the component parts share a common location; and (3) the component parts are experienced simultaneously. The italicized 'currently' above is important, because this sets one limit on unitary perception, namely that when directed attention (i.e. endogenous) is brought to bear on the percept the experience may no longer by unitary, but rather reveal a series of parts. These parts may come in two forms and the term 'part' is used when referring to both. First, where there is a correspondence between a percept and an underlying physical stimulus (e.g. sweetness and sucrose), this correspondence is termed an 'element'. Second, where this is a similarity between a physically present stimulus and some prior experience (e.g. coffee smells similar to certain burning odours, coffee smells similar to certain bitter tastes, etc.), this is termed a 'similarity'. Importantly, similarities do not have to have any direct relationship to the underlying physical properties of the stimulus. These two types of parts are often conflated, but they are not equivalent.

To answer the question of whether parts can be detected in flavour mixtures depends then on what type of part one is considering and the interaction between different types of parts (notably in odour–taste mixtures, i.e. between odour sweetness (a similarity) and tasted sweetness (an element)). Some particularly important studies have tried to determine whether participants can detect elements in mixtures. Here, a *failure* to detect an element could point to a number of possibilities. First, that endogenous attention is largely inoperative in the chemical senses. Second, that fundamental perceptual limits that are unbreachable have been reached. Third, that the element is not detectable for physical reasons (e.g. if a chemical, it may have reacted with another agent). Note that a failure to detect a 'similarity' in a flavour mixture could also be explained by the first possibility, and may be by the second, but clearly not by the third, as similarities are psychological and neural entities alone.

One important way of examining the detectability of parts in a flavour is to determine whether training can improve it. Relatedly, another is to search for individuals who claim special abilities in respect to a particular perceptual task and to determine whether their skills reflect more sensitive perceptual systems or are the result of training and experience—learning/attention. As with Chapter 3, the form this learning may take can be differentiated into that involving semantic knowledge—a framework that can act to direct attention to salient components of the stimulus array and to organize memory—or as a form of learning (or imprinting), in which the ability to perform a particular task is improved by gains that lie in the perceptual domain. These perceptual effects may be further differentiated into those dealing with similarities and those dealing with elements, although these are typically entwined.

This chapter starts by examining the question of the unitariness of flavour. This is followed by an analysis of whether the different component modalities and their interactions can be broken down into parts. In each case, the focus will be on the capacity of participants to identify parts, the limits of the perceptual system and of endogenous attention, and whether learning (experience) can improve performance. For more complex and realistic flavour stimuli—wines, beers, and foods—the literature on perceptual expertise and training will be reviewed, again addressing the same set of questions (as far as it is possible to do so). The final part of the chapter attempts to draw these various findings together and to tentatively address the third question above—how does the mind/brain achieve these feats?

Is flavour a unitary experience?

In the literature on flavour, it is widely held that the experience of eating or drinking is synthetic or unitary (e.g. Lawless 1995, Auvray and Spence 2008). Interestingly, the empirical evidence for this claim is actually rather weak and so the frequency with which this claim is made could reflect its obviousness. By far, the best discussion of this issue can be found in Rozin (1982). The ostensible aim of the Rozin (1982) article was to examine the duality of the olfactory sense—an important question in and of itself that is discussed more extensively in Chapter 6. However, as part of his argument, Rozin (1982) presents a variety of evidence to suggest that people are broadly unaware of the multiple sensory inputs that combine to generate flavour. If they are unaware of the components, then this would be consistent with perceiving flavour as a unitary experience. Whilst the article focuses on taste and smell, the argument can be extended to include the somatosensory component of flavour too.

There are several observations or findings that suggest people are broadly unaware of flavour components. The first concerns what we know about our senses. Children and adults know they need eyes to see and ears to hear, but most people appear to be ignorant of the fact that a nose is needed to appreciate the flavour of food. This observation is supported by the surprise that people reportedly show (even when they are experienced with olfactory and gustatory psychophysics) when asked to pinch—and then unpinch—the nose whilst sampling an odour–taste mixture (e.g. see Murphy et al. 1977, p.210). Nose pinching, of course, prevents retronasal olfaction and results in a marked change in perception of flavour.

A related observation is that people with anosmia commonly complain of an associated deficit in taste perception (Bull 1965). In a review of 750 consecutive patients who presented to the University of Pennsylvania Smell and Taste Center (Deems et al. 1991), nearly 60% of the sample presented with an impairment in *both* taste and smell. However, following a detailed assessment, only 4% of the sample had in fact a detectable loss of taste. These observations are not unique and similar patterns of symptom presentation following olfactory loss have been reported elsewhere (e.g. Gent et al. 1987). As all of these authors note, these findings suggest that patients, along with non-patients, fail to distinguish between the role of taste and smell in flavour perception.

A second observation concerns the words that people use to routinely describe their experience of flavour. That is, first, does the use of this term reflect both an olfactory and taste component and, second, are their words in other languages that do capture the taste and olfactory components of flavour as known to science? Rozin (1982) reported data pertinent to both of these questions. First, he presented students with a list of questions in which they judged whether taste or flavour was the more or less appropriate term (a score of 1 here reflected taste as the more appropriate term; a score of 5 flavour as the more appropriate term). Examples include 'This has a salty _____' and 'I like the _____ of wine'. It was carefully stressed to participants that these judgements pertained to food in their mouth. The sentences included all four basic tastes, and indeed taste was judged the most appropriate usage in these cases. However, of the remaining 12 items, all of which included significant olfactory components (fruit, raspberries, meat, ginger, coffee, spicy, wine, fruity, meaty, fragrant, etc.), only two of these items received a score greater than 3 (i.e. flavour more appropriate). Whilst these findings suggest some limited awareness of an olfactory component to flavour, in the main they indicate that the terms taste and flavour are largely interchangeable in casual use, even for foods that have a clear olfactory component.

The second question Rozin (1982) addressed was whether any other language distinguishes between the taste and olfactory components of flavour. Using a sample of bilinguals who were fluent in English, but who differed in their native tongue, participants were asked to provide synonyms for the terms taste and flavour. In addition, following this task, a more detailed explanation of the distinction between taste and smell in the context of flavour followed, to see whether this might reveal linguistic distinctions not present in English. In seven of the nine languages Rozin (1982) examined, even the distinction between taste and flavour was absent, with Spanish, Czech, German, Hebrew, Hindi, Tamil, and Mandarin speakers identifying just one word that appeared to capture the sensory experience of food in the mouth. Only Hungarian and French were different, with Hungarian being the only language to apparently capture the distinction between the taste and retronasal olfactory components of flavour. Again, the general absence of specific terms to describe the olfactory and taste component of flavour suggests that people are largely unaware of this distinction.

All of the observations/data above could be subsumed under the attentional component of flavour's unitary nature—i.e. a unitary percept is one in which the component parts are not *currently* available to consciousness and so we might infer from the above that people generally do not attend to these parts. In this case, flavour might be unitary by default—that is we do not generally attempt to focus attention on its parts in our day-to-day interaction with food and drink. A further consideration in this regard are conditioned taste aversions, a topic examined in more depth in the next chapter. When an animal or a person becomes sick after eating a particular food, it is the food itself that comes to be the object of their aversion, not particular parts of that food (Scalera 2002), even though the parts (e.g. its smell) may in themselves be sufficient to lead to a later avoidance of it (e.g. Chapuis *et al.* 2007). More broadly, in considering learning about any post-ingestive effect (hedonically positive or negative), the food itself is the key level of description, not its parts.

A further component to the unitary nature of flavour is that olfactory sensations detected in the nose appear to be spatially located to the mouth and, needless to say, experiences in the mouth usually involve simultaneous activation of different sensory channels including taste and smell. The only study to examine spatial localization of smell to the mouth was reported by von Bekesy (1964). Unfortunately, the paper is rather thin on detail. As far as one can tell from reading it, it appears that participants were asked to report the locus of a smell delivered orthonasally, either before, during, or after the delivery of a taste. When taste and smell were delivered simultaneously, the apparent locus of the olfactory sensation moved from the tip of the nose to the back of the throat (see Figure 7, von Bekesy (1964)), but when the odour was presented out of synchrony with the taste, the olfactory sensation remained at the tip of the nose. The data here are very intriguing, and there is probably little doubt that simultaneous presentation plays an important part in co-locating these sensations into the mouth. First, recall that Pfeiffer *et al.* (2005) found that subthreshold taste and smell integration only occurred when the stimuli were delivered simultaneously (see Chapter 2). Second, in the broader multi-sensory perception literature, it is widely acknowledged that simultaneous presentation is a necessary (but not sufficient) condition to obtain integration (e.g. Robertson 2003, Stein *et al.* 2001). However, note in passing (more in Chapter 6) that taste and retronasal olfaction may not be quite as simultaneous as at first appears, as the passage of odourants into the nasopharynx from the mouth may be either delayed until a swallow or is pulsatile in nature (see Chapter 1).

A further issue here is that the von Bekesy (1964) data do not allow us to know whether the reported shift in location occurred as a consequence of the taste or of the tactile sensation that accompanied the taste. There is some data that suggests that it may be the tactile component, but this is premised on the finding that tactile sensations can capture taste. The assumption then is that if tactile sensations can capture taste, perhaps they can also capture smell, and this possibility has been explicitly suggested by Murphy and Cain (1980) and by Green (2002). The empirical basis for the claim that tactile stimulation can capture taste is robust. Todrank and Bartoshuk's (1991) Experiment 1 capitalized on the density of taste receptors located on the tongue tip. The experimenter moved a cotton bud saturated in a tastant in a 3-cm arc from the left fore-tip, over the tip, to the right-fore tip (and vice versa). Intensity ratings consistently revealed that on the start of an arc, intensity ratings were lower, than when the cotton bud reached the tip. Crucially, intensity ratings then *stayed* at the elevated level when the arc was completed on the opposite side of the tongue—i.e. the perception of taste (and intensity) was generalized across the area which had received tactile stimulation (see Figure 4.1).

In addition, Todrank and Bartoshuk (1991) also reported a second study, examining a single case that had lost the ability to taste all but sweet on the left hemitongue. Intriguingly, this participant also demonstrated the same effect

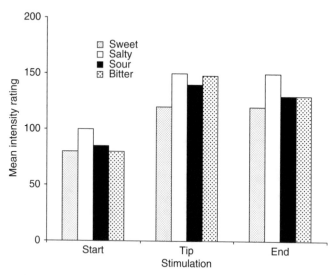

Fig. 4.1 Ratings of intensity for sucrose, salt, citric acid, and quinine, on the start of a traverse (left and right combined), on the tongue tip, and at the end of a traverse (right and left combined) (Data adapted from Todrank and Bartoshuk 1991).

illustrated above. However, in this case, when traversing from left to right, no taste experience was reported on the left side, whilst on traverses from right to left, there was considerable illusory taste reported—a consequence of the generalization of taste experience across the tactile-stimulated area. Further support for the perceptual basis of this tactile capture was provided by Green (2002), who used a more demand-free approach to rule out the possibility that participants gave higher ratings at the end of the traverse so as to be consistent with ratings given on the tip. In sum, these studies suggest that tactile sensation in the mouth locates taste sensation broadly within the mouth (rather than just to areas where taste buds are located). If this finding is extended, we might suggest that concurrent tactile stimulation in the mouth might also capture olfactory sensation and localize this to the oral cavity as well. Thus, these findings would seem to support the latter two aspects of unitary flavour processing, of common spatial location and, as noted earlier, common temporal location.

Our state of knowledge about the unitary nature of flavour certainly leaves much to be desired, but what there is would appear to suggest the following broad conclusion. In general, we do not attend to the component parts of flavour in our day-to-day interaction with food. The component modalities may be bound together so as to be spatially located in the mouth by the tactile sensation that accompanies eating and drinking and by their simultaneous occurrence. This binding of components (more in Chapter 6), especially of retronasal olfaction, results in a flavour percept that is spatially located to the mouth and which is, relatedly, temporally coherent too. To what extent, then, can we consciously experience the component parts?

Wholes into parts

Although we may experience food flavours by default as unitary percepts, it is evident from Chapter 2 and 3 that a capacity to experience parts must exist. How else could we learn, e.g. odour–taste associations and express this learning as an increase in perceived 'sweetness' (or bitterness or sourness) if this taste component was not potentially detectable in the flavour? In Chapter 3, it was argued that we might possess a capacity to detect individual tastes (i.e. elements) in taste mixtures. However, this ability may be far more constrained for smell. This section starts by examining these two senses individually, especially from the perspective of capacity limits, attention, and learning as they apply to detecting parts in mixtures. This approach is then extended to somatosensory perception in the mouth with the focus on texture (this being the most studied component) and then to cross-modal mixtures of taste and smell. Finally, the effects of expertise and training, for wine, beer, and food, are examined, to determine whether experts demonstrate superior abilities to perceive and describe parts, relative to non-experts.

Taste

In Chapter 3, evidence was presented which suggested that participants are pretty good at identifying the elements present in taste mixtures. This conclusion was mainly based on a task in which participants had to identify a single target taste in taste mixtures of varying complexity (Laing *et al.* 2002). Performance on this type of task is likely to be influenced by four factors. First, naive participants may confuse the *terms* bitter and sour. This can create the impression of poor discriminability when, in fact, participants can readily tell apart the percept generated by each tastant (e.g. Robinson 1970). Second, more intense components in taste mixtures are more easily detected, and usually detected first (Marshall *et al.* 2005). Third, bitter may be the most salient taste element under ideal circumstances (i.e. where it is not suppressed by the presence of another taste). For example, Koster *et al.* (2004) gave participants a range of foods for breakfast and then, later in the day, presented them with these same foods or with adulterated versions that contained more or less of certain target tastants. They found that participants were most sensitive to taste adulteration with bitter tastes (i.e. they reported that the adulterated version had not been consumed at breakfast) and least sensitive to changes in sweet taste (i.e. they reported that the adulterated version had been consumed at breakfast). Fourth, tastes are known to differ in their onset latency—bitter being notably the slowest—and these differences in onset, which appear to be preserved in taste mixtures, may also facilitate identification (Kuznicki and Turner 1988).

A particularly interesting set of studies was reported by Kuznicki *et al.* (1983), who examined attentional and experiential variables in a taste-sorting task. This study is informative because not only did it explore, in a different way, the ability to identify elements, but it also examined whether extensive training could improve performance. Experiment 2 in their series looked at the ability of participants to sort taste stimuli into two-quality categories (e.g. sweet vs. salty), when irrelevant but uncorrelated tastants were present. For example, participants might be given salty/bitter, salty/sour, sweet/bitter, and sweet/sour stimuli and asked to sort this series into sweet or salty. This, using Garner's (1974) terminology, is a filtering task as the irrelevant dimension needs to be filtered out to complete it. Participants also engaged in an integration task, in which tastes were again sorted (e.g. sweet vs. salty), but this time the irrelevant taste was always correlated with the sorting dimensions (e.g. sweet/sour and salty/bitter). Finally, a control task was completed in which just the unadulterated tastants were sorted (e.g. sweet vs. salty for just sweet and salty tastes).

The presence of a second taste (i.e. filtering and integration) *slowed* sorting, relative to the control task, and the slowing tended to be most notable when the irrelevant tastes were present at a higher concentration—this being a further factor manipulated in the design. However, whilst sorting time may have been slowed, sorting errors were only notable when sour and bitter tastants were the targets and sweet and salty stimuli the irrelevant tastes. This was especially apparent when these irrelevant tastes were presented at higher concentrations (see Table 4.1). For target tastes 2 and 3 (see Table 4.1) the irrelevant tastes may have suppressed the target-taste qualities, making the uncorrelated task (i.e. filtering) especially difficult (i.e. in the correlated (integration) task

Table 4.1 Mean percent sorting errors (adapted from Table V, Kuznicki, Hayward, and Schultz 1983)

Target tastes	Irrelevant tastes	Errors (%)		
		Control	Filtering	Integration
1. Salty & Sweet	Sour & Bitter	2.4	8.8	7.3
2. Sour & Bitter	Salty & Sweet (weak)	8.8	24.0	7.5
3. Sour & Bitter	Salty & Sweet (strong)	8.6	40.5	17.8

the presence of salty or sweet is predictive of whether sour or bitter is present and so this can be used as a cue for sorting).

Whilst the identifiability of taste components is fairly good (excepting of course for when the target tastants are weak and the irrelevant tastants are strong), to what extent can performance be improved by expertise? Kuznicki et al. (1983) used the same paradigm as above, namely filtering, integration, and control, but in Experiment 4 pitted a group of participants who had received varying levels of descriptive flavour analysis (DFA) training against a group of naive participants. All participants had normal taste and olfactory perceptual abilities. The DFA training involved exposure to parts from all of the modalities involved in flavour, along with the acquisition of appropriate terminology to describe them. In addition, as training progressed, more complex combinations were presented, with the expectation that participants would be better able to break these down accurately into their parts. The results from their study were very clear cut, trained participants performed no better than naïie participants.

A similar null finding was obtained by McBride and Finlay (1989). They compared expert assessors (i.e. a group akin to those used by Kuznicki et al. 1983), who had on average 9 years experience of evaluating various food products, with naive participants. All participants were asked to make sweetness- and sourness-intensity judgements for a range of sucrose–citric acid-taste mixtures. The components of the mixtures were clearly identifiable to both groups. Whilst novices appeared somewhat more sensitive to sour-taste suppression by sucrose, at the highest concentration level, the overwhelming conclusion of the study was the similarity in performance between groups.

The results of both of these 'expert' versus 'novice' studies are analogous to findings from a further experiment reported by Laing's group (Watson et al. 2001). Watson et al. (2001) found that adults and 8-year-old children were equally good at identifying the components of binary mixtures of sucrose and salt. In this case, the analogy is based upon the *assumption* that perceptual experience with tastes increases with age (all other things being equal) and so the absence of an age-related effect may be taken to indicate that taste-part identification ability, when confronted with binary mixtures, is relatively insensitive to the effects of experience or training—if it were not, then the 8-year olds should have been poorer at this task, and they were not.

As will become apparent later in this chapter, expertise involves a combination of perceptual experience with the 'specific' stimuli to be tested as well as conceptual knowledge about the stimuli (this can be generic and specific). It could be argued that both of the naive participants versus experts' studies above do not include participants who really do have *more* perceptual experience with tastes or specific tastes. Indeed, tastes are so frequently encountered that perceptual expertise (i.e. experience) may be close to the ceiling in all participants—naive or experts. Similarly, one could argue that the children in Watson *et al.*'s (2001) study had already acquired sufficient perceptual expertise (experience) for the task at hand. If then a group could be found who really do differ in experience with taste, perhaps they would show evidence of 'expertise'.

There is some evidence that specific perceptual experience may improve taste perception. Japanese people arguably consume and attend more to the taste of MSG in their diet than European or North American people do (after all we use the Japanese term Umami to describe its taste). Consistent with this hypothetical cultural difference, Ishii *et al.* (1992) reported that Japanese participants were more sensitive to MSG than North Americans. A similar increased sensitivity was also observed for sucrose, but not for salt, which somewhat undermines the clarity of this result. However, Kobayashi *et al.* (2006) recently reported that extra (i.e. above normal) dietary exposure to MSG does, indeed, result in enhanced detectability—an effect that is then lost after a period of reduced exposure. A similar conclusion may also be drawn from a far older study by Pangborn (1959), who observed that thresholds for sucrose, quinine, citric acid, and salt all decreased (i.e. increasing sensitivity) over several weeks of intense practice. Whilst all of these effects could result wholly or in part from low-level changes in taste-receptor function, a centrally based effect of experience is suggested by neuroimaging data. Faurion *et al.* (2005) reported that changes in activity in the insular cortex (primary taste cortex) accompanied increased perceptual familiarity with taste stimuli. Together, these findings suggest *the possibility*, that frequent perceptual experience with a particular taste may enhance detectability for that taste. However, whether these threshold changes in sensitivity translate into an improvement in detectability within a taste mixture has yet to be tested.

A further small, but significant, effect on the ability to detect tastes, and presumably individual tastants in mixtures, is that produced by attention. This was investigated by Marks and Wheeler (1998), who assessed participants' sensitivity for sucrose and citric acid using a procedure which tracked trial-by-trial changes in threshold. Attention was manipulated indirectly in three ways. First, individual 'runs', which involved multiple-paired comparison trials where participants were given a taste and water, and asked to indicate which contained a taste, were set-up so that 75% of the comparisons involved just one tastant. Second, participants were forewarned on each run that one tastant would occur more frequently. Third, participants were also provided with the target tastant at suprathreshold intensity at frequent intervals throughout the run. As the manipulation of attention was indirect, it is not possible to conclude whether any effect on threshold is driven by controlled (i.e. endogenous) or automatic (i.e. exogenous) attentional effects, or a combination of the two.

On runs where attention was directed to one tastant, thresholds were significantly lower (i.e. greater sensitivity) for that tastant and the magnitude of this effect did not differ between sucrose and citric acid. Whilst these results suggest that participants can (voluntarily or involuntarily) attend to one particular taste, the effect was small (about 0.2 log concentration steps). This finding has a bearing upon one of the key studies reported by Laing and colleagues in Chapter 3. In their studies, attention was specifically drawn to the target stimulus (by always focussing on one tastant alone), and so their findings are likely to represent the maximum identification ability for this type of task.

In sum, the data here suggest two conclusions. First, even untrained participants are good at identifying individual taste elements in taste mixtures under ideal circumstances (i.e. those which minimize taste suppression). Second, there appears relatively little that one can do to improve this and even where improvements have been observed—the effects are not particularly dramatic. So, in respect to the question as to whether taste mixtures can be broken down into their component parts, the answer would be a definitive 'yes'. Functionally, it could be argued that all of us need the ability to detect potentially beneficial or dangerous elements in food that are signalled by the basic tastes. Consequently, it makes good evolutionary sense to retain an ability to detect them in isolation. A final issue, and one not addressed but assumed in this section, is whether taste parts should be regarded as elements. This assumption appears warranted, because, as indicated in Chapter 1, there are clear associations between tastant, receptor type, and percept.

Smell

Unfortunately, all of the empirical work described below, and hence the conclusions here, rely upon orthonasal presentation. Consequently, generalizations to retronasal olfactory perception assume some level of processing equivalence between these two modes. Whilst this does not appear unreasonable, there are grounds to believe that processing between retronasal and orthonasal olfaction may differ (e.g. see Sun and Halpern (2005), Small et al. (2005), Scott et al. (2007), and see Chapter 6 for a more extended discussion of this issue). With this caveat in mind, the most important finding identified in Chapter 3 was that there is a limit to the number of odourants (i.e. elements) that can be identified in a mixture. This has been most compellingly demonstrated by the techniques developed by Laing's group (see Chapter 3), but also by two other findings. First, that the number of odourants in a mixture (i.e. its physical complexity) is not correlated with the *perceived* complexity of the stimulus (Jellinek and Koster 1979). The underlying logic here is that if the addition of each successive odourant adds an extra detectable part to the mixture, then mixtures with additional odourants should be perceived as having more parts, and thus appear more complex. This serves nicely to support Laing's various findings, which focus on detecting elements (i.e. where the part to be detected corresponds to a physically present odourant, which itself can be a single pure chemical or a mixture of chemicals, such as the elements 'mint' or 'coffee'). In addition, Jellinek and Koster's (1979) results also rather starkly illustrate the difference between 'elements' and 'similarities'. Thus, even physically simple stimuli (single chemicals) can smell complex (i.e. have lots of similarities) and physically complex stimuli (multiple chemicals) can smell simple (i.e. have few similarities)—and vice versa. A second finding that also supports the data from Laing's group comes from a study by Laska and Hudson (1992). They reported that omitting odour elements from mixtures was often not detected by participants. As they too suggest, this reflects our limited capacity to discriminate the elements in an odour mixture.

One possible reason why we may be poor at identifying elements is that we do not have the capacity to focus attention in the olfactory domain, especially as noted before that the olfactory system is unique in connecting directly to the neocortex, rather than relying solely, as the other senses do, on a thalamic link. The thalamus has been suggested as one possible neural substrate of endogenous attention in respect to the other senses (e.g. McCormick and Bal 1994). However, animals and people do appear to be able to direct attention to the olfactory domain. First, in animals, there is good physiological evidence that thalamic-type gating (i.e. selective or endogenous attention) can occur within the primary olfactory cortex (Murakami *et al.* 2005). Second, in humans, whilst there is no definitive physiological evidence, there is clear behavioural evidence in that participants can selectively attend to orthonasal olfactory stimulation versus visual stimulation under conditions which ensured that the olfactory stimulus did not involve tactile or trigeminal cues (Spence *et al.* (2001)). Finally, and of particular interest here, Sun and Halpern (2005) have obtained data which suggest that retronasal olfactory stimuli may obtain greater attentional resources than orthonasal stimuli, under conditions in which participants had to identify two different odourants—one presented orthonasally and the other retronasally. Thus, it is very likely that we can voluntarily attend to odours and, perhaps when the odour arises from the mouth, this may attract attention involuntarily from any concomitant orthonasal stimulation. It would, therefore, appear unlikely that the limits to identification of elements in mixtures are solely a consequence of an inability to attend to them.

The limit on detecting elements in mixtures is further reaffirmed by the finding that it is also present in trained perfumists and flavourists—i.e. experts. Livermore and Laing (1996) took a group of these experts and compared them to a set of control participants who had been trained by the experimenters to accurately label the component odours used in the study. Participants were then presented with various stimuli, from single odours through to five-element odour mixtures, and were asked to identify the elements present in each stimulus. Experts and the experimenter-trained group, crucially, showed the same ceiling effect, with both performing very poorly (at chance) on four- and five-component mixtures. However, experts demonstrated a small but significant advantage over the experimenter-trained group in being better able to identify the components of binary and ternary mixtures. This effect is likely to be a consequence of their expertise.

Apart from Livermore and Laing's (1996) study, no one else has tested whether the perceptual limit on the identification of elements in mixtures can be broken by experts. However, at least three studies suggest that experience with the target odours is an important variable in discriminating elements below this limit. Rabin (1988) presented participants with two stimuli, and they had to make a same/different judgement for the pair. On key trials, a target was presented, followed by the target presented in a mixture with another odour—the contaminant (i.e. a binary mixture). Crucially, the target odour could be familiar or unfamiliar to that participant, as could the contaminant. If experience is an important variable in regulating the discriminability of mixture components, then the best performance should be observed in trials in which both, the target and the contaminant, are familiar, and the worst performance on trials in which the target and contaminant are both unfamiliar. Performance should be intermediate where either the target or contaminants are unfamiliar. Exactly this pattern of outcome was observed, suggesting that exposure (as indexed by familiarity) may act to sharpen the percept (i.e. the target element relative to the background element), thus enhancing its detectability.

A recent neuroimaging study provides some further insight into the neural processes that may underpin these experience-related effects. Li *et al.* (2006) obtained similarity ratings for a target odour versus: (1) a qualitatively similar odour; (2) a structurally similar odour; and (3) a qualitatively and structurally different odour. Participants were then repeatedly exposed to the target odour and, following this exposure phase, the similarity ratings (see above) were obtained again. These ratings showed that the target odour was judged more dissimilar to both the qualitatively and structurally similar odours, post-exposure, with no change in respect to the unrelated control odour. Neuroimaging indiated that two regions were specifically associated with these changes in similarity—the piriform and orbitofrontal cortices (i.e. primary and secondary olfactory cortex)—but only activity in the orbitofrontal cortex correlated with the degree of change observed in similarity scores. These findings suggest that passive exposure may result in changes in perceptual similarity that are accompanied by concomitant neural changes in primary and secondary olfactory processing areas, and it is arguably this type of experience-induced plasticity that improves discriminability of individual elements. This finding also points to an additional conclusion, namely if an element becomes more discriminable, this may manifest as a change in similarity, and this is an underlying assumption in the Li *et al.* (2006) study. It is also a quite justified assumption as significant correlations between measures of perceived similarity and discriminability have been reported elsewhere (e.g. Case *et al.* 2004).

Whilst passive exposure may be important, as with name learning, which can also improve odour discriminability (Rabin 1988), these may not be the only means to alter the way in which participants perceive odour mixtures. Le Berre *et al.* (2008) examined the effects of exposure and exposure strategy on two sets of odourants, composed of a ternary mixture (pineapple) and its components, and a six-component mixture (red cordial) and its components. Of particular interest here was the exposure-strategy task. This, in essence, attempted to manipulate endogenous attention by getting participants to either focus on the component elements that formed each mixture (analytic strategy) or to judge the typicality of each odour in relation to the mixture from which it came (synthetic strategy).

A small, but significant, effect of exposure was obtained, but only for the pineapple odourant. This was detected by examining typicality judgements made in the exposure-strategy phase, by comparing participants exposed to the pineapple components, red cordial components, and to a control group that had not been exposed to the elements (i.e. participants exposed to the components of the pineapple mixture judged the mixture to be less typically 'pineapple-like', presumably because the components were now more detectable in this mixture, thus reducing its typicality). Interestingly, no exposure effect was obtained for the red cordial mixture, presumably because it was a six-component mixture and so was immune to the effects of the exposure strategy as the individual elements were not detectable (i.e. the perceptual limit had been reached).

Of particular note were the findings in relation to the exposure strategy adopted by participants. Participants who engaged in the analytical strategy judged their respective mixture as less typical (i.e. less like red cordial or pineapple) than participants who had engaged in the synthetic task, and these effects were independent of participants' exposure history to the components. The authors suggest that the qualities of the individual elements can remain intact, although not necessarily intact enough to support their identification. This is a contentious claim, as it appears to contradict the more general finding that there is a limit to the detectability of odour elements in mixtures. However, it is of course possible that a more sensitive method might lift this 'ceiling', but if that were the case, one would expect an interaction between exposure and strategy, as both of these should work together to enhance the detection of individual elements and their related qualities; but this was not observed. The authors' conclusion must remain tentative, because we cannot be sure that their effect arose simply from a difference in the number of rating scales being used by participants in this task (recall the discussion in Chapter 2), and whilst the authors argue against this possibility, no empirical data exists as yet to exclude it.

The effects of exposure, naming—and an analytical strategy too, should this be confirmed by further empirical work—may all act to improve a participant's capacity to identify elements in a mixture. However, experience may also act to reduce discriminability. Stevenson (2001) exposed participants to binary mixtures and then tested whether odours exposed together versus those equally exposed, but not together, differed in discriminability on a triangle test of discrimination. Exposure of two odours together significantly impaired discriminative performance, even when in a later study, this was compared to odours that had been exposed alone (rather than in other mixtures; Case *et al.* 2004). The same processes that underpin enhanced detectability may also explain these findings, in that the brain may, by default, encode each olfactory stimulus as a single event (i.e. be it a single pure odourant or a mixture)—a process referred to in the perceptual learning literature as 'imprinting'. This encoding process—e.g. reflected in the neural plasticity observed by Li *et al.* (2006)—may refine subsequent perception of the odourant, improving its detectability in a mixture on the one hand, but reducing the detectability of its components on the other.

The majority of the evidence reviewed here and in Chapter 3, suggests that as the number of odour elements in a mixture increases beyond three, these individual elements become much harder to detect. Limits on endogenous attention do not appear to account for this loss of information, as it applies equally to olfactory experts and novices, and because participants have been shown to demonstrate voluntary orientation towards olfactory stimuli (i.e. endogenous attention). So, in answering the question as to whether a complex olfactory stimulus can be broken down into its parts, for its elements at least, there appears to be a clear perceptual limit and up to that limit the *naive* participant can detect the elements and the expert can do somewhat better.

The presence of this perceptual limit for detecting elements may reflect functional considerations. Organisms need to detect odour objects or deviations from them. These objects are typically complex physical mixtures (e.g. perfume or a burning steak) and there is little functional value in detecting their individual chemical constituents. You need to know whether the smell is a perfume or a burning steak. The ability to detect elements (e.g. perfume or a burning steak) is functionally useful when one element has to be detected against the background of another, such as detecting the smell of burning steak *against* one's perfume or aftershave. In sum, whilst the olfactory system retains a limited analytical capacity, in the main it depends upon recognizing complex blends.

A further issue here concerns the detection of similarities in contrast to elements. Similarities may reflect differences between elements (i.e. coffee has a different set of similarities (qualities) to cheese), but the number of similarities appears to be relatively independent of the physical complexity of the stimulus. As will be seen in the section on wine and beer, and especially for sensory evaluation of food by trained panels, the detection of similarities (qualities) is influenced by training and expertise, and does not appear to have an obvious ceiling in the way that element detection does.

Texture

Texture perception is clearly an important part of flavour perception, and especially so for certain foods (Szczesniak 2002). As a result, there has been considerable interest from the food industry in developing ways of measuring the perceived texture of food (e.g. see Munoz and Civille 1987). However, unlike taste and smell, the study of texture perception is beset with difficulties (see Christensen 1984). As described in Chapter 1, perception of texture is an active process, the food needs to be touched and manipulated to form an impression of its physical properties. As described in Chapter 3, it is also a multisensory process, involving the visual appearance of food (e.g. wilted lettuce), the sound of the food (e.g. crisps), its smell (e.g. fattiness), and, of course, oral manipulation in the mouth. Once in the mouth, texture changes with time as the food is masticated, saliva is added to the food, and changes in temperature occur (e.g. ice cream or chocolate).

For taste and smell, the starting point above was to establish whether participants could identify a particular taste or a particular smell in homogenous mixtures of either tastes or smells ('elements' in the terminology of the introduction to this chapter). It does not appear possible to conduct a directly analogous experiment for texture because it is not possible to independently manipulate texture parts; indeed, no one can be sure as to what the full set of 'texture parts' might be. Instead, a rather different approach is adopted here. The first step is to determine what texture parts participants can identify and whether these reflect 'similarities' to other foods or are specific textural terms that generalize across foods (i.e. more reflective of elements). The second step is then to see whether these parts relate to underlying physical parameters (more reflective of elements). Having then established whether the parts of texture perception more closely resemble elements or similarities, the third step is to establish whether they can be identified in complex mixtures. This may be more likely if the parts are elements (i.e. most like taste).

Szczesniak and Kleyn (1963) asked a variety of participants to generate associations to a large set of foods (using their names) that varied considerably in texture (see below for more details on this study). Their Table 6 provides the 77 words that participants spontaneously generated, which reflected texture-based terms. Of these 77 words, 11 related directly to other foods or objects (i.e. similarities; buttery, chalky, creamy, curdy, doughy, fish eyes, gelatinous, rubbery, sandy, soupy, and starchy), four are marginal (i.e. fatty, spongy, watery, and wet) and the remaining 62 were all specific sensations, that is they refer directly to textural characteristics that might apply across a range of foods (or other objects). Of the 11 'similarities', only one was mentioned with any frequency and that was 'creamy'. As discussed in Chapter 3, creamy may have special status, and this is discussed later below. Notwithstanding, the general conclusion from this study is that participants generate texture descriptors that are tactile-sensation specific in nature (e.g. hard, viscous, slimy, etc.) and this conclusion appears to hold both for other more recent North American samples and for respondents from other countries (see Table 11.2 in Lawless and Heymann (1998)).

Factor analytical studies of texture terms that people use to describe various foods (see Kokini 1985) and the frequency with which texture terms are used (see Szczesniak 2002) have both been used to establish a set of tactile-specific dimensions for texture which are *relatively* independent. These fall into three categories: mechanical-related parts (e.g. hardness), geometrical-related parts (e.g. grittiness), and chemical-related parts (e.g. fattiness). Importantly, ratings of specific terms drawn from all three of these categories have been demonstrated to co-vary, respectively, with changes in the physical, geometrical, and chemical properties of the food stimulus (e.g. Engelen *et al.* 2005, Kokini 1985, Meullenet *et al.* 1998, Vliet 2002). In certain cases, where an adequate stimulus range is used, these correlations are impressively high (e.g. 0.9 for mechanical measures of hardness and hardness perception; Meullenet *et al.* 1998).

The findings above would suggest that there is a clear, but albeit far from perfect, mapping of physical (including here geometrical and chemical) stimulus parameters to percept. This might arguably parallel the mapping of stimulation of a particular taste-receptor type to a particular taste percept. Obtain a particular physical parameter (or stimulate a particular taste receptor) and one will perceive a *particular* texture or taste percept. Consequently, one might predict that if texture perception is primarily elemental in nature, then these elements should be detectable in even relatively complex stimuli— like tastes.

In addressing whether texture attributes can be detected in complex stimuli requires drawing upon both, a limited literature and one that was not explicitly designed to address this question. The place to start is with the 'texture-profile method' developed by Szczesniak *et al.* (1963) as a way of standardizing the verbal descriptions used to describe food texture. Not only does it provide a set of standard foods to represent variations on certain attributes, notably for the mechanical parts (i.e. hardness, cohesiveness, viscosity, springiness, adhesiveness, fracturability, chewiness, and gumminess), it carefully defines each element, and it is prescriptive over when in the ingestion/chewing/swallowing cycle a particular type of attribute rating should be made (Civille and Szczesniak 1973).

It has been suggested that naive consumers do not typically pay much attention to the texture of food, except when their expectations of texture are violated (Munoz and Civille 1987). One might then expect that people who work routinely with food and development of new foods would be more attentive to this dimension of flavour, and this does appear to be the case. In the Szczesniak and Kleyn (1963) study described above, some of the participants were involved in food-technology work, and some were not. Of the total pool of word associations generated towards food, 24% were flavour-related terms. Within this group of flavour-related terms, texture-related words were the most frequent (32%) with food aroma the least (2%). Food technologists generated more texture-related terms (36%) than controls (30%), suggesting that they may, indeed, be more attentive to this dimension of flavour than naive participants—but the difference is not that large, and both groups described food texture in a similar manner, that is with tactile-specific terms.

Cardello *et al.* (1982) investigated whether a group of participants who had received training with the 'texture-profile method' (hereafter experts) would differ from naive participants (hereafter novices) in their ability to assess the texture of a range of foods. The 'differ' can encompass a range of possibilities but as this work was largely exploratory—indeed, it had to be because there is no other work that appears to tackle the issue of textural (or tactile) expertise—it is better to look at the results first and then reflect on what they may mean. In their first experiment, the experts and novices were asked to use similarity scaling for a range of fish fillets that varied in texture. The experts had neither evaluated fish before for texture so they would not be expected to have *specific* perceptual expertise with the stimuli, nor had they used similarity scaling before. The similarity scaling revealed almost identical performance between the expert and novice participants suggesting that they are responsive to largely the same underlying textural dimensions.

The second experiment also involved judging fish, again with both the experts and novices having no difference in perceptual experience with this task. However, this time participants were asked to evaluate the intensity (or degree of presence) of six textural properties and one visual property, for each sample. Correlations between experts and novices, for each rated textural attribute, were all significant bar one (r: 0.55–0.84). However, when the mean ratings for each attribute of the experts was regressed against the mean ratings for the novices, this revealed that, for all of the textural attributes, experts reported a greater range of perceptual experience than novices (i.e. a change of one unit for experts was accompanied by a *smaller* change for novices). This was not the case for the visual attribute where the regression coefficient was around one indicating a similar range in each group.

These findings were confirmed in a third experiment that used a large range of foods differing in texture, different rating scales—namely magnitude estimation (to eliminate any advantage to experts by using the category scale they had been trained on)—and the provision of definitions for each of the textural attributes to be rated. Very good correlations were obtained between experts and novices on all six textural dimensions (all r's: > 0.93), but the regression coefficients for each attribute again showed that experts appeared to experience a greater perceptual range. Finally, in Experiment 4 a selection of breads were rated for texture using magnitude estimation for each of 10 texture attributes, which were again defined for both groups. Two findings are of especial interest here. First, experts revealed somewhat greater independence between the textural attributes than novices. For experts, 42% of the possible correlations between ratings were significant (i.e. non-independent) compared to 53% for novices. Second, instrumental measures corresponding to eight of the textural attributes were obtained and the psychophysical function relating the attribute rating to its corresponding physical parameter was then calculated. In *all cases*, the exponent of the power function for each attribute–physical parameter relationship was higher for the experts than for the novices, suggesting that each unit increase in physical intensity was accompanied by a larger change in perceived intensity for the experts than for the novices (and see Moskowitz *et al.* (1979) for additional data regarding Experiment 4).

Two major conclusions derive from this study. First, novices are clearly good at identifying various textural elements in foods and do not differ markedly from experts in this regard. This is indicated by: (1) the closeness of the similarity scaling results; (2) the significant correlations between experts and novices for various texture attributes; (3) the significant relationships between physical and perceptual texture measures for novices that were obtained in Experiment 4 (range: 0.73–0.88); and (4) the relative independence of many of the textural measures. Thus, as with taste, it appears that novices can readily perceive individual elements that reliably correspond with physical variations in the stimulus.

The second conclusion is that experts, whilst not obviously surpassing novices in their ability to perceive elements (although there is some evidence of a minor benefit here in the greater independence between texture-attribute ratings noted in Experiment 4), have a larger dynamic perceptual range than novices. This might arise in two ways. First, experts may have experienced a broader range of stimulus intensities for each element, so what appears to be a perceptual difference may actually arise from the way in which they scale their responses. Second, experts may truly perceive smaller physical changes in the stimulus as larger. There is certainly evidence from many tactile, perceptual learning experiments that this can occur (e.g. Hodzic *et al.* 2004).

A further, albeit very different, approach to texture perception comes from two studies examining sensitivity to textural change in food (Mojet and Koster 2002, Mojet and Koster 2005). Mojet and Koster (2002) gave participants a meal consisting of a biscuit, pate, and a drink. Later, participants were given a surprise test, in which they were asked to identify which biscuit (pate or drink) they received earlier, from a range of biscuits (pates or drinks), which had had their texture altered. Biscuits varied in fat content, the drinks in viscosity and graininess, and the pate in consistency. Unfortunately, these variations in textural parameters gave rise to some differences in odour and taste, notably for the drinks and biscuits, limiting the conclusions that can be drawn here solely about texture. If participants can detect the target food (i.e. the one they ate before) amongst the distracters, then this would suggest that they could perceive the textural parameter that had been changed. Participants were clearly sensitive to changes in viscosity, fat content, and consistency, and these effects were independent of other changes in flavour (i.e. odour and taste).

In a second study, Mojet and Koster (2005) used foods that varied in texture without appreciable variation in odour and taste. Here, participants were found to be sensitive to changes in crispiness, creaminess, thickness (viscosity), and crumbliness, although fat level was very poorly detected this time. Interestingly, both studies observed that participants were particularly good at identifying foods they had not consumed before, which is perhaps analogous to Munoz and Civille's (1987) observation that consumers are especially sensitive to deviations in texture. More importantly still, it indicates (as must surely by now be apparent) that flavour experiences are routinely encoded into memory.

Whilst most of the texture parts discussed so far appear to be elements, creaminess is clearly something different. It does not have a single underlying physical cause although it can be predicted from multiple physical parameters, although these appear to vary between foods (Frost and Janhoj 2007). More importantly, and unlike almost all other textural attributes, creaminess is a 'similarity', i.e. it asks the participant to determine the similarity between a current experience and a memory of an archetypal stimulus (cream), rather than whether a particular element is present and its degree of presence. As described in Chapter 3, participants, and trained panels, do not appear to have any difficulty in making this judgement, nor indeed do they have any difficulty in rating the textural parameters (elements) that appear to be important in its psychological construction (namely smoothness and viscosity). From this it would appear that participants, be they experts or novices, could readily perceive both the elements that act together to produce a creamy percept as well as the creamy similarity itself.

Whilst the texture literature is far less developed than that for taste and smell, it would appear that naive participants can readily detect various textural elements in complex mixtures—that is in real foods. Perceptual expertise does not appear to extend this ability much—as with taste—although it may extend dynamic range and improve the independence with which each element is detected. In conclusion, participants can detect individual parts of texture, parts that are primarily elements with the notable exception of creaminess, and this ability shows some limited improvement with training.

Tastes and smells

The first question to address is whether there are any limits to the detection of taste and smell elements, when they are presented together in the mouth. Laing *et al.* (2002; Experiment 2) trained participants to identify sucrose, salt, citric acid, and the tasteless odourant octanol. Following this training, participants attended four separate sessions. On each session, their task was to identify (yes/no) whether a target flavourant was present (i.e. sucrose, salt, citric acid, or octanol). Participants received single components, binary, ternary, and four-component mixtures on each session. Identification performance was consistently better for the tastants than for the odourant. Sucrose, salt, and citric acid could be identified above chance in all but four-component mixtures, whilst octanol could *not* be identified above chance in any mixture, although it was readily identified when presented alone.

These findings could, of course, reflect some peculiarity of octanol on the one hand, and on the other might reflect limitations of the particular task that participants were asked to engage in. Consequently, Marshall *et al.* (2006)

conducted a similar experiment, but now including three odourants (cinnamal-dehyde, hexenol, and pentanone) along with the three tastants used previously. Participants were again trained to criterion (85% correct identification) for each stimulus, but this time they had to list all of the components that they believed were present in the stimulus. As with their study above, stimuli were sucked through a straw to prevent inadvertent orthonasal detection. Table 4.2 summarizes the results from this study, in terms of the proportion of tastes and smells identified alone and in combinations of up to six components. Whilst tastes could still be detected at above chance level even in the six-component mixture, reliable identification of the olfactory component was completely eliminated beyond the four-component mixtures.

The data discussed above for odours and for tastes suggest that attention can be selectively directed to each of these respective modalities. However, it was not readily apparent whether this could occur, first, when taste and smell are presented jointly by mouth and second, whether it is possible to direct attention to the olfactory component of a flavour. This second point is especially interesting, because attention may be directed at the mouth, rather than the nose, when a retronasal flavour is presented. Therefore, it is conceivable that even though participants have the ability to selectively attend to the olfactory modality when stimuli are presented orthonasally (i.e. directing attention spatially to the *nose*), they may not have the ability (or at least it may be more limited) when the stimuli are presented retronasally (i.e. they now direct attention to the mouth, even though the nose is needed to identify retronasally presented odours).

These and related questions were explored in an important series of studies by Ashkenazi and Marks (2004). In their first experiment, participants were

Table 4.2 Percent correct identifications based upon the proportion correct out of the total number that were available for identification for that particular stimulus type (adapted from Figure 1, Marshall, Laing, Jinks, and Hutchinson 2006)

Stimulus type	Percent correct identifications	
	Tastes	**Odours**
Single components	100	100
Two components	100	83
Three components	89	33
Four components	58	17
Five components	66	0
Six components	66	0

asked to indicate which of two solutions contained either a target taste (sucrose) or a target retronasal smell (vanilla)—the selective attention conditions, or which out of two solutions contained a flavourant (control condition). Selective attention significantly improved the detection of sucrose, irrespective of whether the distracter stimulus (i.e. the other member of the solution pair) was water or vanillin (see Table 4.3). This effect, as with most of the others here, was independent of stimulus concentration. However, selective attention to vanillin had no effect on detectability, and there was evidence that it actually impaired detectability when the distracter was water (see Table 4.3).

In the second experiment, participants were asked to detect either sucrose or vanilla when they were presented in compound. When sucrose was the target (i.e. sucrose + vanilla vs. vanilla OR sucrose + vanilla vs. water), selectively attending to sucrose impaired detectability, i.e. participants were better at the control task (i.e. which contains a flavour, sucrose + vanilla vs. water). When vanilla was the target (i.e. sucrose + vanilla vs. sucrose OR sucrose + vanilla vs. water), attending to vanilla impaired performance when sucrose was the distracter, whilst there was no significant difference when water was the distracter (see Table 4.3). One possibility here is that the control condition may have been considerably easier in this experiment than in Experiment 1, because of summation of taste and smell, thus boosting detectability. However, even

Table 4.3 Percent correct detections for the target stimulus (vanilla or sucrose), averaged across stimulus concentration, alone (Experiment 1 and 3) or in mixtures (Experiment 2), against various distracters (adapted from Figures 2–4, Ashkenazi, and Marks 2004)

Experiment	Percent correct detections				
Target	Distracter†				Control
	Wat	Van	Suc	Cit	
Experiment 1					
Sucrose	82	82	-	-	76
Vanilla	73	-	74	-	77
Experiment 2					
Sucrose	72	75	-	-	82
Vanilla	80	-	75	-	82
Experiment 3					
Vanilla	72	-	53	63	81

† Wat = water, Van = vanilla, Suc = sucrose, Cit = citric acid

though detection was significantly better for the control in Experiment 2 than in Experiment 1 (see Table 4.3), the reverse pattern held for sucrose detectability on the selective attention task. This was significantly better in Experiment 1 than in Experiment 2. This suggests the decrement in detection ability, under conditions where a taste and a smell are presented together, occurs independently of differences in the control conditions. Similarly, differences in response strategy between Experiment 1 and 2 (i.e. detecting and eliminating the distracter in a mixture rather than solely detecting the target) were also excluded as a possible explanation of the poorer performance in Experiment 2, in a separate control experiment.

In the third experiment, Ashkenazi and Marks (2004) examined whether using the dissimilar tastant citric acid (i.e. all the preceding experiments used sucrose and vanillin which participants regard as being perceptually similar—sweet tasting and smelling) would enable better selective attention to vanillin, when citric acid was presented as the distracter. This was not borne out as vanillin detection was impaired equally, irrespective of whether water, sucrose, or citric acid was used as the distracter. However, as can be seen in Table 4.3, performance was indeed poorest when the distracter was sucrose and, although this did not significantly differ from water or citric acid, only five participants served as subjects in this experiment and so the question remains as to whether a larger sample size may have revealed an even greater impairment when sucrose served as the distracter.

These results are particularly interesting for several reasons. First, they demonstrate that when participants are presented with a single retronasal olfactory stimulus, attempts to selectively attend to that channel impair performance relative to a non-selective control task. Second, whilst detection is improved by selectively attending to the gustatory channel when using a single stimulus in Experiment 1, this did not occur when the taste was presented with a perceptually similar odourant. Third, not only was detection of the retronasal odourant poorer alone, it was also equally poor when combined with a tastant. Needless to say, these differences in performance were relatively modest (albeit significant) and, in general, participants were pretty good (especially when the stimuli were more intense) at detecting either taste or olfactory elements. However, what these results starkly illustrate is that naive participants (if these subjects can be termed as such after their myriad of experimental trials) do not seem to benefit from focussing their attention on the component parts of an odour–taste mixture. Rather, selectively attending to the components appears to impair performance, perhaps as a consequence (in this case) of the perceptual similarity of the taste and the smell employed, especially in Experiment 2.

The failure to find positive performance benefits when attention is directed to either taste or smell in a mixture, as in the Ashkenazi and Marks (2004) study, along with the difficulty that participants encounter in identifying the olfactory components of odour/taste mixtures (Marshall *et al.* 2006) seems to suggest the following. First, that detecting odour elements is even more restricted when they are perceived both retronasally and in combination with taste, than under the orthonasal conditions described earlier in this chapter. So whereas the orthonasal odour-element-detection limit is three or four, retronasally this may be far lower (one or two). Second, taste-element-detection ability is still largely intact, even when odours are present. Given the retronasal olfactory limit and the apparent failure of selective attention to improve detection performance for odour–taste mixtures, one might not be optimistic about finding significant effects of training. Nonetheless, several studies have tried.

An important study in this regards was reported by Bingham *et al.* (1990). In a series of experiments exploring the effects of maltol (a sweet-smelling odourant) on the perception of sucrose sweetness, they reported two key findings. First, that for a trained sensory panel, the addition of maltol to sucrose solution (vs. sucrose alone, maltol alone, and water) did not affect their ratings of sweetness, either when a nose-clip was worn to prevent retronasal olfaction or when the nose-clip was removed. However, when naive participants were used in a final experiment, and given a two-alternative forced-choice task (2AFC)—which is sweeter—5% sucrose and maltol or 5% sucrose alone, 80% chose the sucrose–maltol mixture as the sweeter solution. Whilst, at face value, this suggests that a trained panel may have been able to selectively attend to just the sucrose sweetness, a feat the naive participants were unable to do, two problems arise with this interpretation. First, the tests used to establish the enhancement effect are clearly different. Trained panellists were asked to use time-intensity scaling of sweetness, with and without a nose-clip. Naive participants used the 2AFC task. An ideal comparison would use the same procedure to compare naive and trained participants, and in all fairness this was not the intention of the study. However, the differing nature of the tasks with its potential for differences in test sensitivity (and demand) could equally account for performance difference between naive participants and the trained panel. A second concern is that no details are provided concerning the nature of the training or the level of expertise of the trained panel, nor indeed are any data presented about the naivete of the non-trained participants.

These results prompted Stevenson (2001) to explore more specifically whether training under laboratory conditions might affect the ability of participants to selectively attend to either the taste or olfactory components of odour–taste mixtures and thus to avoid (or diminish) a sweetness taste-enhancement effect. Participants in this study were randomly assigned to either a training or exposure group—the latter receiving the same stimuli as the former, but without any specific instructions being imparted. The experiment began with two tasks that aimed to assess sweetness enhancement—the pre-test. The first was a magnitude-matching task, in which four sweet-smelling odours were presented in sucrose solution, along with sucrose alone, and these were matched for sweetness against a real set of sucrose solutions varying in concentration from 0.36 to 10.7%, in seven 0.8 log steps. On the second task, participants rated the same set of solutions—odour–sucrose and sucrose alone—for sweetness using a line scale.

The next phase of the experiment involved training or exposure. Training participants received two blocks of six solutions—two of the sweet-smelling odours used in the pre-test in water, two of them in sucrose, and two of sucrose alone. Participants were given a brief lecture about the dual nature of olfaction and how taste was different from retronasal olfaction. They then sampled the first block of six solutions, pinching open and shut their nostrils at various times, so that they could see the contribution of retronasal olfaction in the different stimuli (i.e. odour alone, taste and odour, and taste alone). All of this was accompanied by a detailed commentary/dialogue between the participant and the experimenter. On the second block, participants were invited to use these skills (but not nose pinching) to establish the identity of each solution (i.e. taste alone, taste and smell, and taste alone). One week later, participants returned for a second session and the same training regime was repeated as described above. The exposure group received exactly the same stimuli as the training group, however they were just asked to sip and spit, and then judge how much they liked or disliked the stimulus. After the end of the second training/exposure session, participants repeated the two sweetness-enhancement tasks—the post-test. They then filled in a questionnaire to assess their degree of interest in olfaction and the chemical senses. Finally, this was followed by a further repeat of the magnitude-matching task described above. However, this time, participants in the training group were specifically exhorted to use the skills acquired in the training phase and to try and judge the sweetness of just the taste component and ignore any olfactory stimulation. The exposed group did not receive these instructions.

Looking, first, at the change in the size of the enhancement effect between pre- and post-test revealed that training had no effect. More specifically, for the two odours that served in the training (or exposure phase) that might have been affected if training had had an odour-specific effect revealed a similar result—no effect. Indeed, participants in both groups demonstrated a robust enhancement effect on both pre- and post-test for all of the odours, irrespective of the method used to assess it (i.e. rating scale or magnitude matching). However, an analysis of the final magnitude-matching task did reveal an effect of training. For exposed participants, there was no significant difference in the size of the enhancement effect for the exposed and non-exposed odours.

For trained participants, the enhancement effect was significantly smaller for the trained odours than for the untrained odours, and the difference between these conditions significantly exceeded that between the exposed participants for exposed and non-exposed odours (see Table 4.4). Whilst this effect was not large, it suggests that training may produce a *specific* effect, one that does not unfortunately generalize to odours that were not used in training. Finally, enhancement effects were typically smaller in participants who had a greater interest in olfaction and the chemical senses, than those who did not.

The results Stevenson (2001) obtained suggest three conclusions. First, that training may have an effect if participants are instructed to try and use it. Second, that the magnitude of the enhancement effect may be reduced in participants who are generally more attentive to their olfactory experience. Third, that both the first and second conclusion suggest that, by default, participants do not selectively attend to the components of odour–taste mixtures, and that attention to them may only occur either when they are explicitly instructed to do so or when they are more interested in chemosensory-related events. Indeed, Stevenson's (2001) experiment may have found that training had no effect at all if the exposed group of participants had also been instructed on the final magnitude matching task to avoid taking the olfactory component into account, but this would have meant alerting them to exactly the distinction which the training itself was meant to achieve. Of course, it may be that far more prolonged training may work in a way that brief training cannot (e.g. recall Livermore and Laing's (1998) study discussed above). However, whilst Ashkenazi and Marks (2000) found that selectively attending to the components of odour–taste mixtures impaired performance, Stevenson's (2001) findings, and arguably Bingham *et al.* (1990) too, suggest that training *may* produce some limited beneficial effect.

One further reason that training may have been relatively ineffective in Stevenson's (2001) study was that the odours it employed were ones that were already associated with a taste. As discussed in Chapter 3, once this learning is acquired it may be very difficult to disrupt and so the effects on the perception of mixtures may persist even if the participant is valiantly attempting to attend

Table 4.4 Mean score from the final magnitude-matching task (adapted from Stevenson 2001)

Condition	Sucrose alone	Sucrose and trained/ exposed odours	Sucrose and non-trained/ exposed odours
Training	3.0	3.9	4.5
Exposure	3.1	4.3	3.9

to the individual elements. Stevenson and Case (2003) examined this issue in a further study, which focussed on whether training and exposure—of the same sort as described above—would affect the acquisition of an odour–taste association, where the odours used were ones with which the participant had little prior experience. Rather than enhancement effects, the focus of this study was on odour-induced sweetness.

Participants in this study were randomly assigned to either a training or exposure group. All of the participants started the experiment by judging the qualities, using rating scales (e.g. how sweet does it smell?), of four unfamiliar odours—the odour pre-test. The training or exposure phase then began. As before, training involved making participants cognizant of the role of olfaction in flavour perception. This time, however, participants received two of the unfamiliar odours alone in water, sucrose, and citric acid alone, and then one of the odours in sucrose and the other in citric acid. As before, two blocks of these six stimuli were presented, with the same training regime as described above. Exposed participants received identical stimuli, but just made liking judgements. In the second phase of the study, all of the participants received the other two unfamiliar odours, one in sucrose (twice) and one in citric acid (twice). A week later, participants returned to the laboratory and repeated the training or exposure phase, followed by a repeat of the second phase as described above. This was followed by the odour post-test, identical to the pre-test, and an expectancy test, which asked participants to sniff a solution and then predict what taste they thought it might contain.

Training had no effect. However, pre-exposure to the odours did, as both the training and exposure groups failed to demonstrate any change in odour sweetness or sourness, for stimuli that were experienced alone in water prior to conditioning. For the odours presented in phase two (i.e. the untrained/unexposed odours), significant evidence of conditioning—i.e. an increase in perceived sweetness for sucrose-paired odours and of sourness for citric acid-paired odours was observed. Whilst it is difficult to definitively conclude from this that pre-exposure retarded learning, because the design was not optimized to detect this, the results suggest that brief training is ineffective in preventing odour–taste learning.

As noted above, participants may, by default, not try to attend to the component elements of a flavour in the mouth, and this may have been one reason why no effect of training was detected in the study above (Stevenson and Case 2003). This issue has been partially addressed in a study reported by Prescott (1999). Here, participants were exposed to: (1) a sweet-smelling familiar odour paired with sucrose; (2) a sweet-smelling less familiar odour paired with sucrose; (3) a familiar non-sweet odour paired with sucrose; and (4) an unfamiliar odour paired with sucrose. During the period in which they sampled these solutions, participants in one group were asked to judge their overall intensity—the integration group—and in another to judge their sweetness (i.e. the taste component) and flavour (i.e. the olfactory component)—the separation group. A further control group sampled the four odours alone in water, and sucrose alone in water, rating all of these stimuli for overall intensity.

Prior to this sampling period, all participants smelled and rated the four odours, as well as judging their sweetness when dissolved in sucrose. These two tests were repeated following the sampling period. Evidence of odour–taste learning was only obtained for unfamiliar odours in the integration group when assessed via changes in smelled sweetness between pre- and post-test, suggesting that the ratings may have forced participants in the separation group to attend selectively to the taste and olfactory components of the mixture, preventing learning. However, the results from the enhancement test suggest otherwise. Here, *all* of the groups evidenced increased sweetness enhancement on the post-test, relative to the pre-test, and this was most marked for odours that were initially low in sweetness.

These results present something of a paradox for several reasons. First, the enhancement test appeared to reveal evidence of conditioning in every group (if one assumes that odour–taste learning is important for underpinning this effect)—yet the control group never actually received odour–sucrose pairings during the sampling period. Second, no group differences emerged on the enhancement test, yet they did on the odour-smelling test. Whilst it is possible to suggest that conditioning occurred in all groups following the exposure of the odours and tastes together in the pre-test (explaining the first paradox), this fails to explain why group effects should be obtained on one test and not on the other. Nonetheless, these findings do suggest that when participants are forced to engage in an attentional manipulation *during* the conditioning phase of an experiment, there *may* be detectable consequences.

In a further series of studies (Prescott *et al.* 2004), the potential consequences of a synthetic versus an analytical stance were explored. In Experiment 1, participants sniffed two unfamiliar odours and rated their characteristics, including sweetness, as well as tasting and rating these odours dissolved in sucrose. One of these odours was then paired with sucrose and participants were then assigned to the same three conditions described for Prescott (1999)—integration, separation, and a control who did not receive any odour–taste pairs. The post-test followed, and this was identical to the pre-test. This time, a significant change in odour sweetness was observed in all three groups for both odours (contrast with Prescott (1999) where change was only observed in the integration group), but an enhancement effect was now only obtained in the integration group (again contrast with Prescott (1999) where an enhancement effect was obtained in every group). Again, these results suggest that odour–taste learning, this time as indexed by the enhancement test, may be affected by the attentional strategy employed during training, but the inconsistency with the earlier results is quite striking. An additional feature of these results, noted in Chapter 3, was that a final experiment indicated that a single odour–taste pairing may result in learning, with a consequent change in the degree to which an unfamiliar odour smells sweet. This may account for the generality of the odour–taste learning effect in the earlier Prescott (1999) study (i.e. it occurred even in participants who had not received mixtures during the training phase, but in those who had received pairings during the pre-test).

It would be premature at the moment to rule out the possibility that training or attentional strategies may affect odour-induced taste enhancement or odour–taste learning. However, even if they do, they would not appear to be very large effects. If anything, the data that is at hand—the difficulty in identifying/detecting the olfactory element of odour–taste mixtures, the limited ability to attend to components, the limited or inconsistent effects of training and attentional strategies—would suggest two general conclusions. First, when participants, especially naive ones, experience odours and taste together in the mouth, they treat them as a unitary stimulus and that to depart from this state of affairs (i.e. to move towards perceiving the elements independently) is difficult, to say the least. Second, one might tentatively add, that attempting to perceive an odour–taste mixture, as a set of elements may be harder still when the physical components have been experienced before as a mixture.

A final point of discussion, but one that is unfortunately poor in terms of data concerns this last point—experience. Experience of an odour and taste together appears to endow the odour with the capacity to produce a taste-like sensation—i.e. a similarity to a taste. Does the presence of such a similarity make it harder to detect an odour and a taste element in a mixture, than for an odour and a taste that do not share such a similarity? Ashkenazi and Mark's (2002) data come closest to answering this, and there is certainly some suggestion there that it might. A more definitive answer might come from repeating Marshall *et al.*'s (2006) experiment, but using odours that do and do not smell sweet, to compare their detectability. If this type of experiment did indeed confirm that sweet-smelling odours are harder to detect in mixtures containing sucrose, than non-sweet-smelling odours, this would imply that two mechanisms might act to affect the detectability of parts in flavours in general. One mechanism would involve changes in the perception of elements. For example, consider here the results for texture that suggest that experts may have a 'stretched' perceptual space for texture elements (Cardello *et al.* 1982). The second would involve the generation of new similarities (e.g. odour sweetness) that may make elements less discriminable in some cases and more so in others.

Expertise with food and drink—Introduction

As Moskowitz (1996) notes, industrial development and assessment of many foods and drinks involves experts. Expertise, as defined and described below, may come in different forms, and much of the remaining part of this chapter is devoted to the question as to what benefit this brings to the assessment of stimuli within that particular domain of expertise, namely for wine, beer, and food. This literature has a direct bearing upon the questions raised at the beginning of this chapter. First, whether experts are more successful at detecting parts in flavours than naive participants. Second, if they are able to perform better than naive participants, how do they do it?

Wine

Two forms of knowledge and the relationship between them, would appear to underpin expertise with wine (Frost and Noble 2002) and, indeed, with beer and food too. The first is perceptual knowledge. This manifests in the ability to discriminate between wines and, relatedly, to be able to discriminate and detect parts within a wine. The second is conceptual or semantic knowledge. This appears in the ability to: (1) know what makes one variety of wine different from another, so as to guide attention to salient aspects of the stimulus; (2) organize perceptual information into meaningful categories (e.g. by grape variety); and (3) be able to accurately and reliably communicate information about wine to others. As working definitions, conceptual or semantic knowledge can be defined as that acquired by verbal or written means, whilst perceptual knowledge is that acquired by experience with the stimulus.

   These two forms of knowledge have to become connected for wine expertise to emerge, because in theory both forms of knowledge could exist independently but without many of the benefits of 'true' expertise, i.e. regular wine drinkers may acquire perceptual expertise through passive exposure to wine which should assist, e.g. their ability to discriminate one wine from another. Similarly, (but only in theory) a person could study oenology from books and obtain a high level of knowledge about wine varieties and their characteristics without ever tasting a wine at all. Whilst the former clearly exists, the latter is hypothetical and such knowledge would be of little value unless it was linked to the perceptual experience of the former. It is probable that perceptual knowledge of wine is acquired and highly likely that conceptual knowledge is. The caveat of 'probably'for the former is simply an acknowledgement that experts *may* have some initial perceptual advantage over non-experts. Put bluntly, they could be innately more sensitive to perceptual differences between wines than non-experts.

It is very difficult to tell whether wine experts have an initial perceptual advantage over non-experts. First, it is hard to say what such an advantage might look like. It could be better discriminative ability, most notably a higher limit to the perceptual ceiling on decomposing physically complex odour mixtures (say four or five components instead of three). This would appear unlikely given that experts in other olfactory domains do not evidence such an ability (i.e. see Livermore and Laing (1996) and discussion above). Alternatively, it could be greater sensitivity, again especially olfactory sensitivity, which might allow them to detect an olfactory component, which the less discerning nose might miss. However, in all of the studies which have assessed olfactory thresholds in wine experts and novices (i.e. those who lack both perceptual and conceptual expertise), no significant difference in sensitivity for butanol (a chemical commonly used to assess thresholds in clinical studies as it is a relatively pure olfactory stimulant at the concentrations used) has been detected (Bende and Nordin 1997, Parr *et al.* 2002, Parr *et al.* 2004). A far more specific test of this possibility was reported by Berg *et al.* (1955), who assessed thresholds for a variety of tastants and odourants found in wine, in experts and infrequent wine drinkers (i.e. perceptual and conceptual novices). They reported no difference between groups for any compound.

A further possibility is that whilst experts may not exceed novices in their ability to detect odour elements (i.e. the ceiling referred to above), they may be able to detect odour elements more effectively below this ceiling, especially when they are less apparent. That is they could be more efficient at either using a template to search for the presence of a particular olfactory element or be better able to selectively attend to one channel whilst ignoring another. Bende and Nordin (1997) obtained some evidence for this type of effect, in that expert wine tasters were able to detect citral (lemon) at a lower concentration in a fixed concentration of eugenol (clove), than naive participants. Whilst their data suggest this ability of experts may not be a simple consequence of greater familiarity with these odours as only a small proportion of the wine tasters (12–20%) claimed that these odours were wine-related, it is not possible to tell whether any benefit comes from frequent attempts to focus attention on particular components of the stimulus array. Recall that Livermore and Laing (1996) found that olfactory experts performed better than trained novices on identifying the elements in two- and three-component mixtures. This could reflect an acquired attentional skill or an innate advantage—one cannot tell which.

Experts may come to have (or had prior to becoming wine tasters) a better ability to name odours. Naming odours confers a number of advantages; it improves odour discrimination (Rabin 1988), it improves odour-recognition memory (Lyman and McDaniel 1986), and it allows the perceiver to more readily categorize an odour (or wine) based on detected and named character-istics. Whilst Bende and Nordin (1997) found that experts were better than novices at odour-naming this difference was not large, and there was some indication that it occurred for wine-related odours (i.e. suggesting an experi-ential effect). However, Parr *et al.* (2002) found no evidence of better naming ability for wine-related odours between experts and regular wine drinkers (note that these individuals were students of wine and food and so this may be a very conservative comparison).

Experts may also have a better memory for chemosensory events, such that they could more readily encode or retrieve this type of information. This has been explored indirectly by determining if they demonstrate better recognition memory for odours. Parr *et al.* (2002) found that for wine-related odours they demonstrated significantly better recognition memory than did novice partici-pants (note the caveat above about the use of the term novice in their study). In a further experiment they used a much larger set of odours, which were rated for wine-relatedness. Again, using a recognition-memory procedure they observed significantly better odour-memory performance in experts. Needless to say, whilst experts may start out with better recognition memory, the absence of non-wine-related odours here makes it difficult to tell whether any *general* advantage might exist in the experts, because if the benefit was restricted to just wine-related odours then this would point to an effect of experience.

It was noted above that one concern with addressing the question as to whether wine experts have greater 'native' ability was in defining what this ability might be. A second and more pressing concern, and one alluded to above, is that for any comparison of experts and novices that does reveal a dif-ference, it is never possible to tell whether that difference was due to experi-ence or to innate (native) ability. Consequently, the only way to address the native-ability question with any hope of resolving it is either to take a group of novices who have normal perceptual abilities and try to turn them into 'experts' or to follow a large group of people and see whether excellent initial olfactory abilities predict who becomes a wine taster. Whilst the latter is unlikely to ever happen, the former has been tentatively explored in several studies.

Walk (1966) used a set of undergraduate students who were self-selected and who presumably did not differ markedly in chemosensory ability from the remainder of their cohort. These participants then received 10 two-alternative forced-choice (2AFC) trials where two wines were presented and the partici-pant had to say whether they were the same or different. Five dry white wines of different grape variety were employed as the stimuli. Following this baseline assessment, participants were randomly assigned to three groups. All received a further 20 2AFC trials. One group were given feedback as well as being asked to learn an arbitrary label for each wine. A second group just received feedback and the third group just exposure to the wines. All groups then received a further 10 2AFC trials, performance on which was compared to the first set of ten trials to gauge whether any improvement had occurred. Overall, there was an improvement in performance which did not differ between groups, with percentage of correct responses increasing from 62 to 71% and, most markedly, a reduction in errors on same–same trials from 55 to 31%. A similar set of findings was also reported by Owen and Machamer (1979) who used a design much like the one above. At a minimum, these findings suggest that discriminative performance can be improved, apparently with mere exposure. If this possibility is accepted, then one would predict two things. First, that regular wine drinkers might be broadly as good as wine experts at discriminating wines—i.e. both groups have acquired perceptual expertise through exposure, in the same manner as the participants in Walk's (1966) study. Second, that regular wine drinkers and experts would be better at discriminating wines than novices. Note that if the two studies that have addressed these questions confirm that perceptual expertise *can* be equivalent between experts and regular wine drinkers, this would strongly imply that differences in native ability probably do not underpin perceptual wine expertise.

Solomon (1990, Experiment 3) had four novice and four expert wine tasters discriminate between four similar Bordeaux white wines using a triangle-test procedure (three stimuli; two the same and one different—which is the odd one out?). Novice participants performed at chance on this study whilst the experts performed significantly better than chance and significantly better than the novices. This suggests that wine experts are clearly better than novices at discriminating between wines, but what about regular wine drinkers? Melcher and Schooler (1996) selected three groups of participants: novices, regular wine drinkers, and experts. All three groups sampled a target wine. Half of all the participants were then asked to write a description of the wine, whilst the other half completed a crossword puzzle. All of the participants were then offered four wines, one of which was the target. The participants' task was to rate whether or not each of these four wines had or had not occurred earlier (i.e. whether it was the target). Regular wine drinkers and experts who received the crossword puzzle between sampling the target and the discrimination test were not significantly different from each other, but both groups recognized the target significantly better than the novice group. This suggests that perceptual expertise is similar between regular wine drinkers and experts, and is not apparent in novices—the latter finding confirming Solomon's (1990) observation. A further feature of this important study is the effect that writing a description of the wine had on the different groups. For experts, writing a description of the wine had no effect on their discriminative performance, but for the regular wine drinkers this reduced their performance to chance level. Novices benefited slightly from writing a description, but not significantly so (note that these group effects dissipated on a second discrimination trial, a common feature of 'verbal overshadowing'). The effect of writing the description suggests that experts can switch back and forth between verbal descriptions and perceptual experience with little cost, unlike regular wine drinkers. This points to the importance of conceptual knowledge in wine expertise, particularly in experts' ability to match perceptual experience to verbal description and vice versa.

Several studies have explored the ability of experts and novices to match a verbal description of a wine to a real wine. Lawless (1984) compared novice and experts on this task, having both groups sample six wines and prepare verbal descriptions of them. Based upon their own descriptions, experts could match 48% of them to the correct wine whilst novices could only match 28%. This small expert benefit was maintained when matching a description from another participant within their respective group and from matching composite descriptions. Lawless (1984) also found that, for the experts, there was a significant relationship between perceptual discrimination and performance on the matching task. The hardest wines to discriminate were also the hardest to match.

A similar expert benefit was observed by Solomon (1990, Experiment 1). Here, three experts and three novices generated the descriptions. Then novice and expert participants were presented with a series of wines. For each wine they were provided with two descriptions, one of which was correct, their task being to select the correct description. Experts only outperformed novices when the description came from another expert (69% correct), suggesting the importance of identifying the discriminating features of a wine in the description and of then being able to identify these in the wine. Solomon (1990) attempted to assist novice participants with this process in a second experiment by providing them with a checklist of 167 descriptors, but this did not improve their performance. However, as Hughson and Boakes (2002) note, there may have been too many descriptors, and so they could not act to focus the novices' attention to salient aspects of the stimulus. Hughson and Boakes (2002) tested this by providing novices with one of two lists (focussed or a long-list) or no list at all. Novices who were provided the focussed list were significantly better at matching their description to each wine than participants in the other two groups, who did not significantly differ.

Differences in matching ability may become particularly pronounced when the wines to be used are all drawn from the same grape variety. In a further experiment, Hughson and Boakes (2002) found that the same list procedure did not confer any advantage when used on such a sample of wines with naive participants. With experts, the picture is rather different. Gawel (1997) compared regular wine drinkers (who were students of oenology) with established experts, using three similar Chardonnay wines. Half of each group wrote descriptions of the three wines, whilst the other half matched them. On this task, the experts were significantly better (64% correct) than the regular wine drinkers (54% correct), with both performing better than chance. Performance in the regular wine drinkers was enhanced significantly when they were given consensus descriptions provided by a further group of expert wine tasters. Use of these descriptions resulted in 77% correct matching. One difference that was readily apparent in the expert descriptions was the presence of more concrete descriptive terms. Whilst these findings show that experts do consistently perform better than non-experts it is worth pointing out that in none of the cases here did performance approach ceiling. Indeed, as Sauvageot, Urdapilleta, and Peyron (2006) note, there is considerable variation both *within* and *between* experts on their descriptions of the same wine.

As the data above suggest, experts are somewhat better than novices and regular wine drinkers at matching verbal descriptions of wines to real wines. This advantage may derive from their perceptual expertise (i.e. experience with wine) and from two further sources. First, more consistent and appropriate use of terminology, such that only parts that can in fact be detected are used (i.e. concrete terms like astringency), combined with a knowledge of the intensitive range of each term (i.e. an expert has some sense of where on a scale a wine may fall for each part). As noted above, Gawel (1997) reported that experts tended to use more concrete terms than novices, and this has been observed in other studies as well. Solomon (1997, Experiment 1) asked naive participants, regular wine drinkers, and experts to describe wines using the University of California-Davis Wine Wheel. This wheel has three levels of descriptors, broad (e.g. fruity, chemical, etc.), specific (e.g. nutty, earthy, etc.), and concrete (e.g. soy sauce, diesel,etc.). Experts primarily chose concrete descriptors (see Table 4.5), in comparison to regular wine drinkers and novices.

In a further experiment, Solomon (1990, Experiment 4) had novices and experts rank order several wines on a variety of olfactory and flavour attributes. Expert rankings agreed at above chance level on sweetness, astringency, and balance, whilst only sweetness ratings were concordant in novices. These findings, whilst pointing (again) to perhaps less than desirable concordance between experts, suggest that they agree more on both, what a term means and how a wine scales on this term, than naive participants do.

Table 4.5 Mean distribution (percent) of descriptors chosen from the wine wheel by expert wine tasters, regular wine drinkers, and novices (adapted from Solomon 1997)

Descriptor class	Experts	Regular wine drinkers	Naive participants
Broad	17%	31%	25%
Specific	20%	24%	38%
Concrete	64%	46%	28%

A second reason that experts may be better at matching descriptions to wines may come from their knowledge of the perceptual attributes (i.e. parts) that tend to cluster together for each grape variety. In an elegant set of experiments, Hughson and Boakes (2002) explored whether expert wine tasters evidence knowledge of particular clusters of perceptual attributes. Novice and expert wine tasters were exposed to either varietal wine attributes or sets of attributes that were shuffled (i.e. that were not representative of particular varieties but contained parts of two or more). All participants were then given a surprise recall test following these exposures. Whilst experts were superior to novices at recalling the content of varietal descriptions, they were worse than novices at recalling the shuffled descriptions. This difference appears to result from the experts' prior semantic knowledge, as novices were as good as experts when asked to intentionally learn descriptions, but not when learning was incidental. This would suggest that one way in which experts differ from novices is that they can organize perceptual information about wine into categories (by grape varieties). Not only could this knowledge then facilitate a search for parts of the wine that might predict its varietal identity, it would also assist the expert in detecting wines that departed from the expected varietal pattern.

Experts' ability to categorize wines has been studied in two separate experiments. Solomon (1997, Experiment 2) had experts, regular wine drinkers, and novices sort 10 white wines into four groups. Expert assignment to group was reportedly based upon grape variety and region, but not the classifications resulting from the novice and regular wine-drinker groups. Experts' classifications also differed significantly from novices. Solomon (1997) then examined whether perceptual features that were identified in his first experiment (i.e. those summarized in Table 4.5) were more consistent within each groups clustering, than they were between each groups clustering—i.e. did participants tend to cluster the wines in a way that reflected the perceptual features identified earlier? This was the case for novices, regular wine drinkers, and experts. However, experts demonstrated a much tighter match between the features they reported and the groups of wines they formed.

A more recent categorization study by Ballester, Patris, Symoneaux, and Valentin (2008) compared experts and regular wine drinkers. The stimuli here were 10 Chardonnays and 10 Melon de Bourgogne white wines. The participants' first task was to sort the wines into groups based upon their similarity. For this task, both experts and regular wine drinkers produced very similar clusters. This would suggest that similar perceptual information is available to both of these groups of drinkers. However, in the second phase of the study, participants were asked to make typicality judgements for each wine (e.g. how typical a chardonnay is this wine?). Here, experts could readily sort the wines on this typicality dimension and showed good agreement between themselves. However, regular wine drinkers, lacking the conceptual knowledge of wine varieties and their features, revealed no consistent pattern of ratings. This study nicely illustrates—as with the Melcher and Schoolers' (1996) study—the interplay between perceptual knowledge, evident in both groups, and conceptual knowledge, evident in only the expert group, and how experts can use this conceptual knowledge to categorize wine.

In conclusion, wine experts have both perceptual and conceptual knowledge, which is thoroughly intertwined. Their perceptual abilities do not appear to exceed those of regular wine drinkers, but their conceptual abilities allow the perceptual knowledge to be used more efficiently. The stimulus can be searched for particular sets of parts (these may be elements or similarities), and these parts can be reported more accurately. Sets of wines can be categorized and sorted using this conceptual knowledge. Two general conclusions to emerge out of this literature need special emphasis. First, compared with expertise in other domains, where the difference in performance can be quite marked between experts and naive participants, the difference in performance for wines is not especially large (contrast with Biederman and Shiffrar (1987) Myles-Worsley *et al.* (1988)). Second, experts do not appear to have any major advantage in their perceptual expertise other than what is accrued via exposure to wines—i.e. they do not posses preternatural powers of detection or discrimination. What they can sense, we can sense too, if we just consume enough wine.

Beer

The same general statements about wine expertise would also appear to apply to beer, namely that two forms of knowledge predominate—perceptual and conceptual. However, conceptual knowledge here is likely to be more limited because whilst grape varieties are an obvious basis upon which to categorize wines (and indeed are clearly indicated on the label of most wines), beer varieties are less obvious and are not such a conspicuous selling point as they are for wine. In so far as clear distinctions go for beer, two principal types exist—lagers and ales (and possibly lambic too, but this a very rare type of beer nowadays). This distinction arises from the temperature and nature of the fermentation process (and of course the yeasts). Within lagers and ales, there exist several types, notably the Saaz group (e.g. Carlsberg) and the Frohberg group (e.g. Heineken) for lagers. In addition to the more limited typology of beers, there is also the issue of availability and thus exposure to different types. Whilst regular wine drinkers are offered a very broad choice of wines, both within and between varieties, regular beer drinkers are not. Consequently, one might expect that perceptual expertise with beer might also be more limited.

Notwithstanding these differences between wine and beer, somewhat similar findings emerge. First, exposure to beers in true novices, i.e. participants who have almost no experience with beer and who also are initially poor at discriminating between beers, is improved by simple exposure (Peron and Allen 1988). Interestingly, this study found that other forms of training, notably that involving verbal labels for particular qualities that are used to evaluate beer, were not useful. This might suggest that *some* perceptual experience may need to precede conceptual training.

An interesting and important series of studies have been reported by Chollet and colleagues examining the effects of a beer-training program (Chollet and Valentin 2001, Chollet *et al.* 2005, Valentin *et al.* 2007). In their first report, participants had received 11 h of beer training, which included detecting specific odours in beer (these had been deliberately added as adulterants) as well as exposing participants to different beer types (Chollet and Valentin 2001). These participants were then compared to a group of regular beer drinkers. After this short period of training, relatively few differences emerged between the groups. Both groups sorted a set of beers into broadly the same clusters, although some differences emerged on a repeat sorting. Both groups were also equally good on a matching task where they had to describe a beer to another participant within their group and that person then had to select the beer. In fact, both groups used quite similar terminology, but specific concrete terms were the most successful in communicating beer differences in both groups. Note here the similarity to wine tasting, where Solomon (1997) made a convergent observation.

In a further report (presumably on the same group) after 2 years of training, Chollet *et al.* (2005) compared these now 'experts' to a further group of regular beer drinkers. This time, group differences were more apparent. On a discrimination task, the experts were significantly better than the regular beer drinkers on beers the experts had been trained with, and with beers that had been adulterated with the same adulterants used in training. However, for novel, adulterated beers, there was no discriminative advantage in experts, suggesting that their expertise was delimited only to beers they had drunk before. A matching task was also included, in which both the experts and the regular beer drinkers had to produce descriptions of the beers. Then, participants were given a beer, along with two descriptions from within their group, and they had to identify which description matched the target beer. This process was then repeated, but now with the experts receiving the regular beer drinkers' descriptions and vice versa. Overall, matching performance did not differ between groups, but matching was improved in all participants when using the experts' descriptions.

In their most recent report (Valentin *et al.* 2007), the expert beer drinkers had now sampled over 200 different commercial beers, in addition to 2 years of training (44 h in total) and the development of a consensual vocabulary to describe beer. These experts were again compared to regular beer drinkers on a range of tasks. First, participants were asked to evaluate, using eight descriptors, the adulterated beers that had been used in the experts training. The experts were at ceiling on this task and were able to perfectly identify the adulterant in each beer. Second, participants' recognition memory for trained and untrained beers and beer-related odours was tested (trained here, of course, refers to the expert group). For beers, experts were only significantly better for the familiar beers and much of this benefit derived from rejecting familiar distracter beers. However, for beer-related odours, experts were superior for both trained and untrained odours, relative to the regular beer drinkers. Finally, on a discrimination task using trained and untrained beers, there was a marginally significant benefit ($p = 0.08$) to the experts, and both groups were significantly above chance.

To the extent that Chollet and colleagues experts truly are beer experts (in comparison, say, to someone who has completed the German Rheinheitsgebot program) then these individuals demonstrate abilities not dissimilar to wine experts. However, their abilities in comparison to regular beer drinkers are far less marked than for wine experts and regular wine drinkers, perhaps for the reasons outlined in the introduction to this section—less available varieties and more limited scope for conceptual knowledge.

Trained panels

In the food industry, trained panels of participants are used in product development and in quality-control testing, with preference or liking judgements typically made by consumers. For trained panels, their experience may be delimited to one type of food or it may cover multiple food domains. Training, especially for product development, may rely upon one of a number of approaches that have appeared over the last 50 years (e.g. flavour-profile method (Caul 1957), quantitative descriptive analysis (Stone and Sidel 1993), the spectrum^{tm} method (Meilgaard *et al.* 1991), and generic descriptive analysis (Lawless and Heymann 1999). Various specialist-training regimes also exist, such as the American Dairy Science Association scorecard, with its focus on product defects (Bodyfelt *et al.* 1988).

All of these training methods have more commonalities than differences. Most involve: (1) screening out those with poor taste or olfactory function; (2) getting participants to associate particular parts of a flavour with particular verbal labels; and (3) the verbal labels are usually defined in writing and by reference to physical exemplars, which may also be used to indicate the perceptual range for that variable. The group of experts—the panel—reach consensus about the attributes (i.e. parts) that a new product or series of products possess, and then rate the attributes they have identified for each of the products. The proposed end result of training should be a valid and reliable impression of the flavour parts of the product and how (or if) it differs from other products. Participants who have undergone the sort of training described here will be referred to as experts. As with wine and beer experts, it is worth noting again the shared similarity of what is meant by expertise here; perceptual (product-specific experience), conceptual (verbal or written acquired knowledge about the products and how they may vary, and of the chemical senses, etc.), and, crucially, the forming of associations between the conceptual and perceptual domains.

Three types of issue have been addressed in the literature on trained panels. The first is whether they possess any general chemosensory skills that are absent in naive participants, and there is relatively little data on this. The second is whether training achieves its goal relative to naive participants, i.e. do trained panels generate more reliable and valid descriptions of food products and demonstrate enhanced discriminative ability too? This is a very important question because, as Moskowitz (1996) notes again, it is something of an article of faith in the food industry that trained panels *do perform better* than naive participants. Consequently, there has been more work on this question. The third concerns the amount or type of training need to achieve 'expert' or 'trained' status. This is clearly an important applied problem, as shorter training is likely to lower costs. It is useful to consider this literature here as it may provide insights into the process (es) that underpin any improvement in performance.

The first question then is whether experts have any obvious chemosensory advantage over naive participants. Not surprisingly this is a hard question to ask, because at least for trained panels it is, as noted above, routine to screen out potential trainee's who have any olfactory/taste deficit. However, not all experts within this broad area have been trained with the sort of methods described in the introduction to this section. Hirsch (1990) examined chemosensory abilities of a group of culinary experts (chefs) and found remarkably few differences on standardized tests of olfactory and taste sensitivity, recognition, and identification.

Perhaps one could conclude from this that food-related experts may not self-select on the basis of native differences in basic chemosensory abilities. This would also seem to hold for expert wine tasters, too, as described above. A more interesting study (for our purposes) was reported by Lesschaeve and Issanchou (1996) who compared a group of Camembert cheese experts with a group of naive participants. They employed an olfactory recognition paradigm using food-related and other odours. There was no difference in recognition-memory performance between groups, although experts tended to use olfactory labels (i.e. names) more consistently than naive participants. There are not enough data to draw any firm conclusions, but it would seem that experts (as with wine) do not have any obvious chemosensory edge over naive participants.

Several studies have tried to detect differences in performance between experts and naive participants. Of these, a few demonstrate definite benefits; most suggest some very limited benefit and a few no benefit at all. Starting with those that find a definite benefit of training, Ishii et al. (2007) compared regular ice cream consumers with a trained panel. The trained panel had received between 4 and 16 h of training—the training here being exposure to pairs of similar and different ice creams. Over several experiments, they found that differences noticed by the trained panel correlated significantly with differences noticed by the regular ice cream consumers ($r = 0.93$); however, the trained panel were consistently able to detect differences that were not detected by the regular ice cream consumers (see Figure 4.2 below). The trained participants may have attended to features that better differentiated ice creams, by virtue of their training which required them to search for such differences.

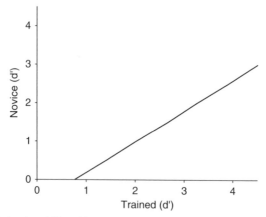

Fig. 4.2 Discriminative ability of ice cream consumers (novices) and trained participants for various pairs of ice creams (adapted from data in Ishii, Kawaguchi, O'Mahony, and Rousseau 2007).

A further successful study was reported by Bitnes *et al.* (2007). They obtained two groups of participants, experts within particular perceptual domains (namely: juice, chocolate, sausages, and beer; hereafter, specialized experts) and experts who had worked on a large range of products but who were not specialists in one particular domain (generalized experts). The specialized experts made a range of taste and odour ratings for a set of foods within their own domain of expertise and for another domain outside of their area of expertise. The generalized experts used the same rating scales as the specialized experts to evaluate each respective set of foods. All participants received brief training with the rating scales used for each class of food product, namely verbal descriptions for each target rating. Performance in this study was assessed by the ability of participants to differentiate the products based upon their ratings, this being assumed to reflect the degree to which the participants could discriminate between products.

The specialized experts were best on their particular foods, demonstrating significant differences for 96% of the ratings, excluding the sausage experts who were notably poor at this task (11%). However, when the specialized experts evaluated products they were not familiar with, they were considerably less discriminating (44%). The generalized experts were pretty good at discriminating between products in all of the domains (83%). Notably, and as with the Ishii *et al.* (2007) study, greater discriminative abilities appear to go hand-in-hand with experience with the product—excluding the sausage experts for reasons that are not clear. However, it is equally plausible that these differences reflect variability in the use of the scaled attributes. Specialized experts evaluating outside of their domain of expertise would have had arguably the least idea of what each attribute meant perceptually (even if it had been verbally described) and would also not have known the range of sensation that might be expected for that attribute. So whilst this study suggests that specialized experts outperform generalized experts in their special domain, it does not tell us definitively how this difference arises.

A larger number of studies find some, but rather limited, benefits from training on performance. Roberts and Vickers (1994) compared three groups: (1) A set of dairy judges who had received the American Dairy Science Association training; (2) A trained panel who had received exposure to various cheeses and who had developed and defined a set of attributes to assess them on; and (3) A group of naive participants. Five cheddar cheeses formed the stimulus set, and all five were readily discriminated by each of the three experimental groups. However, naive participants' ratings tended to be higher and showed less within-group agreement than trained participants—an observation also made in two other such comparative studies using cheese and water, respectively (Gonzalez *et al.* 2001,

Morran and Marchesan 2004). These effects may arise because of the naive participants' unfamiliarity with the attributes to be rated and by their lack of experience with the actual range of each attribute.

Moskowitz (1996) compared an expert panel with naive participants, getting them to rate 24 attributes (drawn from appearance, flavour, taste, and texture categories) for 37 sauces and gravies. In general, experts and naive participants were very similar in performance. The standard deviations for each attribute did not differ between groups and the attributes that produced higher variability for the experts also yielded higher variability for novices ($r = 0.55$). Individual correlations (by attribute) between experts and novices ranged from 0.37 to 0.95, with a median $r = 0.86$. The only tangible difference to emerge was the factor structure of the ratings, which revealed a clearer pattern for the experts than for naive participants. Again, this might be accounted for by the experts' better understanding of the definition of each attribute.

Hersleth *et al.* (2005) compared naive participants with an expert, trained panel in assessing seven different forms of bread. Novices were provided with triads of the breads, and they had to pick out the different one and explain why it was different. From these comparisons, a set of attributes was determined for each novice and these were then used to evaluate the seven breads. The experts used a consensus defined set of 38 attributes to rate the same set of stimuli with. The underlying structure of the data was then examined for experts and for naive participants and the relationship between these structures was determined by regression. There was very good agreement between the two groups, the only difference to emerge was that novices tended to focus on perceptual attributes, whilst experts focussed on their *cause* (e.g. differences in texture versus differences in flour type).

Finally, at least one study has found no difference in discriminative ability where one might be expected. Frandsen *et al.* (2007) compared, indirectly, regular milk consumers against an expert, sensory evaluation panel's ability to detect subtle differences in milk flavour produced by differences in feed type and storage. The experts evaluated the milks using attribute ratings and these revealed differences between the milks on the basis of feed type and storage. The regular milk drinkers undertook two different tasks, a same/different discrimination test and an authenticity test (is this 'Danish' milk or 'foreign' milk?). On the authenticity test, differences between the milks, in terms of feed and storage, were readily apparent unlike for the same/different test. Whilst this paper was primarily focussed on the test differences for the regular milk drinkers, the study illustrates that, with an appropriate test of perceptual discrimination, perceptual experts (i.e. regular milk drinkers) and trained experts (i.e. the panel) may perform at a similar level. This finding agrees with the wine and beer literature (e.g. see Melcher and Schooler 1996).

A question of considerable practical interest is the degree of training needed to benefit performance. At least four studies have examined this. Chambers and Smith (1993) compared a group of experts with between 5 and 7 years of panel experience with a group who had just received 150 h of training. Both groups were tested on a food group that experts had had some experience with (breakfast cereals) and on a food group that neither had any experience with (jams). All groups worked together to generate attributes on which to rate the products. There were few differences between groups and both were readily able to differentiate the products.

Whilst Chambers and Smith's (1993) study used participants with 150 h of training, a more extensive study by Wolters and Allchurch (1994) examined the effects of 15, 30, and 60 h of training as well as comparing these groups to a well-experienced panel. Training here, for the 30- and 60-h groups included all of the facets described above—generating and defining descriptions and practicing these on the foods (orange juices) that were subsequently to be evaluated. The 15-h group received a truncated form of this training. On test, using a set of orange juices, the proportion of attributes that differentiated the orange juice set was identical between groups, and in addition, more training did not lead to greater reliability as one might have expected. In fact, the most striking finding was the similarity between all of the groups, suggesting that training here was redundant (i.e. the attributes would have been readily understood by naive participants) and that all participants already had considerable perceptual experience with the food stimuli used in the study.

Not all such studies have come up empty handed. Chambers et al. (2004) selected seven participants for extensive training. They evaluated, using the same set of attributes, a range of pasta sauces, early, in the middle, and at the end of their training. Training involved exploring the pasta sauces, defining specific reference samples for attributes used to evaluate the sauces, and building consensus within the group. Training reduced attribute variability and increased each attribute's independence. However, all of the products could be readily discriminated initially, and the texture attributes were found to be the most differentiating early on. A similar set of findings emerged from a study by Labbe et al. (2004). Here, participants profiled eight samples of coffee on 20 attributes. They then underwent 21 h of training, involving learning physical references for each attribute and learning to rank and then scale the products by each attribute. Participants were then re-tested. Reliability within the group improved and differences between the coffees were larger on many attributes following training.

The authors suggest that the latter finding may reflect perceptual change, i.e. participants became better at differentiating these stimuli with practice.

Trained panels clearly have some advantages over novice participants, when it comes to evaluating the properties of a food or drink. These advantages may take the form of enhanced perceptual differentiation, which is *suggested* by the Bitnes *et al.* (2007), Ishii *et al.* (2007), and Labbe *et al.* (2004) data, where more 'experience' with the product may result in greater discriminative ability. However, when participants have similar perceptual experience, then differences may be minimal under appropriate test conditions (e.g. Frandsen *et al.* 2007). A further advantage that experts have over novices appears to relate to their conceptual knowledge. Experts may benefit from a better ability to describe their experience verbally (i.e. to know the definition of terms, to link them to percepts, and to know their range). This may result in findings such as better agreement within expert groups (e.g. Roberts and Vickers 1984), a clearer factor structure (e.g. Moskowitz 1996), and greater independence between ratings (Chambers *et al.* 2004). Whilst these perceptual and semantic benefits have been demonstrated, albeit inconsistently, the effects are not large and this would suggest that the limits on breaking flavour into its parts applies to all of us, experts and novices alike.

Expertise with food and drink—Conclusion

A common characteristic for wine, beer, and food experts is that they successfully combine perceptual and conceptual knowledge. This form of distinction, between conceptual (or semantic knowledge) and perceptual knowledge, is widely agreed upon in the broader psychological literature (e.g. Paivio 1986). One thread that was common to preceding parts of this chapter was the focus on elements and similarities. This thread was not extensively picked up for the expert literature above, because in using real stimuli one cannot generally control (or know) what is and what is not physically present in a food or drink. However, in the vast majority of studies included here, and especially those for food, many of the 'attributes' that participants are asked (or choose) to evaluate reflect olfactory-based similarities. In the preceding parts of this chapter, detecting elements was pretty good in naive participants and so one might tentatively suggest that some (if not most) of the expert advantage may relate to more efficient similarity detection of retronasal olfactory stimuli.

Discussion

During routine eating and drinking, flavour is a unitary experience. This appears to be a consequence of not attending to the parts, along with simultaneous experience of the parts and their common spatial location. Whilst there is not an extensive body of evidence to support this conclusion, what there is largely consistent with it. Much of the remainder of the chapter concerned whether flavour can also be perceived as a set of parts. This question was addressed serially, starting with the single senses, then mixtures, and finally with complex real-world stimuli—wines, beers, and foods. For taste, which consist of a type of part termed an element (i.e. where there is a correspondence between a particular taste quality and receptor activity) even naive participants can generally detect most taste elements in homogeneous (just tastes) and heterogeneous (tastes plus one or more modality) mixtures—under ideal circumstances. For texture, which also consists primarily of elements (correspondence here between a particular quality and a physical parameter), naive participants can also readily detect these texture elements in heterogeneous mixtures. Training, for both taste and texture, may result in some limited gains, but these are likely to relate to more reliable verbal labelling of elements (i.e. the name assigned to an element), along with a greater awareness of the range with which that quality can vary. Whether this awareness of range results in enhanced perceptual sensitivity for individual textural dimensions, or is a consequence of the way trained participants use their scales, is not currently known. Thus for the taste and texture components of a flavour, participants, both naive and trained, can generally appreciate most, if not all, available parts or elements as is the case here. This conclusion might reasonably be extended to other perceptual experiences such as irritation and temperature, which also fall under the somatosensory domain. These too would appear to have elemental status (stimulus-receptor-quality mapping) and, at least if the studies described in Chapter 2 are anything to go by, naive participants do not appear to have much trouble in reporting either the temperature of food nor the presence of irritation.

For odour, the situation is more complex. There is a limited capacity to identify orthonasal odour elements in mixtures. Below this apparent physiological ceiling, training does appear to enhance the ability to discriminate elements. This type of effect is mediated by perceptual learning, in that the brain acquires a memory of the glomerular input pattern for the odour, which results in a more distinctive percept when the odour is smelled again either alone or against a background odour (Wilson and Stevenson 2006). However, for retronasal odours, identification of a particular element when other odours, tastes, or textures are present is much harder, although experts may be somewhat better at this than novices, at least for odours they are familiar with (i.e. an analogous situation to orthonasal olfaction). Being directed to attend to the olfactory element in a flavour does not appear to help naive participants detect that element and the evidence suggests that it can impair performance for reasons that have yet to be established, but that may relate to spatial location of attention (i.e. to the mouth rather than to the nose). Thus our ability to detect odour elements in odour mixtures and to detect them in a flavour stands in marked contrast to our ability to detect taste or texture elements in mixtures.

Whilst we may have a limited capacity to detect odour elements, we appear to have an almost limitless ability to detect odour similarities, both to retronasal and to orthonasal stimuli. However, whilst odour similarities are a key part of our experience of flavour, can a similarity be considered a 'part' in the same way that an element can? If an odour paired with a sweet taste gets to smell sweet as a result of this pairing, and if it did not smell sweet before, then whilst this 'sweetness' may be a similarity (i.e. it has no physical basis in the stimulus), it most certainly is a discrete and readily recognizable 'part' of the experience. This would appear to hold especially when such odours are sniffed (here it is arguably the most salient part) and to a lesser extent when they are experienced as part of a flavour (e.g. odour-induced sweetness-taste enhancement).

The situation is perhaps less clear for similarities that are based upon solely olfactory referents. These too are influenced by experience. Common experience of two odour elements together in a mixture can result in them coming to share certain common similarities (Stevenson 2001). After experiencing a mixture of a smoky odour and a cherry odour, the smoky odour comes to smell more cherry-like and the cherry odour smokier, a process that resembles the broader perceptual learning process termed acquired equivalence (Honey and Hall 1989). Experience of odour elements on their own can also act to move each element apart in perceptual space (Li *et al.* 2006). In this case, two odour elements become less similar to each other—i.e. a change in a 'similarity' for each other's respective elemental quality may occur (e.g. lemon odour could become less lime-like and lime odour less lemon-like with passive exposure to each odourant). Both of these effects arguably result from learning an olfactory pattern (imprinting).

Many theories of perceptual learning involve changes in attention. It has been argued that ignoring aspects of a stimulus that are not useful for whatever decision has to be made may be an important part of improving discriminative performance (e.g. Haider and French 1996). Similarly, coming to attend more to parts that are predictive of a difference also improves performance (e.g. Nosofsky 1986). Both of these attentional effects can be seen to be operative in the process of deciding to make a particular similarity judgement—i.e. the participant chooses to compare the target odour (or olfactory component of a flavour) to a memory of a prototypical example of something (e.g. how almond-like does this smell?). In this sense, one could make almost an infinite number of such comparisons, and so here conceptual knowledge may act to limit comparisons to those that maximally differentiate stimuli whilst ignoring those that do not. Training and experience may, not surprisingly, considerably assist the 'choice' then of similarity judgements to make. The skills that are likely to aid this process are exactly those that are common to most expert training programs—exposure to exemplars, learning their names, and learning which similarities tend to co-vary with particular types of stimuli (e.g. in wine this would be grape variety). Learning these patterns of co-variation may then result in the building of particular categories, which do appear to exist as semantic structures in expert wine tasters (Hughson and Boakes 2002).

Clearly then, olfactory referent similarities can be affected by experience, i.e. by learning (perceptual knowledge) and by optimal selection (conceptual knowledge) of the similarity comparisons to be made for a particular stimulus. That these similarities can be used productively, especially by experts, would suggest that they too qualify as parts. However, they are only available if one has the capacity to make the comparison—i.e. the semantic (conceptual) knowledge to decide upon making that particular similarity judgement, the perceptual knowledge of the thing to which the comparison is being made and the link between this perceptual and semantic knowledge. Olfactory referent similarities are then likely to represent the most plastic 'parts' of a flavour, because many similarities are meaningless without the perceptual or semantic knowledge required to make them.

Conclusion

Flavour then, composed of tactile, olfactory, and gustatory modalities, can be perceived as a set of parts. The process of perceiving parts can be almost complete for texture even in complex stimuli. For tastes, this can also be the case under ideal circumstances, but as differences in stimulus intensity grow larger, detection of taste elements will become progressively more difficult. The detection of odour elements in flavour is difficult, even under ideal circumstances, as it is clearly affected by the presence of other odour elements, textures, and tastes. However, for odour, it may be that the detection of individual elements is far less important than the perception of similarities. Many odour similarities are 'potentially' detectable but the ability to realize them depends extensively upon learning and attention. For learning, it may involve the acquisition of a 'similarity' (e.g. sweetness) or the acquisition of a point of comparison to establish the similarity (e.g. judging whether something smells like lychee is not much use if you have not experienced lychee or if you do not know its name).

For attention, it may involve deciding which similarity judgement to make and which to ignore, and this decision process may be deliberate (endogenous attention) or automatic and can be guided by conceptual knowledge. Whilst the questions addressed in this chapter are of interest to psychologists and of immense practical significance to the food industry, the vast majority of people tend to have only one issue at the forefront of their mind when considering what to eat—hedonics. This forms the focus of the next chapter.

Chapter 5

Flavour hedonics

Introduction

This chapter concerns flavour hedonics. The terms hedonic, affect, acceptability, and palatability are used interchangeably here to refer to the subjective experience of liking and disliking (pleasant and unpleasant). For the flavour studies reviewed in this chapter, hedonic response is usually measured by self-report (and less frequently via behavioural measures: ingestion, facial expression, etc.). An important definitional issue here concerns the difference between liking, needing, and wanting (Berridge 1996). Wanting, in the present context, refers to the desire to consume a particular food (i.e. it has both direction *and* force). This may have dissociable explicit (i.e. consciously reportable expectancies and desires) and implicit components. Liking, on the other hand, is generally the direct reaction to the stimulus (e.g. chocolate) or to cues that have become associated with it (e.g. food packaging or the food's smell). This too, it has been argued, can have both implicit and explicit components. Finally, needing here refers to a state of energy deprivation, which loosely correlates with subjective reports of hunger (i.e. desire for food in general). Unfortunately, it has been suggested that self-report, hedonic evaluations may often conflate liking and wanting (e.g. Finlayson *et al.* 2007, Berridge 2004). As noted above, self-report liking has been commonly used as the dependent variable in many flavour studies and so it is, historically at least, hard to know the independent contribution of wanting and liking in many of the studies reported here. However, quite a few studies do examine the interaction between liking and needing.

That flavour has a hedonic dimension is a widely held assumption, but is there evidence to support this? One line of evidence is that flavour liking is a significant predictor of what people choose to eat (Glanz *et al.* 1998, Randall and Sanjur 1981, Tuorila 1990), how much they choose to eat (Hetherington 1996, Sorensen *et al.* 2003), and what they drink (Lanier *et al.* 2005). Another is that hedonic ratings are widely used by the food industry in assessing consumer acceptability of new food products (Cardello *et al.* 2000). As Lawless and Heymann (1998) note '... a product that does not score well in a consumer acceptance test will probably fail despite great marketing' (p.431, *op. cit.*).

If flavour then is affect-laden, one might also expect that its component modalities are as well, and this is indeed the case for odour (Schiffman *et al.* 1977), taste (Steiner *et al.* 2001), texture (Munoz and Civille 1987), temperature (Zellner *et al.* 1988), and chemaesthesis (Rozin 1990). Finally, all of the chemical senses access brain areas that are known to be involved in hedonic processing, including cortical (e.g. orbitofrontal cortex), subcortical (e.g. amygdala), and brainstem structures (Kringelbach *et al.* 2003, Berthoud and Morrison 2008). Together, this would suggest that flavour does have a significant affective dimension.

Hedonic reactions to flavour are functionally important for several reasons. First, they allow us to make decisions about what to eat *prior* to placing food in the mouth. Vision and orthonasal olfaction are key players in this process, as described in the preceding chapters. The visual system primarily accesses semantic knowledge about food (crucially via its identity, i.e. 'that is an orange'). This semantic knowledge will often be important in dictating the affective reaction to that food. The olfactory system works in a complimentary manner by providing information about the food's flavour primarily via perceptual channels, as well as generating an affective reaction. Both channels rely almost exclusively upon learning and memory to generate these types of responses—perceptual, hedonic, and semantic. This is illustrated more generally by the failure of several twin studies (i.e. monozygotic vs. dizygotic) to identify a significant genetic component in food preferences (e.g. Rozin and Millman 1987), excepting certain relationships connected to the taste system (i.e. bitter sensitivity, Krondl *et al.* (1983)) and some small effects of personality variables (e.g. Faust 1974, Yeo *et al.* 1997). In fact, the most innate component of the flavour system is its capacity to learn (Birch 1986).

Once food is placed in the mouth, a second hedonism-mediated function emerges. A decision to ingest needs to be made. Rejection at this stage may be crucial, especially if the food tastes 'bad' or tastes very different from the expectation formed via the eyes and/or nose. In Chapter 4, it was argued that one reason why tastes may be readily apparent in foods (and indeed why they may become associated with odours) is that they allow for rapid acceptance of foods that taste sweet or salty/savoury and rejection of foods that taste bitter or highly acidic. Once food has been accepted and swallowed, a third functional reason for hedonics comes into play. Post-ingestive processes that determine the body's state of repletion after a meal do not operate immediately, and so mechanisms need to be in place to stop ingestion *before* gut-based satiety signals start. One important way that the brain modulates intake during the course of a meal is to alter hedonic reactions to food, from positive to negative, to cease ingestion and also to promote dietary variety. Finally, pleasant feelings of repleteness or unpleasant feelings of nausea that may occur after a meal has finished may become associated with the food's flavour and will be brought to mind when that food is encountered in the future (i.e. to support function one).

What follows in this chapter is arranged by these three primary functions. On consideration, this appears the most natural way of organizing the various hedonic mechanisms that mediate decisions to ingest *prior* to placing food in the mouth (function one), decisions to ingest when food is in the mouth (function two), and decisions about what and how much to ingest (function three).

Function one—Decision to ingest *prior* to oral incorporation

The two senses that are primarily involved in the decision to eat a food prior to placing it in the mouth are orthonasal olfaction and vision. The olfactory system is likely to influence this process via two channels—the perceptual information that it can convey about the likely 'flavour' of the food (e.g. sweet or bitter, savoury, creamy, etc.) and the hedonic response. The hedonic response, especially if negative, would appear to be decisive in preventing ingestion (excepting the effects of context and under conditions of severe food deprivation—more below), and whilst positive responses may be important in initiating consumption these will be moderated by semantic information that is mainly generated via the visual system (e.g. frying bacon *may* smell pleasant to a vegetarian or someone on a diet, but both resist consuming it). If then, olfaction and vision are the principal mediums by which prior ingestive decisions are made, it would follow that neither should be particularly affect-laden at birth—i.e. past experience should be the principal guide in developing hedonic reactions to food.

For olfaction, there is plenty of evidence to suggest that affective reactions develop progressively from birth onwards—i.e. they are characterized by plasticity (see Engen (1982), Moncrieff (1966), Rozin *et al.* (2000) for a similar conclusion). Shortly after birth, newborns show little difference in facial or autonomic responses to smells that adults like (vanillin) and dislike (butyric acid; Soussignan *et al.* 1997). Similarly, Peto (1935) found that under fives did not obviously differ in their affective reaction to odours that adults find clearly different (e.g. lemon vs. faeces). Children become able, by around 3 years of age, to rank preference in a manner similar to adults (Schimdt and Beauchamp 1988). However, as Engen (1974) demonstrated, even when children can appropriately rank the stimuli, the hedonic range of younger children (4-year-olds) is much more restricted than for older children (7-year-olds). Developmental changes in liking continue as children move into their teens. Stevenson and Repacholi (2003) observed that 8-year-olds were indifferent to the smell of pungent male sweat, whilst post-pubescent children strongly disliked it.

Developmental changes are one source of evidence for plasticity. Another is cross-cultural differences in odour preferences. Several examples can be found in the literature: (1) Americans like oil of wintergreen whilst United Kingdom participants do not (Moncrieff 1966); (2) Asians enjoy the fruity/oniony-flavoured Durian and pungent fish-sauce, whilst Westerners do not (Pangborn 1975); (3) Westerners like the rotten odour of blue cheese and the vomitous odour of Parmesan (Jones 2000); (4) Tibetans like the flavour of tea mixed with rancid butter (Moore 1970); and (5) The Dassanetch of Ethiopia like odours associated with cattle and so hands are washed in cows urine, men cover their bodies in manure, and young women enhance their attractiveness by smearing clarified butter onto their bodies (Classen 1992). Similarly, several more formal studies have found that liking tends to differ markedly between cultures *particularly* for odours that are either culturally specific or for those which are not routinely encountered in one culture, but are highly familiar to another (e.g. Ayabe-Kanamura *et al.* 1998, Davis and Pangborn 1985, Schaal *et al.* 1997, Wysocki *et al.* 1991).

The developmental and cross-cultural differences in odour hedonics probably reflect broadly similar processes of familiarization (which is often associated with liking) and associative learning. A further, but rather different, example of olfactory plasticity is the effect of semantic information. Herz and von Clef (2001) found that providing appropriate, but different, names for the same odour led to quite different hedonic responses. For example, pine odour was viewed much more favourably when labelled as 'Xmas tree' than when labelled as 'toilet cleaner'. These effects did not appear to be solely driven by demand, because if e.g. pine was experienced first as 'Xmas tree', then its more positive evaluation affected the later presentation and evaluation of pine when presented as 'toilet cleaner'. The reverse effect was also observed. A more extensive investigation of this labelling effect (verbal context) was reported by Herz (2003), confirming these findings with different odours and labels.

Hedonic reactions to odours clearly exhibit plasticity so they are a *potentially* useful medium for judging whether a food should or should not be consumed (i.e. smells good—consume; smells bad—avoid). What about hedonic reactions to visual stimuli? Here, visual preferences and liking clearly exhibit some plasticity. Liking for relatively neutral objects (these can be faces, fountains, paintings, etc.) can be altered either via passive exposure (e.g. Zajonc 1968) or by association with visual objects that are already liked or disliked (e.g. Field 2006, De Houwer *et al.* 2001). Indeed, variation in liking and preference for visual objects (scenes, buildings, faces, paintings, etc.) can be explained, in part, by reference to experience with that particular target or class of target (e.g. Furnham and Walker 2001)—again suggesting significant response plasticity.

Whilst visual appraisal of food is likely to be affect-laden and a consequence of experience, what may be more crucial is the visual system's ability to immediately invest a scene or object with meaning (Revonsuo 1999). This ability, which flows from the rapid nature of visual object identification, allows us to access a wealth of semantic knowledge about foods—information that also has to be learnt. Whilst the olfactory system is capable of some form of semantic access, this appears to be considerably more restricted than that observed for visual semantic access. Thus it is possible to see the visual and olfactory systems, when appraising food, as a complimentary system: The olfactory system, arguably more affect-laden than the visual sense (e.g. Hinton and Henley 1993, Richardson and Zucco 1989) with an emotive/perceptual reaction to the potential food based upon experience (i.e. reliant upon its plasticity); and the visual sense with its more dominant and rapid access to semantic information about the potential food and the use of this information in shaping an affective reaction to it. Combined, these would provide a comprehensive set of information to make an ingestive decision—i.e. to exhibit preference and liking.

On the basis of the above, one would then want to know what mechanisms dictate the olfactory hedonic response (acquiring affect) and what mechanisms shape the visually derived semantic knowledge about food (which will thus influence preference, liking, and the decision to ingest). Perhaps not surprisingly, these mechanisms fall broadly into one of two categories. Those involving (at least initially) a more conscious cognitive dimension (e.g. acquisition of food knowledge/taxonomy, moralization, over-justification, advertising, etc.) and those, which involve less conscious and perhaps more automatic processes (e.g. associative learning, exposure, neophobia, and current physiological state). Whilst not wishing to make this argument too strongly, the former may have a more direct influence on information processed via the visual channel (with the probable exception of neophobia) and the latter on the olfactory system (with the possible exception of moralisation). Each is considered in turn.

Mechanisms likely to involve more conscious processing

Semantic knowledge about food exerts a profound influence over affective reactions to *potential* foodstuffs. In a series of pioneering studies, Fallon and Rozin (1983) developed a four-part food taxonomy that provides an initial overview of this semantic knowledge base. The first component, distastes, refers to things people expect or know to have unpleasant sensory qualities. Many of the items included in this category are things which generate bitter, sour, or irritant sensations, and these are dealt with in a later section of this chapter. The second component of their taxonomy is dangerous items, which are things that are anticipated to have harmful consequences if ingested. This category of anticipated harms also includes items that people 'believe' are harmful even if they are not. Lee (1989) noted several such examples, including pesticide residues, new food chemicals, and food additives. Food irradiation might also be added to this list (Wheelock 1990), along with MSG, food carcinogens, sugar, and non-natural or processed foods (e.g. Atkinson 1984). These perceptions of harm are very potent in shaping what people may choose to eat. When the media in the United States of America made exaggerated claims about the carcinogen risk of Alar-treated apples, consumption of apples markedly declined, costing apple growers nearly $100 million in lost revenue (Lee 1989). On the other hand, these risks can be very real, such as the transmission of prions following consumption of contaminated beef products in the United Kingdom and the 'possible' and imagined risks associated with genetically modified foods (de Liver *et al.* 2005).

The third category identified by Fallon and Rozin (1983) is that of disgust. This response to certain potential food objects may occur due to actual or believed contamination, such that an otherwise edible food e.g. touched by a cockroach would no longer be classified as 'edible'. This response may also encompass potential foods that are novel. Insects are a good example for North American, European, and non-indigenous Australian populations who do not consume these excellent sources of protein. The Bible sanctions consumption of locusts, grasshoppers, and certain beetles, and around 80% of the world's population knowingly consume insects drawn from some 12–1400 different edible species (Dufour and Sanders 2000). Pets are another set of potential foods that might be subsumed under this category. Owners of horses, guinea pigs, rabbits, and dogs may be disgusted to learn that their favoured animal may form someone else's dinner. Horseflesh is consumed in France and guinea pigs in Peru (65 million a year). Indeed, in Peru, guinea pig consumption is so culturally ingrained that the Cusco cathedral has a painting of the last supper (by Marcos Zapata) that includes roasted guinea pig. Similarly, dog flesh is (and was) widely eaten in the Asia-Pacific region (Olsen 2000). Consuming one's own pet would likely be even worse than consuming a different animal from the same species.

A variety of other things are culturally proscribed as non-foods. The most telling example is the consumption of human flesh. There is some evidence that human flesh was consumed in Neolithic times. This evidence comes from two separate sources. The first is from bone dumps, which contain the *same* bones from humans and animals. More importantly, both sets of bones have the *same* cutting and filleting marks upon them (Villa *et al.* 1986). The second source of evidence comes from genetic studies, which reveal evidence for balancing selection for a heterozygous form of a gene that offers some protection against prion-borne diseases that may follow consumption of human body parts (Mead *et al.* 2003). This may suggest that consumption of human flesh, either for caloric or religious reasons (or both), may have occurred quite routinely in our ancestral past. Clearly today, the prospect of ingesting human flesh is likely to result in a rather strong reaction—a reaction clearly demonstrated in media interest surrounding all contemporary cases of cannibalism.

Within particular groups, there can also be very well-developed sets of rules that govern acceptable and unacceptable sources of food. These can be seen in many religious food prohibitions, including Halal and Kashrut (Muslim and Jewish, respectively) systems, both of which prohibit consumption of pork, restrict the way animals can be slaughtered, and limit which sea and freshwater foods may be eaten. A rather different system is *Ahimsa* (Hindu), which cultivates the notion of non-violence and particularly the sacredness of cattle. For Hindus, in particular, who has handled a food may also be of great significance, particular if the handlers were from a lower caste. The prospect of ingesting any of these prohibited foods for those who hold these beliefs will likely engender disgust and revulsion.

The final category in Fallon and Rozin's (1983) taxonomy are items that are not appropriate to eat, but which are not necessarily dangerous, disgusting, or distasteful. Pencil erasers, grass, chalk, and wax might serve as some examples, but a recent survey-based study suggested that many objects which are clearly 'not foods' and that would be deemed to fall within the inappropriate category may come to generate disgust when people are faced with the prospect of ingesting them, even if they do not normally result in this response (Simpson *et al.* 2007).

Table 5.1 presents a summary of data adapted from Fallon and Rozin's (1983) paper. It illustrates, very clearly, that items from this fourfold set of categories can engender negative affect at the mere prospect of ingestion. Thus affect and knowledge (perceptual and semantic), acquired via experience, affords us the opportunity to eliminate many potential items well before they reach the mouth.

These reactions to *potential* foods are learnt and, at least for those detailed in Table 5.1, this appears to occur during childhood. Rozin *et al.* (1986) examined whether or not children aged between 16 and 60 months would place various objects in their mouths. For the inappropriate category (e.g. crayon, paper, play doh, leaf, sponge, etc.) 62% of these items were placed in the mouth by 16–29-month olds but only 49% by 43–60-month-old children. For the disgust category (e.g. fake dog faeces, hair, grasshopper, fish, etc.), 35% of these items were placed in the mouth by 16–29-month olds but only 12% by

Table 5.1 Self-reported dislike (−ve) for varying degrees of contact with items drawn from the four categories of food rejection (adapted from Fallon and Rozin 1983)

Category	Sight of it	Sight of someone else eating it	Smell of it	Thought of eating it
Distaste	−20	−15	−32	−41
Danger	−21	−50	−19	−76
Disgust	−58	−61	−46	−80
Inappropriate	+2	−20	0	−34

43–60-month olds. For the danger category (soap), 79% of the 16–39-month olds placed this in their mouths compared to only 12% of 43–60-month-old children. Not only do these data illustrate developmental trends in the formation of these food rejections, they also demonstrate again that many decisions about what to eat are made before the potential food ever reaches the mouth (and see Rozin *et al.* (1985) for similar data on food-related contamination sensitivity in children).

The development of semantic knowledge about food undoubtedly both continues into adulthood and continues to shape what we choose to eat and reject. One process that has been identified as particularly important in this regard has been termed moralization, i.e. the conversion of preferences into values (Rozin 1999). Moralization is a powerful force in regards to food (see Belasco 1997) and an excellent example, which has seen some preliminary investigation, is vegetarianism. Vegetarians may avoid the consumption of meat for a number of reasons, however, these can be categorized into two superordinate categories: reasons pertaining to moral perspectives and those pertaining to health perspectives. Of particular interest here is the finding that the more strongly held are the vegetarian beliefs, the more dislike is reported for the smell and appearance of meat and meat-based products (Rozin *et al.* 1997). Thus again, individuals' knowledge of the world of food, particularly relating to the processing of meat, its health implications, and the moral questions concerning the use of animals for food, lawfully influence the way in which they evaluate meat products *prior to* any attempt at ingestion.

The examples above all indicate that affective reactions may be contingent on the possession of particular knowledge, and perhaps not surprisingly this information may also affect the way in which the brain processes food-related information. Grabenhorst *et al.* (2007) presented participants with MSG and a vegetable flavour under conditions in which the description accompanying the food was systematically manipulated (i.e. 'Rich delicious flavour' vs. 'Boiled vegetable water'). Not surprisingly, the verbal label significantly influenced the hedonic rating that participants gave to each stimulus. However, this self-report evaluation was also accompanied by significant differences in brain activity, in that differential activation of the orbitofrontal cortex was related to the change in hedonic response. Of course, this study involved actual ingestion, but the point here is that a mere change in verbal label for the same stimulus resulted in significantly different activity in brain areas that are suspected of being involved in hedonic processing and hedonism-related decision making. It would not then be too much of a stretch to suggest that similar changes may occur when we contemplate ingesting things under conditions in which only our knowledge about them differs.

Semantic knowledge about food can be acquired in several ways—from our parents (see above), from the media, from books and journals, and of course from advertising. There can be little doubt that advertising affects food choices, preferences, and thus liking. A large number of studies have focussed in particular on the effects of food advertising on children. Early studies, such as those of Galst and White (1976) and Goldberg *et al.* (1978), demonstrated quite convincingly that viewing TV food adverts: (1) correlated with children's attempts to persuade their parents to buy these same food products and (2) that even short-term exposure to a particular class of food advert could significantly alter food preferences. These types of findings have continued to receive support in the literature. For example, Chernin (2008) reported that 5–11-year-old children preferred foods that had been advertised, and that food adverts *cause* children to pester their parents into buying what are usually less healthy food products (McDermott *et al.* 2006). It is very likely that food adverts influence adults, indirectly of course through their children, and directly via effects on the adults themselves. This area of 'food knowledge' is one that is currently attracting considerable attention because most of the foods, at least in the US, UK, and Australia, that are heavily advertised on TV (and in other media too) are of poor nutritional quality (Hill and Radimer 1996, Powell *et al.* 2007).

Not surprisingly perhaps, in the light of the persuasive power of TV adverts, parents too may attempt to sway their children's choice of food to encourage consumption of fruits and vegetables. The effect of verbal persuasion and, more importantly, making some reward contingent on consumption has attracted research attention because it appears to be an example of the over-justification effect (Lepper *et al.* 1973). The over-justification effect refers to the cognitive evaluation that may occur after a behaviour is rewarded, e.g. 'If I've got to be offered a reward to eat carrots, then carrots must be horrible'. The reverse effect may also occur. Under conditions where people may search for reasons as to why they took a particular course of action, this may lead to a positive change in preference. One example of this has been described by Peryam (1963). Army recruits on a survival course were offered various incentives for eating a grasshopper, or no incentive at all. Those who did not receive an incentive were most positive about their insect-eating experience.

There is certainly evidence that over-justification effects can occur with foods—at least in children. Birch et al. (1982) gave preschoolers juice with consumption contingent upon access to preferred activities. Preference for this juice fell, suggesting an over-justification effect. However, not all studies have found that contingent access to reward acts to devalue consumption of the target food. For example, Hendy et al. (2005) found no over-justification effect for fruit and vegetable preferences, when consumption was contingent on receiving marks that could be later traded for small non-food rewards.

As the material above amply demonstrates, information about food or about what may happen after consuming it can have a major impact on affective reactions. These reactions may translate into a decision about whether or not to ingest that particular food. Furthermore, the perceptual medium that is most responsible for all of these effects would appear to be the visual system, with its rapid ability to identify an object and its ready access to semantic information about food, acquired recently (via books, TV, etc.) or more distantly as a child.

Mechanisms likely to involve less conscious processing

Several different forms of learning are known to be involved in changing hedonic responses to foods. When a participant is exposed to an energy-dense food, they may come to associate the post-ingestive effect of these calories with its flavour—flavour–nutrient learning. In addition, the pleasant sweet taste of the food (or, for a bitter-tasting food, its unpleasant bitter taste) can also become associated with its flavour (i.e. principally the odour), and this is termed flavour–flavour learning. Certain foods or drinks, such as chocolate, coffee, and alcoholic beverages, have pharmacological effects and these too can become associated with flavour—again mainly odours—and this has been referred to as flavour–drug learning. The most well-documented food-related hedonic change resulting from learning is that which accompanies nausea or vomiting, leading to a 'conditioned taste aversion'. However, in some cases strong aversions may form without nausea or vomiting, or indeed any illness at all, and these may also involve single-trial learning and are termed 'cognitive aversions'. Finally, humans and animals can learn to like (or dislike) a food by observing the reaction of others when they consume the same food—Observational learning. Each of these is considered in turn.

Flavour–nutrient learning can occur in both children and adults. Birch *et al.* (1990) had 4-year-old children drink, on alternate days, a distinctly flavoured high-calorie (maltodextrin) stimulus and a distinctly flavoured low-calorie stimulus. The children came to prefer the high-calorie drink to the low-calorie drink, indicating flavour–nutrient learning. In addition, they adjusted their consumption of subsequent food intake to compensate for the extra calories (or their absence). This 'learned satiety' (i.e. where a flavour cues the likely satiating properties of a food) is a topic pursued later in this chapter.

Kern *et al.* (1993) allocated children to either a learning group, who were exposed to a distinctly coloured and flavoured high-fat (i.e. high calorie) yoghurt on one day and a low-fat (i.e. low calorie) yoghurt on another or to an exposure group who just experienced small quantities of each yoghurt. Children were tested when hungry, and when full, to see if state modulated the appearance of any preference. In the learning group, children only expressed a preference for the high-fat yoghurt when hungry—thus demonstrating state-dependent flavour–nutrient learning, whilst the exposed participants demonstrated some increase in preference for both yoghurts relative to control stimuli (i.e. a mere exposure effect—more below).

Similar effects have also been observed in adults. Brunstrom and Mitchell (2007) had participants consume distinctly flavoured, high-calorie and low-calorie foods on different days. Significant changes in liking were apparent across the course of training, with liking increasing for the high-calorie stimulus. Notably, this study only obtained a change in liking in unrestrained eaters (i.e. those participants not overly concerned with dieting and intake control). Mobini *et al.* (2007) randomly allocated participants to one of six conditions; one stimulus consisting of calories and sweetness, another of no calories and sweetness, and a further one consisting of minimally sweetened, low calories. Participants exposed to these stimuli were either trained when hungry or when full. This is a particularly nice experiment because it can clearly differentiate between flavour–nutrient and flavour–flavour learning, as well as establishing the effects of state on acquisition, especially as all participants were tested both full and hungry. Both types of learning were detected. Greater liking for the sweetened, high-calorie condition was most apparent for participants trained and tested hungry, compared to those trained and tested sated. Flavour–flavour learning, as indexed by changes in liking for the aspartame-sweetened, low-calorie stimulus, was apparent irrespective of training and testing state.

Although most human studies have concentrated on flavour–nutrient learning, in the animal literature there has been considerable interest in whether different forms of nutrient (i.e. carbohydrates, fats, and proteins) differentially support this form of learning. Apart from the work reported above, the only study to examine a specific instance of learning where calories were equated but the foods differed in a specific macronutrient (namely protein) was reported by Gibson *et al.* (1995). They found evidence that flavours paired with disguised protein became preferred when participants had received a protein-'deficient' breakfast—i.e. a state-dependent preference.

Two adult studies have failed to obtain evidence favouring flavour–nutrient learning. First, Appleton *et al.* (2006) examined flavour–nutrient learning under both, 'real-world' and laboratory, conditions. Participants consumed distinctly flavoured yoghurts that were either high or low calorie and these were eaten either when hungry or full. Participants were also tested hungry and full. The location of the training—in the laboratory or in the real world— had no significant effect. However, changes in liking for both the high- and low-calorie-paired flavour was evident, but only for yoghurt flavours that had been consumed when hungry—state at testing (hungry or full) had little affect. Here, the difference in energy may have been insufficient to differentiate the two yoghurts, but sufficient to support flavour–nutrient learning for both. Second, Yeomans *et al.* (2005) had participants consume a fixed quantity of either high- or low-energy porridge, each with a distinctive flavour. On test, liking for the high-energy porridge *decreased*, relative to the low-energy porridge, an effect attributed to the forced-consumption procedure, which appeared to make participants feel slightly nauseous.

Whilst these experiments indicate that adults and children can acquire flavour–nutrient associations, these effects may be moderated by state and restraint, in ways that are not yet fully understood. A further issue concerns the distinction between flavour–flavour and flavour–nutrient learning. Although the Mobini *et al.* (2007) study suggests they are separate entities, it does not definitively demonstrate that flavour–nutrient learning can occur *independently* of flavour–flavour learning. Before examining some of the findings that illustrate flavour–flavour learning, it seems important to indicate that they are dissociable (this having been amply demonstrated in animal studies—Mehiel and Bolles (1988)). Capaldi and Privitera (2007) assigned participants to one of two groups. One group received parings of a bitter-tasting, high-fat food with a distinctive flavour. The other group received an equal number of pairings to a bitter-tasting, low-fat food, again with a distinctive flavour. Thus both of these foods tasted equally unpleasant during training, but differed in the calories they provided. The flavour used in training was then tested in the low-calorie food, but this time with no bitter taste present. Flavour–nutrient learning was evident, in that the group exposed to the high fat–flavour pairing liked the flavour (in the low-fat food) significantly more than participants who had received the low fat–flavour pairing. Thus, under conditions in which only calories differ for an unpleasant-tasting food, increased liking due to flavour–nutrient learning can clearly occur.

The first demonstration of flavour–flavour learning in adult human participants was reported by Zellner *et al.* (1983). In a series of studies, participants experienced unusual tea flavours, with one flavour presented in water and another in sucrose solution. Participants were then tested for both of these target tea flavours (in sucrose and in water) and for two further tea flavours that they had not been exposed to. Liking increased significantly for the sucrose-paired tea, over and above any effect of flavour exposure alone (i.e. mere exposure effect—more below). This flavour–flavour learning effect was also obtained in two further conceptual replications.

Further research on flavour–flavour learning can be divided into two distinct phases. The first, in the 1990s, reflected a resurgence of interest in 'evaluative conditioning' (the learnt acquisition of likes and dislikes) of which flavour–flavour learning appeared to be a paradigmatic example (De Houwer *et al.* 2001). Here, the focus was on the apparently unusual aspects of flavour–flavour learning. Most notably—and akin to certain other forms of evaluative learning—flavour–flavour learning appears to occur with minimal conscious awareness (i.e. participants do not need to know that one flavour has been paired with say sucrose and the other with quinine for learning to occur). Whilst there has been considerable interest and debate about the issue of awareness amongst students of associative learning (e.g. Lovibond and Shanks 2002), there is still a good case for regarding flavour–flavour learning as something of an exception, in that it does appear that people can acquire a liking (and a disliking) for a flavour without readily being able to report either that it has occurred or why it has occurred (Baeyens *et al.* 1990). The argument for regarding evaluative learning—and flavour–flavour learning, in particular—as different from other forms of human associative learning also emerges from the study of extinction (e.g. after pairing an odour with sucrose, the odour is then paired with water). Flavour–flavour learning appears to be markedly resistant to extinction (Baeyens *et al.* 1995). It is also insensitive to contextual modulation, again unlike other forms of human associative learning, in that contextual cues that predict when a reinforcer (e.g. sucrose or quinine) will be present do not modulate liking (or disliking) for the flavour-conditioned stimulus (Baeyens *et al.* 1996). Note the resemblance of this form of learning to odour–taste learning discussed in Chapter 3.

The second, and more recent phase of research, has concerned a rather different set of questions. A particularly important one has been reports that positive flavour–flavour learning, such as that demonstrated by Zellner *et al.* (1985), can be hard to obtain in other laboratories (e.g. Stevenson *et al.* 1995, 1998).

This contrasts with flavour–flavour learning with unpleasant tastes, which is quite robust and has been repeatedly observed. At least three factors have been identified that might explain this discrepancy. First, although most people do not like the bitter taste of quinine or tween-20 (these being commonly used negative unconditioned stimuli), participant's hedonic reaction to sucrose may differ markedly. Indeed, Yeomans *et al.* (2006) found that individual differences in liking for sucrose could readily predict the degree to which changes in liking for a sucrose-paired odour occurred. Second, people's hedonic response to sucrose may change markedly with their state of depletion or repletion. Yeomans and Mobini (2006) observed that liking for a sucrose-paired odour was dependent upon state, in that participants needed to be hungry for a conditioning effect to be observed. Interestingly, liking for a bitter-paired flavour was depressed irrespective of state. Similarly, Brunstrom and Fletcher (2008) found a shift in preference for a saccharin-paired flavour only when participants were trained and tested hungry. Third, participants who are restrained eaters may consistently fail to demonstrate flavour–flavour learning (Brunstrom *et al.* 2001, Brunstrom *et al.* 2005). This may occur because they dislike the taste of sucrose or because they are especially attentive to the experimental contingencies, which then interfere with flavour–flavour learning.

In sum, both positive and negative flavour–flavour learning have been demonstrated—most notably for the odourous component of flavour, with taste serving as the unconditioned stimulus (usually sweet and bitter tastes, but MSG has also served successfully as a positive unconditioned stimulus; Yeomans *et al.* 2008). These effects, like flavour–nutrient learning, occur both in children (Havermans and Jansen 2007) and adults, and seem to have characteristics that differentiate them from other forms of human associative learning.

Both flavour–nutrient and flavour–flavour learning can result in either positive or negative hedonic changes. Taste-aversion learning results in solely negative changes. This name is misleading because, at least in humans, taste aversions are normally formed to whole foods or drinks (e.g. crab or whisky) and should more properly be termed flavour–aversion learning. Flavour–aversion learning can be fractionated into two distinct forms. The first form is strikingly similar to that observed in animals and relies upon an association forming between a flavour and its aversive post-ingestional consequences. The post-ingestional consequences can include food poisoning, physical illness unrelated to food, over consumption (recall Yeomans *et al.* 2005), allergic reactions, motion sickness, and induced nausea (e.g. chemotherapy). This type of flavour aversion can also be generated under laboratory conditions. Cannon *et al.*, (1983) randomly assigned participants who reported rarely

Table 5.2 Design and outcome of Cannon, Best, Batson, and Feldman's (1983) laboratory-based flavour-aversion study

Group	Pretraining	Training	Test 1	
			Drunk (ml)	SR†
Flavour aversion	Orange	Cranberry, Water, APO†	38	2.6
Control	Cranberry	Cranberry, Quinine, SAL†	120	1.3
Interference	Cranberry	Cranberry, Quinine, APO†	63	2.5
Latent inhibition	Cranberry	Cranberry, Water, APO†	100	1.3

† = SR, self-report distasteful; APO, Apomorphine injection; SAL, Saline injection.

drinking cranberry juice (the target flavour) to four experimental groups: Flavour–aversion, Control, Interference, and Latent Inhibition (see Table 5.2 for summary of the procedure and results). During a 3-day pre-training period, the Flavour–aversion group drank orange juice each day, and the Control, Interference, and Latent Inhibition groups drank an equivalent amount of cranberry juice. On the training day, all participants drank a set amount of cranberry juice. This was immediately followed by water in the Flavour–aversion and Latent Inhibition groups, and by quinine in the Control and Interference groups. Then the Control group received an injection of saline, and the Flavour aversion, Interference, and Latent inhibition groups received apomorphine to induce nausea. No adverse symptoms were reported by the Control group, however, 89% of the participants receiving apomorphine reported feeling nauseous and 78% subsequently vomited. Four days following the training period, and then 1 month later, participants were asked to drink cranberry juice again and to rate its characteristics including hedonic ratings.

The results for the first test revealed a significant dislike for cranberry juice in the Flavour–aversion group that was reflected in the relatively small amount consumed and by the their self-report score (1 = not at all, 4 = extremely). In contrast the control group demonstrated no such aversion, and were largely similar to the Latent inhibition group. This finding is important as it suggests that more familiar foods are less likely to be susceptible to the formation of aversions and is also consistent with the associative learning literature (i.e. pre-exposure to a cue with no consequences makes it subsequently harder to associate it with other events). The interference condition should also have reduced the magnitude of the subsequent aversion, but this was not observed. Two more general observations about these results are noteworthy. First, effects in all of the groups, but especially the Flavour–aversion group were attenuated by the passage of time, i.e. the effect was less marked when participants were retested a month later, indicating some forgetting. Second, participants were told (in all conditions) that the injection they would receive might make them nauseous, yet even knowing this did not affect the formation of the aversion.

Several surveys reveal that flavour–aversions are fairly common, and that they have properties similar to those observed in the experimental study described above. Frequency estimates vary. Logue *et al.* (1981) found that 65% of their sample of university undergraduates had one or more aversion. With a similar sample, Garb and Stunkard (1974) reported a 25% rate and there are no obvious methodological reasons for this discrepancy. Logue *et al.* (1981) also reported that, for at least 20% of the aversions, participants were fully aware that the aversive food itself was not the cause of the illness/nausea. Again, similar to Cannon *et al.*'s (1983) data, the longer the time lag since the formation of the aversion, the weaker the aversion was, and aversions were more likely to be formed to unfamiliar foods.

Although flavour aversions are driven by learning processes that appear to be rather insensitive to cognition (i.e. you can *know* that it is alcohol that makes you vomit not the whisky flavour, yet one stills forms an aversion to whisky not alcohol), some examples of strong aversions to food do not conform to this pattern. Indeed, there seems to be some aversions that wholly depend upon cognition for their formation. This has been touched upon already above, where simply negative information can provoke marked avoidance (recall Alar-treated apples), as can contact with disgust elicitors (see Rozin 1976) and enforced consumption of a food (Batsell *et al.* 2002). Survey data suggest that these cognitive aversions may be both stronger and more enduring than those generated via flavour–aversion learning (Batsell and Brown 1998).

Some of the foods and drinks that we consume contain psychoactive chemicals that are able to condition a liking—under certain conditions—for the vehicle flavour. Alcohol is perhaps the most interesting and difficult to study because of the practical and ethical difficulties arising from pairings of alcohol with a flavour (i.e. the participant may become mildly intoxicated). Whilst a large number of studies have explored cue reactivity with mixed results, i.e. whether a cue associated with alcohol ingestion can induce craving, relatively few studies have examined whether a flavour can become preferred following pairings with alcohol. These latter studies have produced mixed results, with some obtaining positive effects and others failing to find an association. At least some of this variability may be accounted for by personality variables and by previous drinking experience (Glautier *et al.* 2000).

Caffeine, another ubiquitous food drug, has been particularly well explored. Regular caffeine consumers, who are acutely deprived of caffeine during training and testing, report liking a caffeine-paired flavour more than a group receiving a placebo-paired flavour (Tinley *et al.* 2004). Similar findings have also been obtained for the combination of pharmacologically active ingredients in chocolate (caffeine and theobromine). Here, liking for a caffeine/theobromine-paired flavour increased over time when trained and tested in a deprived state relative to a placebo condition (Smit and Blackburn 2005). However, although craving for coffee may be driven by caffeine need, at least for chocolate it appears to be its perceptual properties that best alleviate craving rather than its psychoactive ingredients (Michener and Rozin 1994).

Some evidence for the distinct nature of flavour–drug learning has been provided by Yeomans *et al.* (2007). Participants were randomly assigned to one of six between conditions in which a novel tea was either paired with caffeine or with no caffeine, and presented in water, aspartame solution, or quinine solution. Training and testing were conducted under conditions of both food and caffeine deprivation. On test, participants were asked to evaluate both the smell and the flavour of the tea *alone*. Both caffeine pairing (i.e. flavour–drug) and taste pairing (i.e. flavour–flavour) produced independent effects (i.e. no interaction). Participants who had experienced the tea with caffeine liked its smell and flavour more than participants who had experienced the tea with no caffeine. Similarly, participants who had experienced the tea with a sweet taste liked its smell and flavour more than participants who had experienced it with a bitter taste. As with many studies reviewed above, it is notable that the smell of the tea alone (as would be expected based upon the importance of the odour component to the tea's flavour) revealed the same differences in liking (see Table 5.3).

All of the forms of learning reviewed so far have involved direct experience with the stimulus accompanied by an affective state (immediate or delayed)

Table 5.3 The effect of flavour–caffeine and flavour–taste pairing on the rating of the target tea's odour and flavour (adapted from Yeomans, Mobini, and Chambers (2007))

Condition		Caffeine	No caffeine	Average
Sniffed	Water	5.9	−9.9	−2.0
	Aspartame	4.5	−1.8	1.4
	Quinine	−6.4	−20.8	−13.6
	Average	1.3	−10.8	
By mouth	Water	10.0	1.4	5.7
	Aspartame	18.6	1.7	10.2
	Quinine	0.7	−24.3	−11.8
	Average	9.8	−7.1	

produced by drugs, calories, taste (innate like/dislike), or illness. However, animals can rapidly learn to prefer or avoid a flavour by exposure to it on another animal, in conjunction with an appropriate context (Galef and Stein 1985). Conceptually similar findings have been reported in children, adolescents, and adults. Marinho (1942) demonstrated that children could be influenced by a 'leader' child to select the same food as the 'leader' from two equally preferred foods. The resulting preference for one over the other food was still intact 1 year after the initial experimental phase. Birch (1980) also found that a child's preference for a particular vegetable could be modified by placing the child at a table with children who preferred another vegetable. Following four such exposures, the target child's vegetable preference shifted to that of its peers. Adult eating behaviour can also impact on children's food preferences. Harper and Sanders (1975) examined whether young children would place an unfamiliar food in their mouth if a friendly adult or their mother did so, relative to the child just being offered the food. Children were significantly more likely to take the food and place it in their mouth if an adult did so, and especially if that adult was their mother.

Using a rather different approach, Baeyens et al. (1996) asked adolescents to watch, on video, an unknown but similarly aged demonstrator peer sample what appeared to be the *same* set of solutions that the adolescent participants were sampling. Solutions were both coloured and flavoured with orange or raspberry odourants. One colour–flavour combination was consistently paired with the demonstrator emoting a disgust face, the other with a neutral face. Baeyens et al. (1996) found on test that participants came to dislike the flavour paired with the disgust face, but only if the colour context was the same. In a second study, Baeyens et al. (2001) used the same design, but manipulated the adolescents' belief about whether the stimuli they were sampling were the same or different to those being sampled by the demonstrator peer on the video. The belief manipulation eliminated the effect of observational learning in those who were told that there was no relationship between the stimuli they were sampling and those sampled by the demonstrator peer. The other group, however, whilst coming to dislike the flavour paired with the demonstrator's disgust face, did not show the context-specific effect of colour observed in the earlier study.

Observational learning effects have also been documented in adults. Hobden and Pliner (1995, Experiment 2) instructed participants to watch a video of what they were told was a prior participant making a series of choices from pairs of foods. The model chose predominantly familiar or unfamiliar foods (dependent on condition) and then appeared to eat the selected food. All participants, including a control group who did not receive any modelling, were then asked to choose between the same pairs of food as the model, plus five new pairs.

The modelling condition affected participant's choice, but this effect was not clear-cut. For foods that the model had selected, participants who had seen her predominantly choose and consume the unfamiliar foods also tended to choose more unfamiliar foods, and it was likewise for the group that had seen the model choose the more familiar foods. Although neither of the model groups differed from the control, both differed from each other. There was no effect of modelling on consumption of the foods that were not included in the demonstrator phase of the experiment.

Considerable research has been undertaken in animals to examine the neural basis of conditioned flavour aversions and flavour–nutrient learning, but the literature for humans is not so rich. For flavour–flavour learning, a somewhat analogous technique for examining learning using pairings of a food reward with a visual pattern (the food reward is delivered *following* the pattern, so the two events are not experienced simultaneously as in more typical examples of flavour–flavour learning) has been used to investigate whether an intact amygdala is required to form such associations. Interest in this structure was based upon animal findings, which suggest that parts of the amygdala may be crucial in learning associations to emotionally salient events (Zald 2003). Johnsrude *et al.* (2000) compared patients who had had a temporal lobe resection that included the amygdala and contrasted them to controls. The amygdala patients did not acquire a liking for the patterns paired with food reinforcement, whilst the controls did. The relevance of this result for more typical flavour–flavour learning is questionable. First, Brunstrom and Higgs (2002) have also reported that when using this conditioning technique, it is sensitive to concurrent task-load, suggesting that it may be mediated by conscious learning processes, in contrast to those hypothesized to underpin flavour–flavour learning. More strikingly, Coppens *et al.* (2006), using a simultaneous flavour–flavour proce-dure, failed to find any difference between patients with an amygdala lesion and those without. Needless to say, human lesion studies come with many caveats, especially as here lesions were not bilateral (in either study) and so a definitive conclusion for or against the role of the amygdala in flavour–flavour learning remains contested.

Not surprisingly, the orbitofrontal cortex may also be important in acquired likes. Again, using the procedure of food rewards paired with patterns, Cox *et al.* (2005) reported activation in the ventral striatum (more below) and the orbitofrontal cortex when a stimulus was rewarded. However, only the orbit-ofrontal activity was observed when the reinforced pattern was presented alone. Gottfried *et al.* (2002) examined evaluative conditioning between neutral faces and pleasant, neutral, and unpleasant odours. The orbitofron-tal cortex was active during acquisition of both positive and negatively paired faces. Time-dependent changes (over trials) were also observed in the nucleus accumbens, amygdala, and piriform cortex.

Activation of the ventral striatum and nucleus accumbens is not surprising in any conditioning study using pleasant unconditioned stimuli. A consistent finding in humans and animals has been that endogenous opioids mediate subjective states of pleasantness whilst dopamine mediates incentive motivation—craving or wanting (Barbano and Cador 2007, Levine and Billington 2004). However, whilst the use of drugs such as naloxone and nalmafene (opioid antagonists) appears to selectively reduce pleasant affect during eating, whether dopamine pathways primarily subserve incentive motivation alone is more complex. Small *et al.* (2003) reported a significant association between dopaminergic activity and meal-pleasantness ratings. Whilst this could suggest the involvement of this transmitter system in mediating pleasant affective states, it could equally reflect, as noted in the introduction, that wanting many contaminate hedonic ratings. In fact, the neural systems underpinning wanting and liking are inevitably far more complex than the dopamine-versus-endogenous-opioid distinction may suggest. Based upon the far more extensive animal literature, it is quite clear that several other systems are involved in underpinning pleasure, including glutamate, benzodiazepine, and endocannabinoid pathways (Saper *et al.* 2002). In addition, all of these systems interact significantly with neural pathways subserving both wanting and needing (see Finlayson *et al.* (2007) for discussion).

Notwithstanding this complexity, findings in humans suggest that for conditioning phenomena that involve associating reward with a flavour cue, subcortical opioid transmitter systems may be important for the pleasure associated with the unconditioned stimulus. The orbitofrontal cortex may be the neural hub which then acts to associate the conditioned and unconditioned stimulus, store this information, and modulate behaviour based upon it (Berridge and Kringelbach 2008). Presentation of the conditioned stimulus then leads to activation here, and activation of brain structures that mediate reward and/or wanting—depending upon the context. These systems will also be significantly influenced by hypothalamic structures that are involved in energy homeostasis—i.e. in 'needing' (Saper *et al.* 2002).

Observational learning may be mediated by different, but related, structures. For negative observational learning, facial expression may be of key importance in instantiating a feeling of negative affect that then becomes associated with the target flavour. Wicker *et al.* (2003) reported that the same structures (notably the insular cortex) were active in the human brain when participants smelled a disgusting odour, as were active when they passively observed a disgusting face. One inference from this neuroimaging study is that observing other people being disgusted towards a target food may result in the observer *also* feeling disgust towards that food (and possibly reducing its incentive value too). However, the insula may be active whenever an 'emotional' facial expression is viewed or generated, so the aforementioned conclusion must remain tentative (see van der Gaag *et al.* 2007).

For conditioned taste-aversion learning, interest has also focussed on the amygdala as well as other structures such as the parabrachial nucleus in the pons (Reilly and Bornovalova 2005). At least in animals, the role of the amygdala in conditioned flavour aversions is controversial, because lesions to this structure do not produce consistent effects on an animal's ability to form an aversion. Reilly and Bornovalona (2005) suggest that the amygdala, and in particular the basolateral amygdala, may be responsible for neophobic responses in rats. Thus lesions here have the effect of impairing conditioning via a latent-inhibition like process, as the animal may not react to a novel flavour as being novel, thus retarding the formation of an association. Indeed, neophobic reactions to food are of particular importance in regulating consumption and these are considered next.

The judgement of food novelty and its effect on ingestion are arguably best considered here, as a food's novelty will likely be evaluated before the food is placed in the mouth, based again primarily upon visual and olfactory cues. Novelty is generally a disincentive to consume. In many animal species, and especially the rat, avoidance or wariness of new foods is common (Rozin 1978). This also appears to be the case in humans, with unfamiliar foods being reported as typically more disliked than familiar foods (e.g. Hall and Hall 1939). Obviously to be wary of a novel food, it has to be identified as novel. This can be achieved by the provision of misleading or true information about the food or by its actual appearance or smell.

Appearance and smell (alone or in combination) are sufficient conditions to identify a novel food and to mediate avoidance. Tuorila *et al.* (1994) gave participants two very unfamiliar foods and two more familiar foods. These were, in order: (1) viewed, (2) viewed and sniffed, and (3) tasted. For each stage of exposure, hedonic ratings of the foods were obtained. For the unfamiliar foods, viewing alone generated negative evaluations, in contrast to the more positive evaluations of the familiar foods. This contrast was even more marked when the stimuli were viewed and smelled, and even more so when tasted. The important point here again is that viewing and smelling were sufficient to both identify the foods as novel (or familiar) and to mediate a hedonic reaction towards them on this basis. As noted above, information can have a powerful effect on whether one wants to consume a particular food. This has been used to explore neophobia in the laboratory without the problems involved in obtaining genuinely unfamiliar foods. For example, a piece of cooked meat may be described with its correct name, grilled beef steak, or with a false name and description (e.g. grilled langua steak). Misleading labels and descriptions, assuming they are artfully applied, act to reduce participant's ratings of liking and willingness to eat, and increase ratings of novelty (e.g. Pliner and Pelchat 1991).

Neophobic responses to foods in humans are observable from the first presentation of solid foods (e.g. see Birch *et al.* 1998). However, this observation has to be set against infants' willingness to put just about anything into their mouth (e.g. Stanek *et al.* 1998), raising a currently unresolved paradox. As the child matures to adulthood and beyond, neophobic reactions to food tend to diminish (McFarlane and Pliner 1997, Pliner and Loewen 1997). This age-related reduction in neophobia may simply reflect, amongst other things, breadth of experience, so that even novel foods have some apparent similarity to foods sampled before. Neophobic reactions to food also appear to have both state and trait components. For example, exposure to a series of unfamiliar foods (actual consumption) results in higher acceptance for *other* unrelated, unfamiliar foods (Pliner *et al.* 1993). However, trait neophobia appears to be a relatively stable disposition to avoid novel foods, and is accompanied by detectable behavioural correlates such as less vigorous sniffing at food-related odours (Raudenbush *et al.* 1998). When confronted with a novel food, participants appear to avoid it (or be wary of it) for two reasons—they report that they feel it will have unpleasant sensory/affective properties and that it might be dangerous (Pliner *et al.* 1993). Unfamiliar animal-based foods, in particular, appear to evoke a much more marked negative affective response than unfamiliar non-animal-based foods. Humans also appear more unwilling to actually consume novel animal products (Pliner and Pelchat 1991). Increased feelings of disgust towards unfamiliar animal-based foods relative to unfamiliar vegetable-based foods have also been reported (Martins and Pliner 2005).

Neophobic reactions are obviously breachable. Two types of manipulation, both of which almost certainly occur during routine feeding and drinking, have been documented to reduce such reactions. First, simple passive exposure can increase liking and acceptance. This has been most convincingly demonstrated in young infants and children, and may even occur for certain tastes and flavours *in utero* (Rolls 1988). Sullivan and Birch (1994) reported that 4–6-month-old infants fed either peas or beans came to eat more of the exposed food as a function of exposure frequency. In addition, adults who viewed video film of the infants' facial expressions in this study, judged them to have liked the exposed food more than a non-exposed control food. Birch *et al.* (1998), in a more extensive study, also using similarly aged infants, reported that just a single exposure was sufficient to produce a marked increase in consumption and that this could generalize to food with a similar flavour. With slightly older children (two-year-olds), Birch and Marlin (1982) exposed them to different novel cheeses (Experiment 1) and fruits (Experiment 2) any of 2, 5, 10, 15, or 20 times. Increased preference was significantly associated with increasing exposure for both foods. At least then with infants and young children, exposure can enhance consumption and preference for unfamiliar foods.

With adults, the effects of exposure are not so clear-cut. Crandall (1984) reported a study conducted at a remote, Alaskan fish cannery. He arranged for donuts to be served in the canteen over the period of time that the cannery was open. He recorded the quantity of donuts consumed, which was found to increase over time. Whilst this study suggests a 'mere-exposure' effect—i.e. increased liking as a consequence of exposure—it is hard to argue that donuts were an unfamiliar food for the cannery workers, although they may have been unfamiliar *in that context*. Pliner (1982) tested the effects of exposure under more controlled conditions using unfamiliar fruit juices. Participants were exposed to three unfamiliar juices either 5, 10, or 20 times. On test, participants were asked to evaluate liking for these three juices and for a fourth control juice. Liking was found to increase with exposure, but when participants were re-tested one week later, the effect was lost. Bingham, Hurling, and Stocks (2005) examined whether exposure to spinach (a less preferred and relatively unfamiliar vegetable amongst their participants) or to spinach with a cheese sauce (i.e. flavour–nutrient learning) would enhance liking for spinach. No change in liking for spinach was observed, however, when participants were split into those who disliked spinach at the start of the experiment, significant increases in liking were observed for both spinach alone and for spinach and sauce (i.e. both being a probable consequence of exposure). Finally, Levy, MacRae, and Koster (2006) presented participants with orange drinks adulterated with flavourants to manipulate stimulus complexity. They found that repeated exposure to a flavour more complex than an individual's optimum level generated a change in preference in the direction of the more complex stimulus. This finding is of relevance here because stimulus novelty was a key component of judgements of complexity, i.e. more unfamiliar orange-adulterated drinks came to be more preferred with exposure. So whilst there is some evidence that exposure can reduce disliking for previously unfamiliar foods—and indeed this must surely be the case in day-to-day life—the experimental evidence is most compelling in children.

A second method that has been explored to increase acceptance of unfamiliar foods is to use information—an explicit cognitive strategy in contrast to exposure, which appears to work irrespective of whether the participant is aware of the repeated exposures. One reason that participants may choose not to eat a novel food is that they expect it to taste bad. Indeed, people may encourage others to try a novel food by using an information-based strategy, such as 'it tastes like X', X being something familiar and pleasant. Such taste information (i.e. X tastes good) can significantly increase acceptance in teenagers and college students (Pelchat and Pliner 1995) and in older adults too (McFarlane and Pliner 1997). However, these effects are not large and are not always obtained. In the McFarlane and Pliner (1997) study for example, a teenage group did not demonstrate any increased willingness to consume a novel food following the provision of several different forms of information, including taste.

Pelchat and Pliner (1995) observed an interesting and *apparently* anomalous finding. Children, aged 4–7 years, were surprisingly willing (given their general tendency for neophobia) to consume an unfamiliar type of cheese called gjetost. However, this cheese, which has a caramelized appearance, was considered by many children to *look like* candy—consequently, they consumed it. This points to a more general strategy that might be used to overcome neophobia, namely disguise. Locate a novel food in a familiar context, i.e. make it appear to look and smell like something familiar, and this will likely increase acceptance. This important notion was identified by Rozin (1978) and applied to explain the consistency of particular combinations of flavourings used in regional cuisines around the world. Such particular combinations of flavours (see Table 5.4) allow new foods to be introduced into the diet without rejection based upon a neophobic response. In fact, the culture in which a person grows up is likely to better inform one about that person's food preferences than the

Table 5.4 Some examples of typical flavour combinations used by specific cuisines (adapted from the flavour principle cookbook by E. Rozin (1992))

Country	Flavour principle
Japan	Soy sauce, sake, and sugar
Laos	Fish sauce and coconut
Central Asia	Cinnamon, fruit, and nut
Northeast Africa	Garlic, cumin, and mint
Greece	Olive oil, lemon and oregano
Hungary	Onion, lard, and paprika
Mexico	Lime and chilli
Middle east	Lemon and parsley
West Africa	Tomato, peanut, and chilli

food preferences of their siblings and parents (Rozin *et al.* 1984). Culture largely defines the range of foods and flavours that a child and young adult are exposed to.

Hedonic reactions to foods and drinks, irrespective of their nature, will clearly differ depending upon a variety of organism-specific variables. Mood, gender, dieting, pregnancy, and restraint are some such examples. Hunger is likely to have the most profound impact upon food hedonics. Several neuroimaging studies reveal, perhaps not surprisingly, that hungry people demonstrate significant neural activation in flavour-processing-related areas, when exposed to food-related cues. These include the insular and the orbitofrontal cortex (e.g. Porubska *et al.* 2006, Wang *et al.* 2004) as well as the amygdala (LaBar *et al.* 2001, Morris and Dolan 2001). Hunger is very likely to alter hedonic reaction to food prior to ingestion, as well as altering the incentive value of cues associated with food (and see discussion below on alliaesthesia).

There are a large number of anecdotal reports which indicate that, when people are in an especially heightened state of food deprivation, they will likely eat foods that they would not otherwise consume. Laboratory demonstrations of this phenomenon can also be found. People with the developmental disability Prader-Willi syndrome experience constant high-level hunger. However, whilst these individuals have a knowledge of food that is equivalent to normal controls, they report being prepared to eat food that is contaminated as well as unusual food combinations that were not regarded as acceptable by normal or mentally retarded controls (Dykens 2000). These self-report findings are consistent with carers and professional's evaluations of problematic eating behaviour in this disorder, and Dykens (2000) notes that '… their drive for food is so strong that it overpowers their knowledge and otherwise good judgement [about food]' (Dykens 2000, p.164).

Discussion—Function one

As should now be clear, the participant draw both consciously and unconsciously on a large body of knowledge, which then shapes their hedonic response to a particular food. The visual system and the orthonasal olfactory system are the primary modalities involved in this process, with the visual system mediating access to semantic information about the food (which may then shape hedonic responding) and the olfactory system accessing a more immediate and hard to ignore hedonic/perceptual response. Much of this information, both via visual identification and through olfactory hedonics, is gleaned from learning about food and its consequences during and after ingestion.

This ability to acquire food-related information is a fundamental and innate characteristic of human eating behaviour.

Function two—Decision to ingest once food is in the mouth

Once food is placed in the mouth, this is the last chance, bar vomiting, for a decision to reject it. Decisions to reject (or accept) once a food enters the mouth are likely to be made on two different grounds. The first concerns the perceptual properties of the food. Humans and other animals come with some clearly innate preferences and aversions, notably in relation to taste, and to somatosensory activating stimuli that result in pain (i.e. chemical and physical irritants as well as thermal stimuli). Whilst our reaction to all of these types of stimuli can change with experience, their function is arguably a basic one, to prevent harm to the mouth and body. It is for this reason that the *initial* reaction shown to these types of stimuli is rejection. The second reason for rejecting a food once it is placed in the mouth is that it violates our expectations. This can be based upon either prior visual/olfactory appraisal or because the currently perceived flavour differs substantially from sensory memories of prior experiences with that flavour (note that this latter process has a bearing upon certain types of interaction discussed in Chapters 2 and 3, where it was argued that these may be a side effect of learning—more on this below and in Chapter 6).

Innate preferences and aversions, and the effects of experience

There are good grounds for suggesting that humans are born with a preference for sweet-tasting things and with an aversion for bitter and sour tastants—in marked contrast to the general absence of any marked olfactory preferences in neonates (Soussignan *et al.* 1997; excepting odourants with a notable irritant component). Whilst an innate preference for certain concentrations of salt may also be the case, this is more difficult to establish due to the apparently later maturation of salt detection in human infants (Mattes 1997).

In an important series of studies, Steiner (1979), documented the facial and ingestive reactions of various groups of participants to sweet, sour, and bitter tastants. He found that neonates, and neonates born without a cortex, both had similar facial responses to tastants. Sweet tastants produced ingestive facial expressions and sour and bitter tastants rejective ones. The presence of hedonic expressiveness in neonates lacking a cortex strongly suggests that these responses are driven by subcortical structures. In intact human adults, aversive tastes (strong saline) also selectively activate subcortical structures, such as the amygdala, as well as cortical structures involved in affective processing, such as the orbitofrontal cortex (Zald *et al.* 1998). Whilst the latter may be involved in conscious hedonic judgements, the presence of hedonic responsiveness in cortex-less neonates raises some interesting questions about the role of cortical structures in hedonic processing, notably whether their role may be in utilizing this information in decision making (Berridge and Kringelbach 2008) rather than in supporting affective qualia.

Facial expressions to basic tastants in neonates are similar in form to facial expressions generated by tastants in normal adults, blind adults, and mentally retarded participants (Steiner 1979). More detailed studies have also documented different sets of facially ingestive and rejective expressions for sour, bitter, and sweet tastes (e.g. Ganchrow et al. 1983). Whilst naive observers can generally determine whether a taste is 'liked' or disliked' by a neonate, only experienced coders can delineate the difference between reactions to particular tastants such as bitter and sour (Rosenstein and Oster 1988). Although positive hedonic responsiveness to sweet tastes in neonates is well accepted, there may be some additional developmental changes in perception/hedonics for bitter tastants. Some studies have reported increasing negative hedonic reactivity to bitter tastants when neonates are contrasted to infants aged 14–180 days—i.e. although newborns show some reactivity on a variety of measures, including facial expression (arguably the most sensitive measure), this becomes far stronger with some limited maturation of the taste-perception system (Kajiura et al. 1992).

Not only are adult and neonate human facial expressions to basic tastes similar, but there is also a clear phylogenetic continuity as well. The facial and behavioural response of animals such as rats (Berridge 2000) and primates to the same set of tastants is noticeably similar (Steiner et al. 2001). Obviously, however, there are differences in the facial structure and musculature that restrict or alter various aspects of expression in infrahumans. Nonetheless, one can readily interpret the nature of the stimulus that the animal is sampling by observing their facial expression. This synergy between all of these disparate groups for two common facial expression elements is illustrated in Figure 5.1.

In a recent review, Pepino and Mennella (2006) discussed various lines of evidence suggesting an innate preference for sweet tastes. These include increased consumption, especially of sweeter sugars, in neonates, as well as the calmative effects that sucrose can exert on infants. Indeed, sweeteners can produce a sustained reduction in crying, in contrast to the effects of quinine (Graillon et al. 1997). Even preterm neonates respond positively to sucrose, demonstrating an increase in sucking for a sweetened versus an unsweetened stimulus. During development, children and adolescents exhibit a preference for higher levels of sweetness than adults. Whilst this may have biological roots, reflecting perhaps the extra energy needs of the growing body, it is paralleled

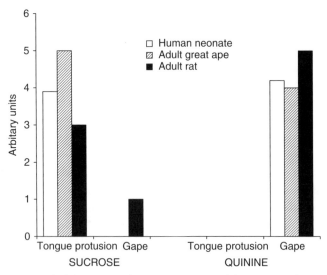

Fig. 5.1 Common facial response elements to sweet and bitter tastes shown by human neonates, great apes, and rats (data adapted from Steiner *et al.* (2001) and Berridge (2000)).

by an increased preference for higher concentrations of sour and salty tastes (relative to adults) as well. This may then point to developmental changes in taste perception rather than specific bodily needs.

Perhaps the most powerful argument for an innate preference for sweetness is to examine the history of sugar production (see Galloway 2000). Two facts are revealing. The first is that without exception, every population exposed to sugar has shown both rapid acceptance and increased consumption of it. The second, and although this is not unique to sugar (e.g. consider the history of pepper and spices), is the insatiable demand for it following exposure. Historically, this demand led to numerous technical advances, as well as labour 'innovations', some of which have had major social consequences (i.e. slavery, indentured labour, ethnic migrations, etc.).

Most things that taste sweet in the 'natural' world are sources of energy. Different forms of sugar vary in sweetness (see Moskowitz 1971). However, there does not appear to be any obvious relationship between the energy that a particular sugar will yield and its sweetness (contrast with increasing sweetness *for a particular sugar* and calories), nor for that matter between the sweetness of a sugar and its frequency of occurrence in unprocessed foods. Salivary amylase acts to breakdown starch, a major energy source, into maltose, which is also sweet. Sweetness then appears to be a generic marker for energy and it is for this reason that humans and other animals probably have an innate initial preference for sweet tastes.

Whilst preference for sweet tastes may be based on their ability to signal the presence of energy, sour and bitter tastes arguably signal harm. Sour tastes at lower concentrations may come to be preferred, not necessarily by neonates, but certainly by children exposed to sour tastes in fruits (Liem and Mennella 2003). However, it is very unlikely that this preference for more intense sour tastes would ever include levels of acidity sufficient to damage the mouth. So whilst sour may indicate the presence of acids (potentially harmful), strong acids would be better indicated by their direct and trigeminally mediated pain response. This contrasts with bitter tastes, as the presence of *any* bitter taste appears to signal the presence of plant-manufactured poisons, notably alkaloids (Maga 1994). In rats, following stimulation with different tastants, 68% of the variance in similarity of neural activity patterns obtained from recordings of cells in the nucleus of the solitary tract can be accounted for by the toxicity (LD50) of the tastant (Scott and Mark 1987). Put bluntly, the neural similarity reflects bitterness, and bitterness reflects toxicity. In humans, as part of a larger study examining the underlying relationships between the physical and perceptual characteristics of basic tastants, Schiffman and Erickson (1971) asked participants to judge how poisonous they thought each tastant might be. Judgements of poisonousness correlated 0.86 with the rank order of poisonousness (LD50) derived from the Merck index. Both of these relationships—in rats and humans—demonstrate a close correspondence between things that taste bitter and the degree to which the chemicals that generate the bitter taste are poisons. This relationship is also expressed in the relative tolerance for bitter tastes in animal diets. Animals that consume primarily vegetarian diets are more tolerant of bitter tastes (i.e. they trade off risk against necessity) in contrast to animals that primarily consume other animals for food (Glendinning 1994). There are then good grounds to believe that an evolutionary explanation for innate rejection of bitter tastes, based upon their likelihood of signalling poison, is correct.

Certain tastants, notably salts and acids, some odourants and some specific chemicals (carbonic acid, capsaicin, zingerone, piperine, etc.) are also innately aversive because of their ability to stimulate the trigeminal system (Rozin 1990). Chemical irritants produce a typical physiological reaction when applied to the mouth, nose, or eyes. They will induce copious salivation, running nose, and tearing, presumably to dilute or wash out the irritant. Not surprisingly, preference for foods that contain irritants is the province mainly of adults, suggesting that children will typically avoid ingesting foods that contain these irritants, and indeed, foods that contain bitter tastants, too. This raises an important point, namely that whilst humans may start out with innate preferences (sweet) and aversions, even these may be modified by experience.

Preference for sweet tastes is markedly different between adults (Conner *et al.* 1988) and even amongst teenagers and children who share the same genes (i.e. Greene *et al.* 1975). Adults appear to demonstrate four different types of relationship when liking/disliking for sweetness is plotted against increasing sweetener concentration (Duffy *et al.* 2006). The first is the inverted 'U' response, in which increasing concentration is accompanied first by increased liking, which then plateaus, followed by a decline into disliking. The second is a monotonic increase in liking with concentration. The third is the reverse of the second, a monotonic decease in liking with concentration. Finally, a fourth group demonstrate almost no hedonic response to sucrose solutions of any concentration. Some of these differences in responsiveness may be explained by dietary exposure to sweet tastes (e.g. Bacon *et al.* 1994); a further proportion of this variability may be explained by genetic factors such as sensitivity to certain bitter tastants (Duffy *et al.* 2006).

The ability of some individuals to detect PROP and a related chemical PTC, and for others not to be able to do so, was first noted in the 1930s by the chemist A.L. Fox. For safety reasons, modern research on this topic has used the related but less harmful chemical PROP. Threshold detection tests reveal two distinct populations, 'tasters' and 'non-tasters'. Tasters can be further divided into 'tasters' and 'supertasters' based upon superthreshold intensity judgements of PROP's bitterness. Supertasters find PROP extremely bitter tasting (Bartoshuk *et al.* 1994) as they do certain other bitter tastes—but not all. Two consistent correlates of supertaster status are an increased density of fungiform papillae and female gender. The presence of more taste buds and hence taste receptors has a number of knock-on consequences for perception and hedonics. First, as the free-nerve ending receptors that detect chemical irritants are located around the base of taste buds, PROP-sensitive individuals tend to be more sensitive to chemical irritants such as capsaicin than non-tasters (Bartoshuk 1993). Second, several studies have revealed consistent differences in perceptual and hedonic responsiveness to sweet tastes between PROP tasters and non-tasters. Looy and Weingarten (1992) found, for both adults and children, that sweet likers tended to be PROP non-tasters, showing a monotonically increasing liking response for sucrose. In contrast, PROP tasters tended to show the reverse pattern. These self-report ratings were also mirrored in their facial expressions. These differences in responsiveness are particular to sweetness (and bitterness), in that they are not observed for salt. They also generalize to reactions to sweet tastes in more naturalistic stimuli as well (Looy *et al.* 1992). A third consequence relates to the finding that increased tactile sensitivity may accompany increased PROP sensitivity, leading to potentially greater sensitivity to fats (Bartoshuk *et al.* 2006). Indeed, evidence is emerging that people with reduced PROP sensitivity may be more at risk for weight gain, than supertasters.

Not surprisingly, PROP (and PTC) sensitivity will also influence the potential for acquiring a liking for bitter-tasting foods (e.g. brussel sprouts, cabbage, olives, etc.) and several studies have demonstrated such relationships to food preferences (e.g. Glanville and Kaplan 1965, Fischer *et al.* 1961). Although PROP sensitivity may be one factor in developing a preference for bitter-tasting foods, experience is likely to be important too. London *et al.* (1979) observed that in rat pups exposure to bitter and sour tastes led to an increased preference for these tastants. Dietary exposure in humans may have similar effects. Moskowitz *et al.* (1975) found that Karnataka Indian labourers, who consumed large quantities of the sour and bitter tamarind fruit in their diet, reported liking the bitter and sour tastants quinine and citric acid considerably more, and at higher concentrations, than comparable controls from the same region who subsist on different diets (medical students at a local university). These differences could not be readily attributed to variations in scale use, as there were no consistent differences in salt- or sucrose-liking judgements between groups. Conversely, the south American group, the Aymara Indians, who have a notably bland diet, show far less liking for salty, bitter, and sour tastes, but not sweet tastes, relative to control groups exposed to more varied diets (John and Keen 1985). Presumably, the differences in responsiveness between all of these groups are driven, at least in part, by dietary experience.

The effects of dietary experience have been explored quite extensively in respect of the chilli pepper. People clearly develop a preference for its burn, as plots of liking/disliking versus perceived intensity show different patterns for individuals who report frequent versus infrequent consumption. Frequent users show an inverted 'U' response, liking increasing with intensity to an optimum, and then progressive reductions in liking with further increases in intensity. In contrast, infrequent users show progressive disliking as perceived intensity increases (Stevenson and Yeomans 1993). Clearly, desensitization to the effects of capsaicin cannot wholly explain this difference in response. The participants who report frequently using capsaicin, although clearly less responsive to the same concentration than infrequent users, like capsaicin *because* of its burn, not despite it. However, they only like it when it is restricted to the mouth—not in the eyes or on some other part of the body (Rozin and Shenker 1989).

Several possible explanations for how participants come to like the burn of the chilli pepper have been advanced and all may play a part. Chilli's use in traditional diets is often associated with foods that are bland and relatively unpalatable. Chilli not only provides a rich source of vitamin A and C, but it also actively promotes salivation, making unpalatable bland diets much easier to consume (Rozin 1990). Actual study of preference development in naturalistic settings suggests that social modelling may be important in initiating use. Rozin and Schiller (1980) noted that no overt pressure was ever put on Mexican children to consume chilli, however, chilli condiments were always available at mealtimes and adults routinely used them.

Once initial exposure has taken place, how can one explain the ability to like a burning sensation? The burn that capsaicin produces is a 'false-alarm' as it is not accompanied by tissue damage. Only experience with it (and seeing others consume it without negative consequences) can demonstrate this. Indeed, associations between constrained risk and sensation seeking, and a liking for the chilli burn have been noted (Terasaki and Imada 1988). Learning to *interpret* the burning sensation as pleasurable and harmless may be the key to understanding how liking for it develops following initial exposure. Several studies in different domains have demonstrated similar effects that may arguably apply to chilli. Salkovskis and Clark (1990) had participants hyperventilate following two divergent sets of instructions, one of which emphasized the interesting and positive nature of the resulting state (altered state of consciousness) whilst the other concentrated on a more negative interpretation. Perhaps not surprisingly, participants given the positive interpretation reported the hyperventilation experience as pleasurable—unlike the negative interpretation group. Similar findings have been obtained with other stimulus materials (see Anderson and Pennebaker 1980). So whilst humans may enter the world with a limited set of innate preferences and aversions, even these can be modified by experience.

Violated expectations

Day-to-day experience with food and drink allows us to acquire a large body of knowledge about them. We know, e.g. that tea should be served hot, and drinking water cold, and when these expectations are violated—in this example, expected temperature—the stimulus is generally disliked (Zellner *et al.* 1988). Apart from acquired knowledge, information about a food or drink may come from two further sources that were discussed above, specific information about a product (e.g. information on a restaurant menu or product packaging) and from the visual appearance and odour of a food that one is about to eat. Not surprisingly, colouring foods or drinks in a way that leads to a particular expectation about it's flavour can lead to dislike and rejection of that food if this expectation is violated when it is subsequently ingested. This is only likely to occur if the flavour experienced in the mouth is notably different from what one expected (e.g. DuBose *et al.* 1980, Zellner *et al.* 1991).

When a food or drink is manipulated in some way so that its appearance (or the information provided) is misleading, two possible hedonic outcomes may occur, and both have been documented in the literature. Under some conditions, a participant may demonstrate assimilation, in which the hedonic rating of the violated food or drink 'moves' towards the hedonic expectation. Under other conditions, a participant may demonstrate contrast, in which the hedonic rating of the violated food or drink 'moves' away from the hedonic expectation. Finally, when expectations are confirmed, there should be little change in hedonic ratings. Before examining theoretical considerations, namely the conditions that may dictate assimilation or contrast, examples of both will be reviewed.

Several studies that have manipulated participants' expectations have obtained assimilation effects (e.g. Cardello *et al.* 1985, Schifferstein *et al.* 1999). Cardello and Sawyer (1992), Experiment 2, selected a tropical fruit juice that was found to be hedonically neutral in a large-scale prior pilot test. Four groups of participants were then formed, one received accurate information (most people were indifferent to this drink), a second group received negative information (most people disliked this drink), a third group received positive information (most people liked this drink), and a fourth group were not given any information. Each group then examined the drink and estimated how much they thought they would like or dislike it. These ratings confirmed that the participants' expectations were in line with the experimental manipulation. They then sampled the drink and gave hedonic ratings of its acceptability. Some evidence for an assimilation effect was obtained, but only for the group that received the positive information, as their actual hedonic rating of the juice was significantly higher than that obtained in the accurate information and no information groups. Negative information had no effect.

In a further experiment (E3), participants were asked to sample a range of cola drinks and rate how much they liked or disliked each one. Then participants were assigned to one of six experimental groups (see Table 5.5 for design and results) and sampled colas either disguised as ones they had previously repoted

Table 5.5 Design and results for the cola expectation experiment (data adapted from Cardello and Sawyer (1992))

Group	Brand expected	Hedonic expectation	Brand *actually* tasted	Prior hedonic rating	Hedonic rating obtained
1	Bad	3.8	**Good**	**7.8**	6.4
2	Good	6.1	**Bad**	**2.4**	6.0
3	Neutral	5.3	**Good**	**7.8**	6.1
4	Neutral	5.3	**Bad**	**2.2**	5.5
5	Bad	5.2	**Bad**	**2.2**	5.6
6	Good	6.5	**Good**	**7.8**	7.4

as liking or disliking, or the actual liked or disliked colas from the pre-test. In all of the cases where expectations were manipulated (Groups 1–4 on Table 5.5), assimilation was evident, in that where the expected rating was lower than the prior hedonic rating, then so was the obtained rating (i.e. Groups 1 and 3). Similarly, where the expected ratings were higher than the prior hedonic rating, then so was the obtained rating (i.e. Groups 2 and 4). Note that Group 5's expectations were somewhat anomalous when compared to their actual ratings obtained on pre-test. As discussed later, this may imply that the actual differences here (i.e. between 'bad' and 'good' colas) may not be large, and this, as will become apparent, may be one determinant of whether assimilation or contrast occurs.

Two more recent sets of experiments have also demonstrated contrast effects. Zellner *et al.* (2004) assigned participants to three groups. One group was told that they would be asked to taste a mouth cleanser, a second that they would be asked to taste a Japanese candy, and a third group was not given any expectancy information. Based upon prior experimental work, Zellner *et al.* (2004) knew that participants tend to like candy, but not mouth cleansers. They hypothesized that whilst participants may report that they would *expect* to like Japanese candy, there should be significant uncertainty around this expectancy, which should then lead to more attention towards the stimulus and thus a greater awareness of the discrepancy between their prior expectation and the flavour of the stimulus. This prediction was confirmed, in that the candy group reported the stimulus as significantly more unpleasant, than the other two groups—i.e. a contrast effect. Zellner *et al.* (2004) then replicated this effect with a fruit drink, again labelled in such a way as to induce sufficient uncertainty about the expected hedonic value so as to promote attention to the stimulus. In a further two experiments (3a and b) participants were given information about ratings obtained from American participants who had previously evaluated the stimulus (the stimuli being the same as used above). In this case, Zellner *et al.* (2004) argued, participants should be sufficiently confident about the ratings and so should not pay undue attention to the stimulus. Consequently, an assimilation effect would be expected, and this was obtained.

Yeomans *et al.* (2008) provided a further demonstration of contrast using a food that had the same visual appearance as a sweet and fruity ice cream, but which in fact was a savoury salmon-flavoured ice cream. In their Experiment 3, participants were instructed to examine the stimulus, which was labelled either as ice cream, savoury mousse, or came with no label. After providing their expected hedonic ratings, participants were asked to sample the stimulus and to provide hedonic ratings again. The pre and post hedonic ratings are presented in Figure 5.2. It is readily apparent that expecting 'ice cream' leads to

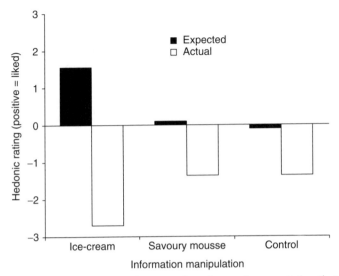

Fig. 5.2 Hedonic ratings of salmon ice cream based upon the expectation that it is 'ice cream' (i.e. sweet and fruity), a savoury mousse, or with no information (data adapted from Yeomans *et al.* (2008)).

a positive expectation that is clearly violated when participants actually sample the stimulus. In this case, there is nothing that might unduly affect participants' certainty about their expectancies; rather, here it is the stunning perceptual difference between the actual taste and the expectation (which was ascertained to be sweet and fruity in the ice cream label group) that results in the observed contrast effect.

In a particularly cogent discussion of expectancy effects, Zellner *et al.* (2004) suggested drawing upon the wider literature (i.e. beyond food) on hedonic context effects as a means for understanding the conditions under which assimilation and contrast occur. According to Wilson and Klaaren (1992), contrast effects will be more likely to occur when a participant notices the discrepancy between their expectation and the stimulus (i.e. see Yeomans *et al.* (2008) result above). In addition, when participants are certain about their expectation, they will likely pay less attention to the stimulus and so be more likely to demonstrate assimilation (i.e. Zellner *et al.* 2004, E3a and b). Relatedly, with greater uncertainty more attention will be devoted to the stimulus, thus increasing the possibility of noticing a discrepancy and hence a contrast effect (i.e. Zellner *et al.* 2004, E2a and b). Finally, ambiguous stimuli will more likely be prone to assimilation effects. This is consistent with Cardello and Sawyer's (1992) cola study, where the colas were probably quite similar (recall the shifts in liking for Group 5 when asked to re-evaluate the least-liked colas), and thus, in some sense, more ambiguous and hence prone to assimilation effects.

Finally, there are instances where a food is placed in the mouth, but the resulting flavour is appreciably different to how the food tasted before. Needless to say, all of the examples above involve some form of contrast (i.e. flavour in the mouth vs. expectation), but the point of contrast in these examples may be generated semantically (i.e. 'I expect this to taste sweet and fruity'). However, there may be another point of contrast based upon flavour memory. Flavour memory *could* play a role in the forms of contrast described above—i.e. participants' expectations could activate flavour memory and it is to this that current flavour perception is compared. In addition, flavour memories could be redintegrated by the retronasal olfactory component of the currently present flavour. Any difference between the percept and memory could result in attention being directed towards the stimulus and rejection. This type of comparative process might be a further contributor to the cross-modal interactions discussed in Chapters Two and Three (i.e. the retronasal olfactory component of flavour redintegrates a flavour memory that includes a sweet-taste component).

Discussion—Function two

There appear to be two principal mechanisms that can act to prevent (or promote) ingestion once a food has been placed in the mouth. The first of these relies primarily on innate preferences and aversions—preference for sweet and aversion for sour, bitter, and irritant sensations. However, whilst these reactions may be innate, they are clearly modified by both experience and other genetically based predispositions, notably sensitivity to bitter-tasting PROP. The second mechanism relies upon participants' expectations of how a food will taste. Violation of these expectations may lead to rejection when the discrepancy is large (and negative) or where the participant is carefully attending to the stimulus and perhaps *looking* for grounds to reject it.

Function three—Decisions about how much to ingest

Once a food or drink is in the mouth and a decision to ingest has been made, a food may taste initially very appetizing (the appetizer effect), promoting intake, then less appetizing (sensory-specific satiety), reducing intake, and finally after the meal is complete the smell of more food may be mildly aversive until hunger ensues and food-related cues start to evoke positive hedonic responses again (alliaesthesia). Other hedonism-related factors may also modify ingestive behaviour during a meal, notably specific appetites which may make certain foods especially appealing, as well as the consequences of learning the satiating effects of a particular food (i.e. using its flavour as a cue to its satiating effects). All of these factors contribute (along with *many* other processes that deviate to far from the core areas of this book) to function three.

Appetite promotion

Most of the processes considered in this section relate to reducing intake. However, there is good evidence that at the start of a meal there is an initial increase in hunger over the first 25% of it, *if* the food is highly palatable (Yeomans 2000; see Figure 5.3). Yeomans (2000) has termed this the appetizer effect and it is only observed, all other things being equal, if the food consumed is actually liked by the participant; if it is not, then hunger ratings tend to fall linearly with the amount consumed (see Figure 5.3). The role of flavour hedonics in this process is exemplified by the effect that opioid antagonists have on the appetizer effect. As noted above, several authors have suggested that endogenous opioids are involved in flavour hedonics. If the appetizer effect is driven by meal palatability, then opioid antagonists such as naltrexone should selectively affect the linear increase in hunger observed over the first quarter of a meal. Just such an effect has been observed in human participants (Yeomans and Gray 1997; see Figure 5.3).

Both prior to a meal, and during a meal, specific foods may be chosen and consumed over others, so as to meet particular dietary needs peculiar to that person at that time. There has been a long interest in this issue and it has taken

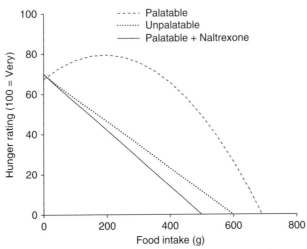

Fig. 5.3 Hunger ratings over the course of a meal, by food intake, for a palatable and unpalatable food, and for a palatable food following administration of naltrexone in human volunteers (data adapted from Yeomans (2000) and Yeomans and Gray (1997)).

several forms. One form concerns 'specific appetites', i.e. whether a preference may develop for a food that contains a particular micronutrient. Another is whether people or animals under ideal conditions will *purposefully* choose a diet that meets all of the bodies needs. In general, the evidence for such specific appetites, especially as it applies to particular micronutrients, notably vitamins, is not convincing. The contemporary perspective is that neither humans nor animals can reliably detect foods that contain vitamins for which they have a deficiency (Galef 1991). Indeed, examining, e.g. the history of scurvy or any of the other nutritional deficiencies, exemplifies how difficult it has been to relate the physical consequences of vitamin deficiencies to food, rather than to some other cause (see Gratzer (2005) for the fascinating history of this topic). However, note that the flavour system does contain a powerful process to boost dietary variety, namely sensory-specific satiety, and the role of this process in regulating intake is discussed further below.

One clear exception to the general statement above, are specific appetites for salt. Salt need is complicated to study in humans as discretionary salt use (i.e. the salt shaker) does not actually account for much of the salt that is consumed in our diet. However, there is certainly evidence in humans that liking for salt is affected by the climatic conditions under which people live. Leshem *et al.* (2008) studied female Bedouin participants who still lived under relatively traditional circumstances in the Negev desert, relative to Bedouins and Jewish women who lived in towns (i.e. access to climate control, running water, etc.). Leshem *et al.* (2008) found that not only had the traditional Bedouin women experienced more episodes of dehydration than the other two groups, they also had significantly higher liking ratings for more concentrated salt solutions than controls.

Exercise can also produce somewhat similar effects. Leshem *et al.* (1999) examined differences in preference for salt in soup, before and after exercise in one group, and over the same interval, but without exercise in a control group. Preferred level of salt in the soup was elevated by around 50% following exercise, but without any change in the control group, or in both groups' preference for sugar in tea. These results are similar to those obtained in numerous animal studies, and arguably reflect hormonal influences (aldosterone and angiotensin) on salt preference driven by dehydration.

Intake regulation

Two hedonism-related mechanisms contribute to regulating food intake during the course of a meal. The first of these concerns learned satiety. This is arguably composed of two facets—a hedonic one relating to a state-dependent affective reaction to the target food's flavour (positive when energy depleted and negative when sated) and a regulatory one, relating to reduced consumption of either the target foods, or other foods, based upon knowledge (implicit or explicit) of the foods satiating value. As already discussed, there is good evidence for flavour–nutrient learning, however the evidence for learned satiety is not so compelling, with some positive demonstrations in adults (Booth *et al.* 1982, Booth *et al.* 1976), and children (Birch *et al.* 1990), along with at least two cases in adults where the effect was not be obtained (Brunstrom and Mitchell 2007, Shaffer and Tepper 1994).

The second mechanism, sensory-specific satiety, is very well supported and is arguably an important mechanism for ceasing consumption prior to the operation of regulatory signals emanating from the gut (Hetherington 1996; but see Mook and Votaw (1992)). The effects of sensory-specific satiety are demonstrable by measures of intake and hedonics. Rolls *et al.* (1981) gave female participants in one experiment access to either sandwiches with just one sort of filling, or to sandwiches with four different types of filling. Participants given four fillings ate approximately 380 g of sandwiches, compared to the 290 g eaten by those with access to just one sort of filling. Similarly, in a second study using yoghurts, participants with access to just one flavour ate around 620 g compared to 730 g when given access to three successive flavours (note here the relationship to promoting *variety* of intake). Hedonic ratings of a food's odour also reveal parallel effects. Rolls and Rolls (1997) had participants in Experiment 1 eat banana to satiety on one test day and chicken to satiety on another. Liking ratings were obtained for the odours of both of these foods, and control foods, before and after each meal. As is readily apparent in Figure 5.4

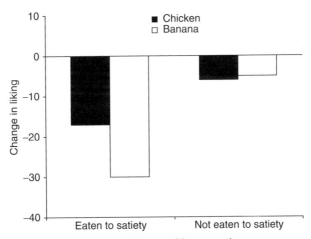

Fig. 5.4 Mean change in liking for chicken and banana odours across a meal composed of either chicken or banana (data adapted from Rolls and Rolls (1997)).

hedonic ratings of the food consumed to satiety reveal a larger negative shift in liking than the smell of foods not eaten to satiety. Both sets of findings, the consumption and hedonic data, suggest these effects are complimentary.

Not only can changes in liking be observed for the odour of a food eaten to satiety, but other characteristics of the food are also subject to the same affective shifts, notably its taste, texture, and visual appearance, independent of any actual perceptual change (Sorensen *et al.* 2003). These changes also appear to be both, independent of the calories consumed during a meal (Rolls *et al.* 1988) and independent of the type of macronutrient that constitutes the target food (Johnson and Vickers 1993). Although these conclusions about independence from energy and macronutrient type are consistent with the theoretical model of sensory-specific satiety (i.e. intake control prior to post-ingestive physiological signals) and most data, there are some reports that both caloric load and macronutrient type can affect it (Johnson and Vickers 1993, Johnson and Vickers 1992). However, if such influences exist they are probably small, as sensory-specific satiety can be obtained by repeatedly smelling certain foods, or by chewing them rather than ingesting them (e.g. Rolls and Rolls 1997). Indeed, in studies where ingestion does take place, it may be more sensitive to volume consumed (i.e. physiological signals from the stomach) than to calories (Romer *et al.* 2006). Finally, the relatively rapid onset of sensory-specific satiety, following the start of ingesting a target food, would also argue against a primarily energy-based effect.

Several studies have explored the neural correlates of sensory-specific satiety. In animals, where the same sort of effect can also be obtained, it appears that endogenous opioids may have a role in underpinning changes in palatability—at least in as much as these effects are indexed by consumption in rats. Wooley *et al.* (2007) established that for a pre-fed flavour, opioid receptor agonists could act to increase consumption (i.e. reduce sensory-specific satiety) whilst opioid receptor antagonists could act to reduce consumption of a recently consumed flavour (i.e. not an effect of neophobia, but arguably of induced sensory-specific satiety). The drugs in these experiments were administered directly to the nucleus accumbens, a structure that has been implicated previously in supporting orosensory reward (Berridge and Kringelbach 2008). In humans, several neuroimaging studies have specifically implicated the orbitofrontal cortex as the structure whose activity corresponds most closely to the changes in liking observed for food-related stimuli (O'Doherty *et al.* 2000, Kringelbach *et al.* 2000, Small *et al.* 2001). As noted above, it may be that this structure is the point of decision, in which affect-related signals from subcortical regions (and signals relating to incentive salience—wanting) are integrated into the final behavioural and affective response shown by the participant.

Sensory-specific satiety commences fairly rapidly and is operational before post-ingestive signals (excepting possibly gastric ones) indicate the energy content of the food consumed. However, another system relies wholly upon energy-based physiological signals. Cabanac (1971) has described the role of such internal signals in modifying hedonic response to motivationally relevant stimuli (e.g. sweetness in respect of hunger/satiety), a process that he has termed alliaesthesia (change of sensation). Alliaesthesia, as it applies to foods, has been explored in two basic ways, response to sweet tastes, and response to food and non-food odours. When people are hungry, some at least, will enjoy the sweet taste of sucrose. Following ingestion of energy, the enjoyment of sucrose will diminish, to be regained progressively as the state of energy repletion declines and depletion ensues (e.g. Cabanac and Fantino 1977). The same effect has also been documented for food-related odours—these may be markedly pleasant before consuming energy, and significantly less pleasant after consumption, returning progressively to a positive hedonic reaction as depletion increases (Duclaux et al. 1973). There are no equivalent depletion-sensitive changes for non-food odours.

It is apparent that these changes in affective responding to the same stimulus under different states of depletion are dictated by calories and not by the volume of material ingested (Cabanac and Fantino 1977). Similarly, it is not repeated exposure to the taste of sweetness that is important in generating the effect, but the consumption of energy, as alliaesthesia to sucrose can be produced following delivery of sucrose directly to the stomach via a nasogastric tube (Cabanac and Rabe 1976). This apparent dependence on calories and thus post-ingestive signals is further strengthened by the observation that alliaesthesia develops gradually over a period of 45 min to 1 h following a meal and then recedes (Cabanac and Fantino 1977). Alliaesthesia also has a more rapid onset if the calories are delivered to the small intestine rather than to the stomach, and the finding that mannitol, a sugar which can not be absorbed by the small intestine, can also generate alliaesthesia suggests that the effect may be mediated by receptors in the small intestine that are sensitive in some way (directly or indirectly) to carbohydrates (Cabanac and Fantino 1977).

The probable hard-wired nature of alliaesthesia is evidenced by its demonstration in 3-day-old human infants (Soussignan et al. 1999) and its observation in animals, where activity in the ventral pallidum correlates closely with the rats' ingestive behaviour for salt solutions under conditions of deprivation (salt-appetite) or non-deprivation. However, it also needs to be noted that many investigators have failed to convincingly demonstrate an alliaesthetic effect (e.g. Mower et al. 1977). In humans, at least, there may be several individual differences that affect whether or not it will be obtained, including gender and the participant's initial hedonic response to sucrose (e.g. Laeng et al. 1993).

Not surprisingly, and as described above, the brain's response to food-related cues under fasting and sated states differs. Whilst this does not directly address the neural mechanisms that may underpin alliaesthesia, it suggests structures that may be important. Hungry participants, shown pictures of foods versus non-food objects, demonstrate selective activation in the insular and left orbitofrontal cortex (Porubska *et al.* 2006). Similar results were obtained in hungry participants, when they were both shown and were able to smell food—i.e. activation in the insular and the orbitofrontal cortex (Wang *et al.* 2004). However, when the same participants are compared hungry versus sated to visual images of food or non-food objects, the amygdala is identified in such a contrast (LaBar *et al.* 2001). Likewise, Morris and Dolan (2001) reported that enhanced recognition memory for food-related pictures, when hungry versus sated, was differentially associated with amygdalar activation. In addition, this study also observed a role for the right lateral orbitofrontal cortex in selectively processing food-related stimuli in the hungry state, as well as increased activity in the nucleus acumbens to food-related stimuli in this state. Unfortunately, none of these studies include hedonic ratings of the food-related pictures, but it seems fair to expect that pleasantness ratings of food-related images would be higher before a meal and fall after. As all of these studies only look at short intervals *after* a meal, they are of less use in detailing the type of structures that might underpin the downwards shift in hedonic ratings that is allaiesthesia. However, the fasting condition used in all of these studies is revealing, and suggests a similar neural network to that outlined earlier. Hedonic sensations generated in response to food-related stimuli by subcortical structures (e.g. nucleus accumbens, amygdala, etc.) with cortical structures, notably the orbitofrontal cortex, integrating this output.

Discussion—Function three

Clearly, the body has at least three hedonism-related processes that are involved in appetite regulation. Palatable food may stimulate hunger in the early part of a meal, whilst a particular food will become less pleasant with more exposure, before post-ingestive cues start to operate (with the additional effect of promoting dietary variety). As the post-ingestive consequences of a meal come on line, hedonic responses to food and its smell become more negative. This reverses as hunger again ensues. Obviously, other factors too may influence hedonic response to particular foods and thus affect the amount ingested. For example, dysphoria has been suggested to promote consumption of carbohydrates, arguably to up-regulate serotonin and thus reduce negative mood. However, the evidence for these sorts of effects is inconsistent (e.g. Schlundt *et al.* 1993, Patel and Schlundt 2001).

General discussion

In this chapter, the principal argument has been that flavour hedonics contribute to three discrete functions: (1) acceptance or rejection of food prior to ingestion; (2) acceptance or rejection of food once it is initially placed in the mouth; and (3) regulation (partially at least) of the quantity and type of food ingested during a meal and following a meal. Two points are pertinent for discussion. The first concerns the extent to which hedonic states that are arguably involved in these three functions are consciously used in food choice (i.e. functions one and two) and in appetite regulation (i.e. function three). The position adopted here is that conscious decision making, involving affect, is important, but this comes with a significant caveat, in that many unconscious influences, psychological and biological, impact here as well (e.g. see De Castro 1996). As noted in the introduction, food choice can be significantly predicted, albeit imperfectly, by participants' reported food likes and dislikes (e.g. Glanz *et al.* 1998, Randall and Sanjur 1981, Tuorila 1990). The existence of this relationship suggests that hedonic states, which accompany thinking about, viewing, or smelling a food, are probably used in conscious decision making about which foods to eat. Therefore, function one is likely to entail a significant conscious component. The same is undoubtedly true for function two, especially if aversive stimuli can automatically engage attention—and thus enter consciousness (assuming here, as many do, that the focus of attention is synonymous with the current content of consciousness; see Velmans 1991).

It is the third function, namely regulating food intake, where there is likely to be most debate about the role of conscious processes. However, even here there are good grounds for thinking that conscious control is important. Theoretically, this is reflected, e.g. in the boundary model of food intake (Herman and Polivy 1984), which suggests that physiological factors only exert control, for healthy individuals, when hunger or satiety is relatively extreme. Empirically, one type of study, in particular, offers strong support for conscious regulation of appetite in the short term. Rozin *et al.* (1998) found that amnesic patients would readily accept and consume a second identical meal if this was presented shortly after consuming a first. A more recent study has replicated this finding (Higgs *et al.* 2008) and in addition observed that sensory-specific satiety is intact in such amnesic multiple-meal eaters. This new finding implies that sensory-specific satiety may not be an especially potent regulatory mechanism. In sum, conscious use of hedonic signals is probable for functions one and two, and whilst there are good grounds for conscious contribution to the regulation of food intake, hedonic influences may be less important here.

The second point for discussion concerns the distinction between liking, wanting, and needing as it applies to the three functions outlined in this chapter. The first function concerned acts prior to ingestion and so should involve significant inputs from wanting and needing, as well as liking. Needing can clearly be one factor in energizing the search for food, but there are likely to be many others that can also result in a state of hunger or a general desire to eat (e.g. temporal cues, TV adverts for food, etc.). For visual cues in particular, with their greater access to semantic information about food, it would be tempting to suggest that explicit wanting may be more strongly reflected in this modality, in contrast to orthonasal olfaction which may reflect more implicit wanting (i.e. paralleling the mechanisms argued to underpin the formation of hedonic reactions). The incentive salience of both, visual and olfactory, food-related cues will depend upon experience—i.e. the degree to which the associated foods were enjoyed in the past, so there should normally be concordance between the degree of wanting and liking for a flavour-related cue (i.e. what is liked is wanted, and what is wanted is liked).

As for the second function, this would appear to be more purely hedonic. Here acceptance or rejection is governed by the direct sensory properties of the food, its flavour. For function three, wanting for a particular food being eaten may initially increase, but only if the food is palatable. Wanting may then wane over the remainder of the meal. The initial increase in appetite for a palatable food (appetizer effect) would seem at least one instance of where wanting and liking are visibly dissociated in the current literature. Whilst hunger ratings (which may represent a specific wanting for the target food) increase linearly for a palatable food during the first part of a meal, liking ratings (or attractiveness ratings) do not (e.g. Yeomans 1996). Interestingly, the genesis of this effect, as described earlier, would appear to be hedonic, in that the appetizer effect is eliminated following opioid blockade. This would suggest that it is liking which engenders a second and separate process—wanting for that specific food.

Once a meal is underway, the particular foods being eaten appear to decline in pleasantness, which it has been suggested plays a role (but arguably not a particularly powerful one) in terminating the meal before any post-ingestive signals become available. Here one might suggest that it is not the hedonic tone of the food that is changing, but rather the desire to eat it. This may be conflated by participants in their ratings of pleasantness. According then to this perspective, a particular flavour should have a fixed level of pleasantness—a product of past experience with that food. This can act to cause wanting if it is liked, and once ingestion starts, it may increase wanting when the food is initially consumed. However, as the food is eaten, wanting may decrease independently of liking, but these two constructs may not be readily dissociable to participants. Finally, after the meal is complete, and post-ingestive satiety signals from the small intestine come into play, the absence of needing may reduce (but not eliminate) the ability of any rewarding food to induce a specific wanting.

The type of model advanced above could be stated as follows. Needing may up- or down-regulate the ability of any food to induce wanting. The ability of a food to induce wanting is based upon the degree to which it is liked. The degree to which the food is liked is primarily dependent upon experience, and baseline liking for a food's flavour may be that occurring under conditions that obtain prior to a meal (i.e. in a state of mild food deprivation or hunger). More specifically, this type of model, which obviously draws heavily upon three basic constructs—wanting, needing, and liking—assumes that it is a food's baseline level of liking which is responsible for inducing wanting. Based upon the various pieces of physiological evidence presented here, these three processes are each mediated by separate, but interacting, neural circuits that are then integrated into a final, consciously available decision by the orbitofrontal cortex.

Chapter 6

Flavour theory

Introduction

This chapter has two aims. The first is to present an integrative functional model of the flavour system derived from the preceding empirical chapters. The second aim is to examine three theoretical issues that arise from this functional model. The first concerns flavour as a perceptual system. The term is not used in the strict sense that Gibson (1966) defines it; rather, here it implies the idea of anatomically discrete sensory modalities cooperating to achieve particular functional goals (e.g. obtaining food, avoiding poisoning, etc.). This perspective has been championed, in varying degrees, by several recent reviews of flavour psychology and neuroscience (e.g. Abdi 2002, Auvray and Spence 2008, Small and Prescott 2005).

The second theoretical issue concerns the claim made in this book (and to varying extents elsewhere) that flavour is a preservative emergent property. There are three aspects to this problem: (1) Do two modes of flavour perception actually exist (i.e. unitary versus component)? (2) How are transitions made between these perceptual modes? (3) How do the mind and brain bind the anatomically disparate input from various sensory systems to produce the unitary flavour percept? All of these questions have been touched upon in earlier chapters, but the binding problem (question 3) has seen the least discussion and so occupies the most space here.

Several issues concerning binding are discussed. Binding may have both, a local aspect—namely binding of mouth-based receptor output—and a central aspect—the binding of the latter with smell. This distinction has been made by Verhagen and Engelen (2006), and they refer to it as that between peripheral and central multisensory integration. Whilst flavour represents one central binding problem, there is a second: namely how odour-induced tastes (and other redintegrated flavour percepts) are bound to the exteroceptive sense of smell, rather than to the mouth (Stevenson and Tomiczek 2007). Two related issues follow on from this discussion. The two forms of central binding involve, respectively, retronasal (flavour) and orthonasal (redintegrated flavour) olfaction. This distinction may be of considerable explanatory importance for flavour binding and the broader implications of perceptual differences between these two forms of olfactory stimulation are examined. A further concern is the 'potential' cost of binding. If odours (either orthonasally or retronasally) can redintegrate memories of prior flavour experience, this has the potential to interfere with current perception of events in the mouth. How does the flavour system resolve this problem, and is it a problem at all?

A third issue is whether a food's flavour can be considered as a form of multimodal object. A related problem is also examined, namely the variation in the flavour stimulus encountered over the course of a typical meal. For example, let us say one is eating a prototypical British dinner of meat, gravy, potatoes, and 'two veg'. During the course of ingesting this meal, the content, and thus the flavour, of individual mouthfuls of food may vary considerably; meat and gravy; potatoes and gravy; meat and vegetables, etc. This input variability, has potential implications for both viewing flavour as an 'object' and for the notion that the 'function' of binding (or multisensory integration) is to promote recognition, identification, localization, etc., these being the usual benefits accrued by bringing together anatomically disparate sources of information. Instead, for flavour, the functional benefits of binding are delayed, rather than immediate, and the implications of this are discussed.

Functional approach to flavour

The first part of this section presents a functional approach to the flavour system from a psychological perspective. The second part examines the putative neural substrates of these functions.

Psychological perspective

Based upon the earlier parts of this book, five different functions of flavour can be identified. These functions are organized here as a cycle, starting and ending with the search for food.

Function one—locating, identifying, and selecting food

The first function involves locating, identifying, and selecting food. Whether or not we consider ancestral (i.e. hunter–gatherer) or modern environments, a person has to locate food, identify whether or not the located items are food, and then select from such items those that are to be eaten. All three of these activities rely principally upon the eyes and the nose (i.e. orthonasal olfaction). Visual information can readily access both, semantic memories about a potential food source (e.g. was it tasty, is it safe, is it novel or familiar, is it nutritious, etc.) as well as yielding an affective reaction based upon its appearance and this knowledge. Negative affective reactions are likely to result from deviations from the norm (e.g. green sponge cake, unripe fruit, etc.) or from visible signs of decay or contamination. Most notably, the visual system enables rapid and accurate identification of food.

The nose also generates an affective reaction to potential foods, but in contrast to vision, the information which it accesses is primarily perceptual in form rather than semantic. Orthonasal odour perception draws upon prior experience with food by automatically redintegrating its flavour. Not only does this lead to an immediate sense of whether the item is a food or non-food, but it also provides a perceptual experience of its likely flavour, including its taste and possibly textural attributes such as fattiness. Orthonasal odour perception (as with retro-nasal perception) is especially sensitive to deviations from prior experience. Not only are these deviations experienced perceptually, i.e. a food may smell qualitatively different, but this will also be accompanied by negative affect—and similarly if the food had made one sick. However, if the food being sniffed had a pleasant taste before and was associated with energy or drugs, this should lead to a positive affective reaction, based again upon prior learning and memory. Together, visual and orthonasal olfactory information are complimentary. Not only do they act to locate, identify, and select food, they underpin the decision as to whether or not to place a food into the mouth. For this reason, and in this context, both vision and orthonasal olfaction have to be regarded as part of the flavour system, as both are 'users' of flavour-based information—semantic, perceptual, and affective—gained during previous bouts of feeding.

A prior requirement for function one (i.e. the context) is the presence of a suitable motivational state to initiate the search for food or drink—hunger or thirst. This motivational disposition is reflected both in whether food- or drink-seeking behaviour is initiated, and in the reaction that ensues when exposed to food- or drink-based cues that are encountered in this state (see e.g. Changizi and Hall 2001). Thus following a meal, an organism will experience reduced hedonic responsiveness or indeed, negative affect, to food-based cues—alliaesthesia. Once this state has dissipated, motivation to eat returns, and this will be one factor in the complex chain of events which leads to food-seeking behaviour. Then, when a food that was affectively pleasant before is encountered, or cues related to that food, this can engage a specific desire for that food—wanting. Wanting may then dictate the food item(s) that are ultimately selected for ingestion. Perceptually, all of these processes rely upon orthonasal olfaction and vision (and to a lesser extent audition too, this being functionally here more like vision).

Function two—harm detection in the mouth

The second function of the flavour system is to detect harmful food or drink when it is placed in the mouth. There are two components to this function.

The first relates to our general ability to detect the constituent taste and somatosensory parts of a food's flavour (i.e. the 'preservative' part of the preservative emergent property—flavour). This is, as argued earlier, of great functional significance. First, it allows the detection of essential micro- and macronutrients in new foods (i.e. sweet, salty, fatty, umami, etc.). Second, because it allows for the ready identification of a number of harmful situations—bitter tastes, burning sensations generated chemically or by hot objects, intense cold, the presence of hard or sharp physical contaminants (e.g. grit or glass), choking hazards (e.g. doughy and stringy), etc. Identification of these situations would lead to rejection of the food. In all of these cases, the reaction is based upon information drawn from the 'individual' senses that contribute to flavour. Many of these affective reactions are likely, initially at least, to be innate (i.e. bitter taste, oral pain, partial choking, etc.), and the presence of any one of these unimodal sensory signals may demand attention.

The second aspect of this function is the detection of deviations from the norm (i.e. prior experience)—i.e. where the flavour percept (i.e. the emergent property of both peripheral and central binding or multisensory integration) is a detectable mismatch with the expected experience. This can occur in two ways. First, the flavour of the food in the mouth may redintegrate perceptual memories of similar flavour experiences and where there is a mismatch between them, this *can* result in conscious awareness of a deviation. It is important to note that the threshold for this deviation detection is likely to be dependent upon a number of factors, most notably how much attention is being paid to the flavour. It is likely that tolerance for this form deviation is normally quite broad (after all, the flavours of natural foods do vary).

The second way in which this can occur, is where the appearance of the food leads to an expectation, which is then violated when the food is placed in the mouth. Whilst this second process is also based upon learning and memory, it likely involves a significant semantic component. For example, in the savoury ice cream experiment reported in Chapter 5 (Yeomans *et al.* 2008), participants clearly expected something sweet and fruity—and, of course, this was not what they got. It would seem unlikely that the visual appearance of the ice cream induced a fruity–sweet perceptual expectancy (although it may have primed one), but rather a semantic expectation that could be readily described in words. Irrespective of whether the expectancy violation is semantically or perceptually mediated (or both), the function is the same—to prevent ingestion of harmful or potentially harmful foods.

Function three—encoding experience with flavour

The third function of the flavour system is to encode and store flavour experience. This has two aspects to it that reflect the operation of a more conscious associative process and a less conscious encoding process. The former involves abstracting and converting perceptual experience into words and associating this semantic information with the visual appearance and name of the food. Thus, drawing again upon the example above, participants in Yeoman *et al.*'s (2008) experiment knew (i.e. this information was readily verbalizable and to hand) that ice cream of this colour normally tastes sweet and fruity, that it should be cold and smooth, and that they like or dislike it. The formation of this sort of semantic knowledge about food is important for the reasons identified above, and may assist in both Function one (identification/selection of food) and in Function two (detecting potentially harmful food). Not only is this semantic information obtained directly from experience with food, it is also acquired from a multitude of other sources, including observation of other consumers (and during development, one's parents and siblings), cookery books, TV advertising, etc.

The second encoding system relies upon the output of the flavour-binding system, which is then encoded as a flavour memory (dependent upon familiarity) in a form, which largely reflects the perceptual experience of that flavour. This type of memory formation process, although clearly a form of learning, is quite different from the type of learning that was described above. Flavour experience learning does not appear to require attention to the parts (i.e. you do not need to *know* that sweet and strawberry occurred together to acquire this flavour combination), it is rapid and resistant to change. As well as encoding the perceptual aspects of the experience, which like the original flavour itself is open to introspective analysis of the parts (i.e. taste, fatty, etc.), the encoding process also includes a significant affective component.

This affective learning process, which has been termed flavour–flavour learning (e.g. associating the pleasant affective property of a sweet taste with an odourant) whilst having similar properties (i.e. minimal need for conscious awareness of the parts, fast, and resistant to change) differs in that its output is sensitive to motivational state, whilst the output of perceptual flavour memory is not—i.e. a sweet smell will smell sweet when sniffed, irrespective of whether one is hungry or full, but ones hedonic reaction will be state-dependent. It would seem parsimonious to regard these two forms of encoding as identical, with both relying upon the same mnemonic system. The difference emerges in the way that motivational state operates upon *either* the recollected affect *or* upon the way that the perceptual flavour memory reengages hedonic systems.

Function four—regulating food intake

The fourth function of the flavour system concerns the regulation of food intake. This encompasses both the initial boost to intake generated by an affectively positive food (the appetizer effect) and the intake retarding effect of sensory-specific satiety. The former mechanism is likely to be partially dependent upon flavour/affective memory, as flavours that were associated with satiation (i.e. the product of flavour–calorie learning) are likely to be regarded as especially pleasant. Interestingly, the consequence of flavour–flavour (or CTA for that matter) are more likely to be important to Function One, as here the whole food is in the mouth, and thus the taste, somatosensory, and olfactory components are all present, and thus may generate affect 'directly' (e.g. sweet taste, creaminess, etc.). For this reason, affect that relates to positive post-ingestive consequences can probably exert an additional hedonic effect, beyond that directly produced by the stimulus.

For sensory-specific satiety, whilst this clearly relies upon the flavour, it does not appear to rely directly upon mnemonic processes—i.e. the gradual reduction in affect afforded by a particular flavour(s) is a likely consequence of a variety of factors, including initial hedonic response (e.g. very rich foods, whilst very palatable, appear to decline in pleasantness rather rapidly whilst bland foods do not), complexity, variability, and dynamic contrast. Whilst some of these factors may be affected by experience or motivational state (notably initial hedonic response), sensory-specific satiety would appear to be an innate intake regulatory mechanism that operates to modulate the amount consumed prior to the start of physiological satiety cues. In addition, it may also serve to promote dietary variety.

Function five—delayed consequence learning

The fifth, and final function of flavour, is one that occurs after a meal has ended and may not involve any direct conscious experience of flavour. This function, which clearly occurs (i.e. conditioned aversions, and calorie learning are well-established phenomena) must involve some form of intermediate memory store that retains a trace of the preceding ingestive episode (flavour memory) over the hours following the end of a meal. Whilst recency must be important to the content of this store, it is likely that more novel, but less recent, components of a meal's flavour could act to displace familiar but more recent items, allowing the more novel flavour to become associated with subsequent events (i.e. sickness or calories). This form of intermediate flavour memory store can be seen to parallel features of Wagner's (1981) SOP model, in which recent stimulus information is retained in an activated state, but is not available to consciousness. The content of this intermediate store may then be associated with post-ingestive events that primarily include drug effects, the satiating value of the food (i.e. flavour–calorie learning), and any nausea or vomiting that ensued after the meal.

Information on recent flavour experience is then displaced when the person consumes their next meal, and the associations formed during the prior inter-meal interval are retained and integrated into perceptual/affective flavour memory. Whether the post-ingestive events have to be consciously experienced for them to become associated with the activated flavour in the temporary memory store is not currently known (vomiting or nausea would suggest so, but what about post-ingestive effects of energy or drugs?). Whilst flavour–drug, flavour–calorie, and flavour–aversion learning appear to have properties that are similar to flavour–flavour learning (and to encoding of flavour experience), i.e. they are rapid (i.e. one or two trials) and require minimal conscious awareness of the event contingencies, the precise nature of these processes is poorly understood in humans.

Discussion

Two general observations can be made about this functional account. The first is to note its heavy reliance upon learning and memory, themes that have emerged throughout this book. This should not be surprising in context of the task facing an omnivore, namely lots of potential foods, making learning about nutritious and safe foods an essential component to successful dietary choice and hence survival and reproduction. The second observation is that flavour has to be both analysable and integrated—but more on this below.

Biological perspective

The following section considers some of the candidate neural systems that underpin the functions described above.

Function one—locating, identifying, and selecting food

The neural correlates of locating, identifying, and selecting food (Function One) are not directly known. However, it is possible to infer from similar processes a general picture of how this function may be instantiated by the brain. Two general statements can be made about accessing of semantic memories of food. The first, based upon meta-analysis of neuroimaging data, is that left frontal regions, notably the pars triangular of the inferior frontal gyrus and related areas (BA44-46) will be involved in semantic retrieval, along with other frontal (e.g. BA10) and temporal regions, too (Cabeza and Nyberg 2000, Buckner and Wheeler 2001). The second is that semantic information pertaining to food is likely to be stored in cortical areas directly adjacent to those involved in its perception or action components, as this appears to be a rather general feature of semantic memory storage. This is illustrated rather nicely by a recent neuroimaging study in which participants were simply asked to read olfactory-related words. This was found to activate the olfactory cortex (Gonzalez *et al.* 2006).

In terms of the ability of odours to redintegrate previous flavour-related experiences of which they were a part, the literature is more restricted. As detailed in Chapter 3, Stevenson *et al.* (2008) obtained evidence that to experience an odour-induced taste required an intact taste system—i.e. participants with defective taste perception (due to brain injury) or with known lesions in primary taste cortex (the insular) or the insula–amygdala circuit, were found to be impaired in their experience of odour-induced tastes, but not odour perception in general. Similarly, suggestive findings have been reported by Leger *et al.* (2003). This type of finding is consistent with redintegration, whereby a part (the odour) can recover a whole (the flavour). Whilst this perceptual redintegration may not be unique to olfaction in that there is evidence that something *similar* may occur when one tries to recall vivid visual or auditory experiences (e.g. Wheeler *et al.* 2000), it certainly is unique in that the process is both automatic and is not accompanied by any conscious awareness that it is an 'act of retrieval' (there are other features to that make olfactory redintegration unique, but more below). The nature of the neural processes underpinning this redintegration suggests that it may involve reactivation of the same neural networks that were active when the flavour itself was originally experienced. If it did not, then it is hard to explain why a damaged taste system should impair perception of odour-induced tastes.

The account above leaves three specific questions to be resolved. First, how does network reactivation take place? Second, how does the brain bind this reactivation to 'the nose' rather than to 'the mouth'? Third, do these processes occur automatically? Before addressing these questions it is necessary to raise a further one pertinent to Function One, namely how is affect integrated into this scheme, assuming here (as throughout) that the neural processes driving affect are down-stream of the initial perceptual processes. This point will be discussed later in this section.

Dealing first with network reactivation, this process is initiated via orthonasal olfactory perception. Following the generation of a glomerular-based activity pattern, unique to that odourant, the pattern passes largely intact to the piriform cortex—primary olfactory cortex. It is the output from this structure, which appears to have properties that are the first to most closely parallel conscious experience of smell (i.e. eliminative and affected by prior experience). It has been suggested that the piriform cortex may be one structure in which multimodal associations can be stored (Haberly 2001). These associations may not represent the experience *per se*, but rather act as pointers to other neural networks whose activation does result in conscious experience of redintegrated flavour. Thus the full associated flavour experience may be recovered by inputting the piriform output into a number of other neural networks, the same networks that were active when the original flavour was experienced.

There is an equally compelling alternative. In this case, rather than the piriform acting as the basis for locating the pointer (i.e. directing its output), the orbitofrontal cortex acts in this role. This structure has been repeatedly identified as a hub in flavour processing—both affective and perceptual—and it fulfils this role in Rolls' (2006) diagrammatic neural model of flavour processing. As there is good evidence that piriform output is largely preserved in form in the orbitofrontal cortex (Schoenbaum and Eichenbaum 1995), it is equally plausible that it is this structure which acts to point such output towards neural networks in other cortical areas (i.e. somatosensory and taste).

If this reactivation account is correct (irrespective of whether the orbitofrontal cortex or the piriform is its hub), the question arises as to how this redintegrated flavour is treated as a part of an odour, rather than belonging to the mouth (i.e. a flavour). Several mechanisms are possible and these are discussed later below when the issue of central binding is examined. A third and related question poised above concerned automaticity. It is important to note that automaticity is an assumption, but at least introspectively, certain odours *just* seem to smell sweet, i.e. one is not aware of having to make any effort to recollect whether or not the odour related to a sweet taste. One explanation for this immediacy may relate to the way in which olfactory information can directly access the neocortex, in contrast to all other sensory systems that relay first through the thalamus (Ray and Price 1992). This ability to obtain direct cortical access and reactivation of flavour-neural networks may be the neural parallel of automatic redintegration.

The final issue that was raised concerned the processing path for affective experience that accompanies both the sight and smell of food. Dealing with smell first, the assumption here is that affective reactions follow the initial perceptual processing outlined earlier, which is believed to occur in the piriform cortex. There is, however, an alternative view. Odours may engage two recognition processes, one primarily for perceptual purposes and another for affective processing. The reason why only one is assumed here (i.e. affective processing following initial perceptual processing) is to preserve parsimony. However, there is one interesting study, which implies that this may not be correct. Perl *et al.* (1992) found that patients with advanced Alzheimer's disease demonstrated appropriate facial expressions to foul smells. Many studies have found that Alzheimer's disease significantly impairs olfactory perceptual abilities, notably sensitivity and discrimination, so these results would appear to suggest an intact affective recognition system under conditions where no perceptual recognition system would be expected. Although this is an intriguing finding, it will take several similar results before a dual-route model looks likely.

If affective processing is downstream of the piriform, this could also be dependent upon reactivation of structures that underpin affective processing for flavour, as well as for smell (e.g. the amygdala). The most likely structure subserving this function is the orbitofrontal cortex, which has a well-established history of involvement in affective processing (e.g. Kringelbach *et al.* 2000). Integrating this with the perceptual processes described above might suggest the following. The piriform points its output towards structures that underpin the perceptual components of flavour, whilst the orbitofrontal cortex fulfils the same function for the affective components of flavour.

Obviously, the sight of food can also generate a positive (or negative) affective response. Output from the inferior temporal visual cortex (the 'what' stream) enters both the orbitofrontal cortex and the amygdala. Not only may this be important when considering how flavour-based learning is instantiated in the brain, it may also be crucial in accessing hedonic experiences connected with the food being viewed. However, one would note again, that introspection suggests a rather different form of affective reaction to a smell than to a visual stimulus, at least in respect to food. The smell of sour milk, e.g. 'feels' much more like a direct contact with the stimulus—and it is a more evocative and compelling experience—than the sight of curdled milk. It may be that whilst the orbitofrontal cortex can act to recover affective associates for visual input, the nature of what is recovered may be tangibly different, or at least less affect-laden.

Function two—harm detection in the mouth

The second function concerns detecting harmful (or beneficial) substances within a food and rejecting food on the basis of a mismatch between what is expected and what is experienced. Data from humans and animals suggests that the detection and rejection of bitter tastes can occur without a cortex (e.g. Bermudez-Rattoni 2004). Similarly, nociceptive behaviour can also be demonstrated in decerebrate animals—which will include responses to oral somatosensory stimuli produced by chemical, tactile, and thermal stimuli. However, whilst these responses may be intact, at least in humans it is likely that the conscious experience of aversive or painful stimuli requires an intact somatosensory cortex (for pain) as well as intact taste-based circuitry (i.e. amygdala–insula). As with all forms of aversive stimulation, these are likely to demand conscious attentional resources, and result in rejection of the oral stimulus.

There are at least two forms of mismatch detection, one based upon semantic knowledge and another based upon the actual flavour of the food versus flavour memory. The former is likely to be a conscious process and will probably rely upon similar circuits to those identified above for semantic retrieval (i.e. fronto-temporal) and visual identification (i.e. what stream) pathways into the orbitofrontal cortex. The latter may function automatically, and the result of the comparison process may be reflected in the percept. The percept of a mismatched stimulus may feel unusual—allowing its novelty or difference to become noticed (i.e. attention demanding) and this is also likely to be accompanied by negative affect. The larger the discrepancy, the more attention demanding and the more unpleasant the stimulus becomes. The same processes that were presumed to operate for redintegration of hedonic and affective circuits are also likely to be operative here (see above). Notice how detection of discrepancy is likely to attract attention and thus predispose the organism to learn about a novel stimulus. This, of course, raises a thorny issue. If flavour learning requires minimal conscious awareness, but learning only occurs with novel combinations, novel combinations are arguably attention demanding, apparently contradicting the observation that learning requires minimal conscious awareness. There is no easy answer to this paradox. It maybe that the stimuli used in laboratory studies of flavour learning are *just* novel enough to support learning, but not novel enough (i.e. attention demanding) to lead to conscious involvement in this process. Of course, in the real world such considerations may be irrelevant, especially if flavour learning of a novel compound engages both conscious processes (increasing the store of semantic knowledge) and those not dependent on awareness (increasing the store of perceptual knowledge).

Function three—encoding experience with flavour

The third function is learning; semantic, perceptual, and affective, before and during the experience of a food's flavour. For semantic learning, this will likely involve a range of structures, from the piriform to frontal structures known to be involved in associative learning. For perceptual learning, this will depend first of all upon stimulus novelty. This may not be such an important limitation for learning the name and properties of a food and its flavour (semantic learning) as this will often be a controlled process and thus the learner can voluntarily direct attention to relevant parts of the stimulus array. For encoding of flavour—perceptual learning—as noted earlier in Chapter 3, this seems to occur with minimal conscious awareness. The structures involved in learning a flavour are not fully understood. Verhagen and Engelen (2006) discuss a number of possible auto-associative neural networks that are candidate structures to support learning and, relatedly, the recovery of information following learning from the network. Many of the candidate structures are ones already highlighted in this discussion, including systems primarily located:(1) within the olfactory system (olfactory bulb, piriform cortex, entorhinal cortex, etc.) and insular, amygdalar, and orbitofrontal cortex; (2) hippocampal–orbitofrontal networks and; (3) perirhinal–entorhinal–hipoocampal networks. A similar picture is also likely for changing the affective properties of flavours, and their associated olfactory components.

Function four—regulating food intake

The fourth function concerns the promotion and regulation of ingestion. One potential mechanism for supporting the appetizer effect, i.e. increased consumption and hunger ratings with a pleasant food, was concomitant release of endogenous opioids in the nucleus accumbens, and this was discussed in Chapter 5. Similarly, in Chapter 5, mechanisms underpinning sensory-specific satiety were also identified, and these have been rather closely tied to the orbitofrontal cortex—to the extent that changes in hedonic ratings across the course of consumption for a specific food are found to correlate with activity within this structure. Whether activity within the orbitofrontal cortex directly supports affective qualia associated with sensory-specific satiety or with the use of affective information in decision-making processes remains to be determined.

Function five—delayed consequence learning

The fifth function of flavour involves delayed learning between a food's flavour and its post-ingestive effects (both good and bad). Logically, this requires two things. First, some form of tagging, activation, or storage is required for the most recently consumed food/flavour. Second, the degree of tagging or activation, or the maintenance of a flavour memory within a storage system, will be a function of food/flavour novelty. As noted above, at least as far as associative learning models go, the capacity to store information in the medium term is acknowledged to be a necessity to explain several learning phenomena. In terms of structures that might support this process, one possibility again is the orbitofrontal cortex; however, whilst it has been suggested that this might have a short-term storage capacity (Rolls 2006), an intermediate capacity has not been directly suggested. An alternate view is some form of subthreshold (threshold here referring to awareness) activation of the neural network pattern that encodes the flavour representation. Interestingly, in this case, one might expect to find evidence of reactivation of this pattern as post-ingestive information comes 'on-line'. However, neural activity during the aftermath of a meal has not been extensively studied.

Discussion

The central structures involved in supporting flavour perception and affect are quite well established, and these have been extensively reviewed in several recent articles (e.g. Rolls 2006, Verhagen and Engelen 2006). There seems little doubt that the orbitofrontal cortex occupies a central position in this regard. However, there are at least three areas in which there are clear shortfalls of knowledge. The first, and the most striking given its centrality to the flavour system, relates to the neural basis of flavour learning in humans. The second concerns the neural substrates that underpin flavour binding and orthonasal redintegration of flavour. The third involves the relationship between perceptual, semantic, and affective flavour processing. Whilst the second and third have seen some important initial work, notably with neuroimagining, the first is largely untouched in this regard. More generally—and as argued below—neuropsychological approaches to flavour, which are currently a rarity in the literature, may offer considerable insights into the nexus between brain systems and behaviour, as they have in several cognate areas (see Farah 1990).

Issues arising

The following sections deal with questions that arise out of the functional perspective on flavour presented above. This is organized into three sections. The first deals with the appropriateness of proposing a flavour system. The second deals with flavour as a preservative, emergent property. The third deals with multimodal objects, and the stimulus variability problem.

Flavour as a system

There are at least three ways in which one can conceptualize the organization of flavour. The first is to regard it as a disparate set of sensory modalities (taste, smell, somatosensation, etc.) whose output has to be bound together to yield the conscious experience of flavour. The second is to regard flavour itself as a discrete sensory 'modality'. The third is to regard flavour as a sensory 'system' that is organized to achieve a particular set of biologically significant functions. This third perspective is the one that is currently dominant within the literature (e.g. Abdi 2002, Auvray and Spence 2007, Small and Prescott 2005).

The first-mentioned alternative is grounded in sensory physiology. It also receives a lot of empirical support in that naive participants can readily identify many of the parts (individual tastes and somatosensation) that comprise flavour (and certain similarities for smell). However, even though we have this capacity, what we may perceive is typically more than just a collection of parts—there is an emergent property, one that is largely preservative in form to use Kubovy and Van Valkenburgs (2001) terminology.

The second-mentioned alternative, that flavour itself is a discrete sensory modality, does not have much to commend it. Viewing this from the perspective of sensory physiology, a sense is defined principally on the commonality of the receptor system it deploys (see e.g. Boring (1942) or indeed most (if not all) modern perception textbooks). Clearly, for flavour, these are diverse. Thus on the grounds of lack of commonality amongst receptor systems and given participants' naive ability to identify the taste and somatosensory components of flavour (and some olfactory similarities), this alternative looks decidedly unattractive.

The third-mentioned alternative, a flavour system, based loosely upon a Gibsonian perspective, has more to recommend it in that it focuses on how sensory input can be used to achieve particular functional goals. It does not seem at all inconsistent to regard flavour *both* as a functional system, whilst at the same time acknowledging that it is made up of discrete sensory systems (i.e. the first alternative above). In this view, the brain's and mind's task is to integrate (or not as the case may be) information from discrete sensory systems to achieve particular functional goals.

Two issues arise from this perspective. The first concerns delineating the extent of the 'system'. The view here is that *both*, orthonasal and retronasal, odour perceptions are central to the flavour system, with learning acting as a bridge between the two. This seems to be an inescapable consequence of the role of orthonasal olfaction in locating, identifying, and selecting food long before it goes anywhere near the mouth. The value of this process seems hard to ignore, as it allows ingestive decisions to be made without the risk of placing something that might be harmful in the mouth (Verhagen and Engelen (2006) make much the same point).

The visual system also contributes to this function in an equally important manner, by its superior ability (relative to smell) to draw upon semantic information via rapid object identification. The flavour system envisaged here thus encompasses both orthonasal and retronasal olfaction and visual processing as it relates to food (as well as, of course, taste and somatosensory input from the mouth). This system perspective also calls for a rather different take on the reason for generating a multisensory flavour percept in the mouth, which appears to be primarily for mnemonic purposes. Indeed, activities that occur prior to ingestion have typically been ignored, with the focus instead on events within the mouth. This perspective can be highly deceptive, because it leads one to consider events within the mouth outside of the broader context of ingestive behaviour—i.e. one might conclude that multisensory perception of flavour 'in the mouth' functions to assist identification and/or recognition of food. Well, in a strict sense it does not, because the visual system is probably far superior in regards to recognizing and identifying food, and the olfactory system, with full access to flavours past, can give a good guide to what sort of flavour experience may eventuate if the food is placed in the mouth. The closest to identification and recognition that flavour in the mouth might get, is probably in detecting mismatches between what is in the mouth and what one expected. But this is clearly a different function to that which emerges if you think that flavour in the mouth is used solely to identify or recognize a food.

The second issue arising from a systems perspective concerns the consequences that flow from taking a 'strong' approach to perspectives one (independent systems then binding) or three (functional system). A strong Gibsonian approach to flavour, or indeed to perception in general, places little emphasis on cognitive operations and internal states and considerable emphasis on invariant information directly available in the stimulus array. More recent Gibsonian perspectives on perception (e.g. Stoffrgen and Bardy 2001, O'Regan and Noe 2001) echo these themes. Direct pick-up of information from the stimulus array is not a tenable position to adopt in attempting to explain how the mind and brain execute the various functions described above. To know whether a food is good or bad requires inference based upon experience.

A point of outright conflict with a neo-Gibsonian approach emerges when considering dreams, imagery, and synaesthesia—where there is clearly perceptual experience either in the absence of stimulation or in the presence of an inappropriate stimulus. Not surprisingly then, the view that a food's odour may result in a percept that is flavour-like (e.g. something smells sweet) is incompatible with a strong version of this theory, but accumulating evidence, much of it reviewed in earlier chapters, leads inescapably to the conclusion that; (a) orthonasal olfaction can lead to percepts that contain inferential information and (b) that this information is of functional value. The real value then of Gibson's approach is to focus on function. This can be seen as a healthy counterweight to an overly zealous physiological approach with its emphasis on discrete sensory modalities. Function and thus perception require a different form of organization, one that is achieved by artful combination of inputs (binding), attention to components, learning, and memory.

Wholes, parts, and binding

In the introduction to this chapter, 3 questions were raised in respect of flavour perception—(1) Do two modes of perception actually exist? (2) How are transitions made between these perceptual modes? (3) How do the mind and brain bind the anatomically discrete input from various sensory systems to produce a unitary flavour percept? The claim has been made in this book that flavour is an example of a preservative emergent property. This statement presumes that there are two modes of perception—flavour (the emergent property) and parts (the preserved components). There is substantial evidence that taste and somatosensory parts can be perceived (see Chapters 3 and Four), even by naive participants, which would suggest that the latter contention is correct. The same can be extended to olfactory parts, but as discussed in Chapter 4 these are of a different type to taste and somatosensory elements. Olfactory parts are typically similarities, mnemonic constructs rather than reflecting more direct correspondences between stimulus and percept—elements. Is there a flavour (or unitary) mode of perception? The evidence that there is such a mode (examined in Chapters 3 and Four) is consistent with this idea, but the evidence base is rather indirect: (1) anosmics identifying themselves to medical professionals on the basis of loss of 'taste', not smell; (2) linguistic considerations, namely absence of smell-related words relating to experiences in the mouth; (3) processing considerations, namely temporal contiguity and commonality of location; (4) consequences of flavour, notably odour–taste learning and interaction effects; and (5) functional considerations that argue for the presence of this processing mode.

The second question that was posed concerned how transits are made between these two modes of perception. Clearly, participants can voluntarily shift their attention to the parts of flavour (see Chapters 2, 3, and 4) as they do when they make ratings of particular component elements or similarities. However, the default mode may be unitary perception—flavour. Whilst the empirical evidence for this may not be well developed, one can mount a good functional argument for this, based on the necessity to encode a general picture (i.e. the flavour) of the oral experience with a food, so that this overall impression can be accessed via the orthonasal olfactory system at a later point in time. This is discussed more extensively below when considering the functional benefits of binding. More importantly, a capacity to detect parts, particularly taste and somatosensory elements, is unambiguously important (see Function Two above) notably in detecting beneficial and harmful components. In this case, attention may be directed involuntarily to the components, especially if they produce negative affect.

The third question concerned binding. Revonsuo (1999) has identified two different binding problems. The first concerns the phenomenal unity of conscious experience, and so here, e.g. this would reflect our perception of flavour during routine eating and drinking. The second concerns functional binding, at either a cognitive or biological level of explanation. Here, e.g. this might reflect the temporal synchronization of taste, olfactory, and somatosensory stimulation, which functionally binds together these three modalities and which provides one 'possible' mechanism to account for the phenomenal unity of flavour. The assumption will be made here that the phenomenal unity of flavour experience arises directly from functional binding (whatever the mechanism/s may be responsible for this). In respect to the level of explanation, this rather depends upon the particularly type of binding that is under consideration, because as noted in the introduction to this chapter there is a potentially important distinction between peripheral and central forms (Verhagen and Engelen 2006).

Binding has been most extensively studied in the visual system, and it is quite apparent that several different mechanisms contribute to the phenomenal unity of visual experience (e.g. Robertson 2003, Humphrey and Riddoch 2006). Before turning to flavour binding it is useful to briefly examine these, as it would be rather surprising if there were not some commonalities between these mechanisms and those that the brain/mind deploys for flavour. Revonsuo (1999) has provided a very succinct typology of binding forms: (1) Gestalt laws, including simplicity, similarity, continuation, proximity, common fate, and familiarity, along with some more recent additions such as common region of space, connectedness, and temporal synchrony; (2) feature integration, such as colour and form, dependent upon focal attention; (3) semantic-conceptual binding, in which perception of a (typically) visual object automatically makes available knowledge about that object; (4) location binding of various visual objects to particular spatial locations within a scene; and (5) event binding, in which objects retain their identity and coherence as they transit in space and time. All of these forms of binding are demonstrably independent. This is most potently illustrated by specific neuropsychological deficits (N) or by experimentally induced performance deficits (E). For the five types of binding noted above, these are respectively: apperceptive agnosia (N), illusory conjunctions (E), semantic dementia (N), Balint's syndrome (N), and akinetopsia (N).

For flavour binding, there are several related issues that need to be considered—three different situations in which binding or binding-like processes appear to occur—and two considerations that are relevant to these binding operations. The first form of binding may occur at a peripheral level between the various taste and somatosensory receptors located in the mouth. The second form of binding is that between retronasal olfaction and orally based taste/somatosensory input, and this is presumed to have principally a central basis (e.g. Shepherd 2006, Simon *et al.* 2006). The third form of binding is that between redintegrated flavour percepts and orthonasal olfaction. After discussing these three forms of binding, two related issues are considered.

First, the distinction between orthonasal and retronasal olfaction and its neural correlates, and the effect that experience has on this distinction. Second, how for the second form of flavour binding (retronasal odour—oral input), the system manages or not to: (1) delineate redintegrative flavour from stimulus-generated flavour and (2) compute mismatches between redintegrative flavour and stimulus-generated flavour.

Peripheral binding-like processes of mouth-based modalities

A number of investigators have noted that multisensory integration can occur in the peripheral nervous system for the mouth-based senses (e.g. Verhagen and Engelen 2006, Simon *et al.* 2006). In many instances, binding and multisensory integration are synonymous, i.e. whilst binding problems have typically been restricted to considerations within a particular modality (notably vision), multisensory integration effectively refers to similar types of function, but which occur across the senses (see Robertson (2003) for a similar argument).

The claim of peripheral binding rests upon a number of interactions that were considered in Chapter 2. Notable intermodal examples are interactions between temperature and taste (thermal tastes), and taste and irritation (taste suppression of sweet and bitter). Intramodal examples include bitter and sweet tastes (suppression) and temperature and irritation ('hot' and 'cold' irritants). These types of interactions may rely upon common receptors for uncommon stimuli, such as the ability of chemaesthetic agents (e.g. capsaicin, menthol, etc.) to interact with receptors whose function is ostensibly to detect thermal energy. Alternatively, they can occur downstream from the receptor, such as where temperature affects TRPM5 ion channels, leading to depolarization of the taste receptor cell and an action potential (i.e. thermal tastes). Although it has been argued that these processes reflect peripheral integration, it is hard to see what functional benefit they yield. The general nature of coding of somatosensory and taste inputs appears to be based around preserving information about identity, because this has distinct value (avoid bitter tastes, avoid very hot or very cold, sharp, or gritty foods, consume sweet, fatty, salty, proteinaceous food, etc.). These interactions appear to add noise to the brain's ability to detect such parts and the absence of any obvious functional benefit (apart, of course, from that pertaining to cuisine where these are heavily exploited) suggests that they probably should not be considered as a form of functional binding.

Flavour binding (retronasal olfaction and oral inputs)

The flavour-binding problem is how the brain puts together the sensory information from olfactory, somatosensory, and taste inputs to produce the emergent property of flavour. This is, as repeatedly noted, a partially preservative process, in which individual taste and somatosensory components are available, although whether they are noticed depends upon the locus of attention and the presence of aversive stimuli, the latter automatically invoking attention. An immediate observation here is the role of attention. Attention is central to visual feature integration. If form and colour are presented outside of focal attention, this can result in illusory conjunctions—i.e. participants appear to bind colours and shapes in a manner different to that obtaining in the physical world (Treisman and Gelade 1980). In contrast, focal attention to the flavour stimulus maybe more likely to result in the perception of individual parts, suggesting that focal attention is not necessary to produce a unitary flavour percept. As discussed in Chapter 3, it rather appears that the default mode for perceiving flavour is the absence of focal attention, and focal attention occurs naturalistically only when something particularly aversive occurs or perhaps during psychophysical or sensory evaluation-like tasks.

Semantic-conceptual binding also appears to be conspicuous by its absence. Indeed, one of the reasons for focussing on the important role of vision in the initial selection and so on of food is its ability to readily access just this sort of information. It is interesting in this regard to consider the interactions between the visual system (and this applies to some extent to the auditory system too) and the chemo-somatosensory perception of flavour described in Chapters 2 and 4. Rather than being a perceptual interaction, vision's role may be crucial in setting an expectant context or frame of reference, in which the chemo-somatosensory information is evaluated. This is of course what was discussed above, namely the formation of semantic expectations.

The two principal explanations discussed in Chapter 3 to account for the unitary nature of flavour experience were common location and time, both of which can be subsumed under the Gestalt 'laws' of perceptual organization. Clearly temporal synchrony is important, as suggested by Von Bekesy's (1964) experiment, in which subtle asynchronies between taste and olfactory stimulation altered the apparent location of smell from the mouth to the tip of the nose. The neural basis of temporal synchrony could be achieved by the physical similarity in timing that must exist between events in the mouth and nose—i.e. once food is placed in the mouth, sensory output from olfactory, taste, and somatosensory receptors will become active at around the same time, and information from these senses will similarly converge at around the same time in multimodal cortex. Temporal synchrony would then appear to be important because it preserves information across the stimulus/receptor divide. Indeed, there are theories of binding that place considerable emphasis on temporal synchrony and these have been notably championed by Singer

(1996), who argues that temporal coherence of activated neurons is ultimately responsible for functional and phenomenal binding.

One potential problem for a temporal synchrony account is the intermittent or pulsatile nature of retronasal olfactory stimulation (see Chapter 1). Pulses of volatile-laden air are dispatched to the olfactory epithelium either after swallowing or during exhalations whilst chewing. Interestingly, there does not appear to be much conscious awareness of any waxing or waning in the olfactory component of a food's flavour. There could, e.g. be persistence of volatiles in the olfactory mucosa for sufficient time to preserve perceptual continuity or there may be some form of 'filling-in'. This makes understanding the precise dynamics of retronasal olfaction an important research question. Nonetheless, synchrony *might* be adversely affected by the pulsatile nature of retronasal perception.

A further consideration is common location. As we know introspectively, flavour is experienced in the mouth, not in the nose. Any mouth-based stimulus, even sugared water, will activate taste, temperature, and tactile receptors—these have both common physical timing *and* a common physical location. As described in Chapter 3, oral somatosensory stimulation that accompanies taste appears to distribute taste perception across the surface of the mouth. Information about physical location is likely to be represented in the brain by the 'mouth part' of the sensory homunculus in the somatosensory cortex. Similarly, information about taste will be represented in the insular cortex amongst other regions. Both taste and somatosensory input will also activate specific regions of the thalamus, as both access the cortex via this structure. There are several ways in which this spatial *and* temporal information could be used to bind *just* somatosensory and taste input: (1) the thalamus could act to index the common arrival time of information from the different senses; (2) the first point of multimodal convergence could act to index common arrival time; (3) activation of the sensory homunculus mouth area 'in conjunction' with (1) or (2) might then result in binding; (4) activation of the insular (primary taste cortex) 'in conjunction' with (1) or (2) could also result in binding.

The next step is the crucial one in considering the flavour-binding problem. Whilst olfactory, taste, and somatosensory stimulation all originate in the mouth, retronasal olfactory perception draws upon the same receptors as orthonasal olfactory perception—so how is retronasal smell perceived as being located in the mouth? There are at least three mechanisms that seem worth considering. The first is that a somatosensory distinction between orthonasal and retronasal odourant delivery, respectively, disables or enables binding, as long as the conditions described above are fulfilled (i.e. common oral timing and concomitant oral taste/somatosensory input). Nasal physiology lends some support to this hypothesis. The anterior portion of the nose, which is exposed to odourants during orthonasal olfaction, is more sensitive to chemical irritation than the posterior part of the nose (Frasnelli *et al.* 2004). Recall that most odourants are also irritants. Conversely, the posterior part of the nose appears to be more sensitive to mechanical stimulation (e.g. pulses of odourized air passing from the mouth into the nose). Thus differential somatosensory input, accompanying orthonasal and retronasal delivery, might provide information that either engages (posterior mechanical stimulation) or disengages (anterior chemaesthesis) binding.

A 'sole' dependence upon such somatosensory cues is unlikely to be the case. A series of currently on-going experiments in my laboratory has explored this. Participants are asked to judge whether an odour is located in a fluid they poured into their mouth, or in a fluid that they simultaneously sniff. On every trial, they exhale, pinch their nose, pour in a fluid (which in fact *never* contains an odourant), unpinch their nose, and sniff a fluid (which is either an odourant or a water blank). After they have inhaled, the nose is pinched shut, and the participant then exhales through their mouth. The key task is then for participants to judge whether the 'smell' they perceived came from the cup (i.e. in the mouth) or from the jar (i.e. in the nose). This judgment is made on a seven-point category scale from 1 (definitely in the jar) to 4 (unsure) to 7 (definitely in the mouth). For our purposes here, the results from several such experiments suggest that odours in the jar *can still be localized towards the mouth* even when active sniffing takes place. This would suggest that whilst differential nasal somatosensory input may contribute to binding, it is clearly not essential.

A second possibility is that any olfactory stimulation that is concurrent with the presence of oral stimulation (somatosensory alone or somatosensory and taste) will engage the binding process. Again, preliminary findings from the procedure described above suggest that somatosensory stimulation alone (achieved with mouth movements of varying vigour in one experiment and with stimuli of varying viscosity in another) will at best produce only a small shift in perceived location from jar to mouth. In contrast, stimulation with a taste (that obviously also includes oral somatosensation) produces a much more definitive shift. These results suggest that taste *and* somatosensation are more important than somatosensory stimulation alone for localizing an odour to the mouth (i.e. binding).

One apparent problem with this second possibility arises from the consequences of lesions to the insular cortex, which because of their effect on taste perception should result in impaired flavour binding. Whilst several studies have examined the impact of such lesions on taste perception (e.g. Cereda *et al.* 2002,

Mak *et al.* 2005, Pritchard *et al.* 1999, Stevenson *et al.* 2008), no investigator has yet reported that patients spontaneously describe gross abnormalities in flavour perception (i.e. binding failure). Needless to say, deficits in flavour binding in insular-lesioned patients could be subtle, i.e. they may only appear on tests such as the one described above (jar vs. mouth), and this needs to be tested. Alternatively, lesions, which damage the oral part of the sensory homunculus could also reveal flavour-binding deficits, but this does not appear to have been investigated either.

A third possibility concerns airflow direction over the olfactory mucosa. Several recent studies have examined the effect of delivering gaseous phase odourants either to the anterior or posterior nares using endoscopically placed catheters (Heilmann and Hummel 2004). Airflow rate is kept constant, so that the only major difference is between the release of odourants in the anterior nares (orthonasal) versus release in the posterior nares (retronasal). Several investigators have reported that this difference in delivery is sufficient to generate the localization illusion, such that odourants delivered to the anterior nares are perceived as coming from the external environment and those from the posterior nares as coming from the mouth (e.g. Hummel *et al.* 2006). Using this technique, Small *et al.* (2005) suggested that the crucial distinction might lie in the direction of odourant-flow across the olfactory mucosa. Indeed, Hummel *et al.* (2005) reported that whilst participants could not detect whether a pure odourant (i.e. one with *no* irritant properties), in a continuous air-stream, was delivered to the left or right nares, they could reliably detect whether it was delivered to the 'mouth' (i.e. retronasal—posterior delivery) or 'nose' (i.e. orthonasal—anterior delivery).

These findings suggest that odourant flow direction is detected by the olfactory epithelium, and this information *in and of itself* is sufficient to bind the stimulus to the mouth or the nose. Some preliminary evidence for this conclusion is provided by the observation of Small *et al.* (2005) that retronasal odour delivery (using the catheter procedure) resulted in differential neural activity (using fMRI) in brain regions associated with supporting the somatosensory representation of the mouth—in contrast to orthonasal presentation. This conclusion is tentative for two reasons. First, because the effect was not present for all of the odourants, yet all of the odourants were apparently perceived as being localized to the mouth in the retronasal (i.e. posterior delivery) condition. Second, as described above, sniffed odours can still be perceived as coming from the mouth even though the airflow direction in these experiments is clearly an orthonasal one.

To summarize, flavour binding appears to depend upon temporal synchronization and localization. Temporal synchronization is common to taste, smell, and somatosensory stimulation—i.e. it is a property of the stimulus and this information is likely to be preserved and used by the brain/mind. Location, on the other hand is more complex. Physically, taste, smell, and somatosensation all result from the stimulus in the mouth that is present during eating and drinking. Assignment to the mouth of taste and somatosensory stimulation may be readily accomplished as taste sensation is restricted solely to this physical location and will always be temporally correlated with somatosensory stimulation. The tricky problem is how the brain/mind identifies whether the odourant detected by the olfactory receptors comes from the mouth or the environment. There is only one set of odour receptors (disregarding left vs. right sides), but two potential origins for chemicals reaching the receptor surface. Three suggestions are currently tenable. First, that it depends upon somatosensory differences between orthonasal (higher chemaesthetic sensitivity) and retronasal (higher mechanical sensitivity) delivery. Second, that it depends upon temporal synchronization of *any* olfactory stimulation with oral stimulation, especially taste. Third, that the direction of odourant flow across the olfactory epithelium results in localization to the mouth or nose. These are not mutually exclusive possibilities and all are probably employed during routine flavour perception.

Flavour binding—functional considerations

So far the focus has been on mechanism, but it is also important to consider the functional and phenomenal consequences of flavour binding. First, functionally, binding results in: (1) a neural state that *can* be preferentially encoded into memory as a single event as well as (2) be compared (automatically) to prior flavour events. Notice that this distinguishes the learning (or encoding) process from the binding process. This assumption is based upon the observation that learning seems to occur preferentially for unfamiliar stimuli, yet binding appears to occur for all stimuli in the mouth. It would be preferable to have some firmer evidence upon which to draw this distinction and it *may* be that the two processes are far more entwined than is made out here (after all temporal contiguity was once thought to be the basis for associative learning and it is argued above that it is an important mechanism for binding).

Whilst there is plenty of evidence—much of it discussed at length in this book—that suggests that the product of binding is encoded into memory (i.e. learnt), there are far less data on the effects of disrupting the binding process. Would it, e.g. affect what is learnt and thus later redintegrated (remembered) or would it more directly affect the learning 'process', rather than the content of what is learnt? In other words, is there a functional cost for not binding? One means of disturbing the binding process might be to selectively attend to a part of a flavour. This would result in a percept dominated by the attended part. As discussed in Chapter 4, there is some evidence that this may disrupt learning *or* its content, but it is not a very consistent effect nor a very strong one.

A more recent piece of evidence, albeit from rats, suggests that retronasal delivery of an odourant results in the formation of a stronger conditioned-odour aversion than orthonasal presentation (Chapuis *et al.* 2007). This would suggest that there is a functional advantage to co-presentation in the mouth, but it does not tell us where this advantage is (and, of course, these findings are from rats, not humans). However, this advantage is not overwhelming in magnitude because a conditioned odour aversion could also be obtained by orthonasal means, but this required a shorter interval between presentation and poisoning, and even at shorter intervals, it was not as strong as conditioning obtained by retronasal delivery.

Phenomenally, binding results in a conscious unitary experience—flavour. Evidence for the unitary nature of this experience was reviewed in Chapter 4 and briefly described above. Earlier, in discussing Revonsuo's (1990) typology of binding, it was noted in passing that neuropsychological cases, and their observed pattern of deficits, had been instrumental in defining different forms of binding. It is striking how little data we have about the experience of flavour in neuropsychological populations and, as far as I am aware, there are no published articles at all dealing with flavour-binding failures. Of course, part of the problem is knowing what to look for and this may be a difficult task, especially if multiple mechanisms (as suggested above) contribute to it. Notwithstanding this, flavour-binding failures should still have detectable functional and phenomenal implications. Functionally, it might result in faulty encoding of flavour experience, so that, e.g. odour–taste learning might no longer be possible, even though both the olfactory and taste components of flavour would be perceived. Phenomenally, flavour experience might be fragmented. This is hard to imagine, but it could take the following form in which it would be difficult to simultaneously experience all of a flavour's elements, i.e. taste might dominate, then smell, then tactile stimulation. Alternatively, retronasal odour might be poorly localized to the mouth or easier to mis-localize to the tip of the nose than in an intact participant.

Flavour binding (orthonasal input and redintegrated flavour)

As discussed in Chapter's 2 and 3, an orthonasal odour that once formed part of a flavour can redintegrate the original flavour experience, such that the participant experiences, e.g. a 'sweet' and 'fatty' smell. In this case, the binding problem is how distributed activity within the brain—similar to that when the flavour was originally experienced—results in 'an olfactory experience'—i.e. one localized to the tip of the nose rather than to the mouth. Although it may sound ludicrous to suggest that orthonasal redintegration of flavour might lead to an 'oral' experience rather than, as it does, to a nasal experience, a moment's thought about redintegration should clarify why attribution to the nose *is* a problem. If the recovered flavour memory is complete, it should also logically engage the oral sensory homunculus, which according to the discussion above might then result in mouth-based binding—it does not, so why?

Two possibilities may account for nasal localization (or binding). The first, again, is the direction of airflow across the mucosal surface, which as discussed earlier may be of significance in dictating where an olfactory stimulus is perceived. The second possibility, and the two are not mutually exclusive, is thalamic activity. Redintegration of cortical activity—somatosensory and taste—will not obviously result in concomitant thalamic activity, because the cortical structures are not being accessed this way. It has long been acknowledged that one unusual anatomical feature of the olfactory system is its dual route to the cortex—directly from the piriform cortex and bulb, to the orbitofrontal cortex, and indirectly, via the mediodorsal thalamic nucleus (MDNT), and thence to the orbitofrontal cortex (Ray and Price 1992). Stevenson and Tomiczek (2007) suggested that it is activity in the MDNT, but not in thalamic nuclei that cater for taste and somatosensation, in conjunction with activity in somatosensory and taste cortex, that results in the experience of flavour attributed to the nose, rather than to the mouth.

The binding that results from these hypothetical processes generates a redintegrated flavour experience perceived as: (a) coming from the nose and thus from an environmental source and (b) more as a smell, than a flavour. Two implications flow from this account. The first is that if it is correct, it implies that thalamic activity may be important in the binding of taste, somatosensory experience, and odour to produce flavour. The second implication concerns synaesthesia in which stimulation of one sensory modality results in an experience in another (e.g. smell vanilla, experience vanilla *and* a sweet-taste-like sensation).

At least two definitions of synaesthesia can be found in the literature (Stevenson and Tomiczek 2007). The first, termed phenomenal synaesthesia, may result from the consumption of hallucinogens, sensory deprivation, or brain damage. In contrast, a second form of synaesthesia, which has attracted considerably more research attention (see Ward and Mattingley 2006), appears to result from neurodevelopmental causes, is likely to be neocortically based, is continuously present, and usually of a quite specific form (e.g. a particular word induces a particular flavour). In addition, it is readily identifiable by the observer and appears to require attention for a synaesthetic effect to occur. This is quite different from the type of experience that occurs when an orthonasal odour induces a taste—arguably another form of synaesthesia. Here it does not appear to require attention, it may not solely be a neocortical phenomenon, and it is not readily noticeable. In addition, and most strikingly of all, nearly everyone appears to experience odour-induced tastes, whilst phenomenal synaesthesia and neurodevelopmental synaesthesias are relatively rare. The implications of this are discussed further in Chapter 7.

The orthonasal and retronasal distinction

In the context of the arguments advanced above, one could crudely term orthonasal olfaction the 'retriever' and retronasal 'olfaction' the learner. Clearly, this is not an absolute, as there is extensive evidence that the olfactory system demonstrates plasticity via the orthonasal system, with some authors even going as far as to suggest this may be a fundamental component of olfaction (e.g. Wilson and Stevenson 2006). Nonetheless, for an odour that has been experienced as part of flavour, the orthonasal system allows the retrieval of sense and hedonic impressions of which that odour was a part. Similarly, we have the capacity to encode flavour experiences, which include a retronasal olfactory component. From this perspective, one might then expect some differences in the way that the brain responds to orthonasal and retronasal odourants—i.e. the former might be expected to more strongly engage retrieval processes for a flavour-related odour, and the latter to engage learning processes, especially for a more unfamiliar odour.

Two studies have tested the distinction between orthonasal and retronasal olfaction using fMRI and the delivery technique pioneered by Heilmann and Hummel (2004). Gerber et al. (2003) reported a small study using two non-food odours, but found relatively few differences between orthonasal and retronasal perception, with the insula having higher activation in the orthonasal condition. A more in-depth study by Small et al. (2005) examined responses to one food (chocolate) and three non-food odours. In comparisons of chocolate versus the other odourants, predominant activity with orthonasal stimulation (subtracting out retronasal), revealed enhanced thalamic, insular, orbitofrontal cortex, hippocampal, and amygdalar activity—all were more active when sniffing chocolate odour. Conversely, for retronasal perception (subtracting out orthonasal), activity was observed more definitively in the orbitofrontal cortex, along with activity in a range of structures (temporal gyrus, temporal operculum, periegnual cingulate, etc.) that may be associated with food reward. The major conclusion drawn by Small et al. (2005) was that these different patterns of activation reflect the operation of 'wanting' (orthonasal) and 'liking' (retronasal)—the amygdala representing anticipation of food reward and the temporal gyrus and others reflecting the receipt of food reward.

As discussed in Chapter 5, food hedonics is extremely important, and is reflective of the same basic processing distinction noted above—retrieving (orthonasal, anterior delivery) and learning (retronasal, posterior delivery). Learning, is of course, not well reflected in these data, as chocolate was likely to be highly familiar to all participants. Thus it is perhaps interesting to reflect on the structures active during 'sniffing' chocolate and so see the structures that may be differentially involved in retrieval (redintegration). From this perspective, three observations can be made about this study. First, the activity in the insular cortex under orthonasal conditions is interesting as this may relate to the redintegration of taste-based information (after all, chocolate is likely to smell sweet). Second, activity observed in the hippocampus and the orbitofrontal cortex under orthonasal conditions are also important, as these have been identified before as structures likely to be involved in the auto-associative networks that may underpin the retrieval or redintegrative process (Verhagen and Engelen 2006). Third, thalamic activity is especially noteworthy, as this may be an important component in binding orthonasally redintegrated flavour to the nose.

A further issue concerns whether orthonasal and retronasal stimulation of the olfactory mucosa, by the same odourant, results in a similar percept. Several investigators have reported that retronasal identification of odourants is more difficult (e.g. Pierce and Halpern 1996). In addition, thresholds and intensity-concentration functions may also differ (e.g. Diaz 2004), with typically greater sensitivity for the orthonasal system. Moreover, it appears, based upon animal work, that these differences in performance may owe something to the chemical nature of the stimulus, with the greatest difference (ortho vs. retronasal) in electrophysiological response between hydrophilic chemicals (Scott *et al.* 2007). Two points are raised by these findings. The first, is that subtle differences (or perhaps not so subtle differences in the case of polar chemicals) in neuronal activity patterns between the same odourant presented orthonasally versus retronasally, or indeed more generally, could be a further cue to the source of the stimulation (i.e. mouth vs. environment)—in addition to those of detecting the direction of odourant flow across the mucosal surface and so on.

Second, whilst the differences identified above are indisputable, it is important to note that the similarities in performance between orthonasal and retronasal perception are predominant. If this were not so, then transfer of knowledge from what is learned in the mouth to what is detected by the nose would be impeded and this does not seem to be the case. Indeed, a brief review of the evidence readily suggests that there is substantial transfer of knowledge between these two modes of olfactory presentation. For example take: (1) the many successful demonstrations of sweetness enhancement and odour–taste learning reviewed in Chapters 2 and 3, respectively, all of which require such positive transfer; (2) orthonasal identification predicts performance on retronasal identification (Chen and Halpern 2008), that is odours that are hard or easy to name in one mode are, similarly, hard or easy to name in the other; (3) retronasal identification itself is well above chance suggesting it must draw upon prior orthonasal name learning (e.g. Sun and Halpern 2005, Chen and Halpern 2008); and (4) there is significant positive transfer of identification learning between the two modes of presentation when tested experimentally (Pierce and Halpern 1996). So, whilst differences clearly do exist between these two modes of presentation, these differences may only exist to the extent that they are functionally useful. This functional value may be reflected in their contribution to localizing an odourant to the mouth or nose (environment).

A final distinction is between the way in which we react hedonically to the same odourant when presented either orthonasally or retronasally. Rozin (1982) identified this difference in regards to certain specific foods, such as strong-smelling blue cheese that may be appealing in the mouth (retronasal olfaction) but unappealing when sniffed (orthonasal olfaction). Although such differences may exist, there does not appear to have been any systematic exploration of them, and one might be tempted to suggest that they may be the exception rather than the rule. Indeed, in the few studies so far that have examined whether flavour-based learning can be detected using orthonasal and retronasal routes, Yeomans et al. (2007) found that flavour–drug (caffeine) and flavour–flavour learning were detectable via both modes of presentation. For unpleasant odours, such as that of the Durian (at least to Western noses), Stevenson et al. (2007) also found substantial transfer of the effects of presentation context between orthonasal and retronasal routes of delivery. That is, participants who sniffed durian odour (and then tasted it) after an unpleasant orthonasally presented olfactory context, liked it more in both modes (sniffed and tasted) than participants who had experienced a pleasant orthonasally presented context. Yet again, it would appear reasonable, from a functional perspective, to preserve hedonic responses across presentation modes for the same odourant, and this does appear to be true. Finally, and as suggested by Small et al. (2005), there is the issue of correspondence between orthonasal and retronasal stimulation, and wanting and liking. Perhaps, the engagement of neural systems underpinning either odour-driven wanting or liking also rests upon the mechanisms that assign an olfactory percept to either the mouth or nose.

Delineation and matching

Although it may be functionally advantageous for an orthonasally presented odour that was once part of a flavour, to be able to redintegrate that flavour, this could be *potentially* problematic if a retronasally presented odour were able to do the same. This is because it might interfere with veridical perception of flavour in the mouth. Indeed, to some extent this does appear to be the case, as with sweetness-taste enhancement and subthreshold integration of taste and smell, which were, of course, examined in Chapters 2 and 3. However, as noted in Chapter 3, sweetness-taste enhancement appears to be a less robust phenomenon than that of odour-induced tastes. Most notably, odour-induced tastes occur largely irrespective of how they are rated (single vs. multiple scales), yet sweetness-enhancement effects are quite sensitive to this manipulation. Moreover, enhancement effects are relatively modest, and it is notable that whilst sniffing odourants such as caramel, the apparent sweetness can be quite striking, but this effect appears much diminished in the mouth when combined with a real sweet taste or even water.

Two points need to be made about these observations. The first is to consider the role that experience with a flavour may have on the 'binding' processes. It is certainly possible that experience results in a more unified percept (stronger binding), the implication being that discrimination of individual parts might become more difficult. The only evidence that comes close to supporting this is from Ashkenazi and Marks (2004)—see Table 4.3 (and this was only indicative *and not statistically significant*)—but the issue has not been well explored. The second point concerns the apparent shift in magnitude of odour-induced tastes when experienced in the mouth versus in the nose. One possibility (albeit with no empirical support as yet) could be a suppressive effect on the redintegration process under conditions of retronasal stimulation, or when somatosensory and taste stimulation are present. Irrespective of the mechanism, this could function to reduce the impact of redintegrative flavour on the perception of real flavour.

Stevenson and Boakes (2003) suggested that for orthonasal odours, perception crucially depended upon a pattern-matching process. Even if the pattern was incomplete, it could act to retrieve the missing parts. What is perceived, according to this view, is as much an act of memory as of perception. Under conditions where the input pattern failed to match anything available in odour memory, learning takes place resulting in the encoding of the new pattern. This leads, behaviourally, to enhanced discriminative ability, as observed in a number of human and animal studies. Largely the same principles can be applied here to flavour. Take, e.g. a novel combination such as lychee (odourant) and sweet (sugar taste), presented retronasally. This input combination is bound and compared to past experience. The combination is novel and so it is learnt. For a familiar odour–taste combination, presented in the mouth, the combination is bound and compared to past experience. This comparative process may result in a match, a match that can then produce, e.g. the type of sweetness-taste-enhancement effects discussed earlier. However, this matching process may crucially act to detect departures from the norm—the norm being prior experience. Whether or not this departure demands attention may be a function of the discrepancy—and greater discrepancies will both be unpleasant (like an artificially flavoured orange juice) and attention demanding. This capacity to demand attention for larger discrepancies may be important for two reasons. First, it provides a ready mechanism for rejecting foods. Second, it may explain the apparent failure to demonstrate extinction-like phenomenon with odour–taste learning. Unless the discrepancy is sufficiently large, the participant may not be able to engage in consciously mediated associative learning, because if the discrepancy is not noticed, then the flavour system may not have the capacity to automatically learn the deviated combination— because it is a close enough match to prior experience to retard encoding.

Multimodal objects and flavour variability during a meal

A major functional benefit of multisensory perception is enhanced detection, recognition and location of biologically important stimuli (e.g. food, mates, predators). For example, in the second paragraph of the Introduction to the *Handbook of Multisensory Processing* (Calvert *et al.* 2004) the authors state 'There can be little doubt that our senses are designed to function in concert and that our brains are organised to use the information they derive from their various sensory channels cooperatively in order to enhance the probability that objects and events will be detected rapidly, identified correctly, and responded to appropriately' (op. cit., pg. xi). This view is wholly correct for visual and auditory interactions—such as, e.g. the ventriloquism or McGurk effects. But for flavour perception, which is clearly multisensory, and clearly perception, these types of functional attributes, detection, identification, and response appropriateness may be of far less immediate relevance (with the notable exceptions of 'creaminess' and 'auditory-texture' interactions—see Chapter 3). Rather, it is the capacity to generate a discrete output, flavour, from a multisensory input, and to then encode this, which represents the primary functional goal of this form of multisensory perception. Thus, whilst 'detection' of food, 'identification' of food, and decision to ingest ('response appropriateness') via orthonasal redintegration of flavour *may rely upon the outcome of earlier multisensory processing*, they are not functions that are relevant to flavour in the mouth.

The reason for raising this issue of functional benefit of multisensory processing is to tackle the question of whether flavours can be considered as multimodal objects. This question appears to me to be closely tied to a problem that has been shied away from in this book, namely the considerable variation in flavour that may take place within a meal. Before considering this issue and its implications, it is necessary to do two things. The first is to establish a working definition for multimodal objects. The definition used here for an object comes from Kubovy and Van Valkenburg (2001). They define an object as that which is susceptible to figure–ground segregation. This definition does not preclude the object being composed of parts that are derived from multiple sensory systems. The second is to examine whether or not flavour variation is a real problem and this is dealt with next.

If it is assumed that the flavour perception evolved to facilitate better nutritional choices (i.e. more calories, less poisoning, etc.) one way to assess the potential impact of flavour variation involves examining what our ancestors ate. This is premised on the assumption that ancestral diets shaped our current flavour system. Two general approaches to this are available. One is to look at the remnants of our ancestors, their bones, teeth, middens, and fire places, and from this infer things about their diet. The second is to draw upon anthropological research on modern hunter–gatherers, with the assumption (albeit with many caveats) that their dietary behaviour is 'broadly' reminiscent of our distant hunter–gatherer past. From the archaeological record, it is known that our early diet (*c.* 1.5 million years ago) was probably composed of scavenged (not hunted) meat, roots, nuts, and fruit (Larsen 2000). With the advent of the use of fire, and the use of this for cooking, which is estimated to have occurred some 0.5–1.4 million years ago, preparation of basic mixtures may have started—cooking in leaves, stomachs (haggis-like), etc. (Tannahill 1988).

A more revealing picture emerges from the anthropological record. For example, the Hadza, a hunter–gatherer group who live near lake Eyasi in Tanzania, eat food items in a sequential manner. That is, whilst out collecting berries or roots, the particular food item collected is consumed sequentially during collection, with only the excess (if any) brought back to camp—the same goes for game (Woodburn 1966). This might suggest that 'meals' typically contain relatively few, specific food items, and that those items are eaten in that 'sitting'. As more complex methods of food preparation require more ingredients, as well as more effort, this strategy of foraging and consumption *may* be an indication of the sort of dietary patterns for which the flavour system evolved—namely one with little variation *within* a meal.

Needless to say, with the shift from hunter–gathering to farming (around 7000 years ago), and the growth of villages and eventually towns, considerable dietary change occurred. In the main, there was a decline in the nutritional quality of the diet, with less variety and more reliance on specific staples (Ortner and Theobold 2000). Wide availability of food types and cooking methods, for the general populace, is (in First World countries) a very recent phenomenon, owing much to the development of food-storage technology, new farming methods, and a market economy (Fogel 2004). Thus a modern diet, with its emphasis on high within- and between-meal-flavour variety, and its use of cooking, is in evolutionary terms, a very recent development.

For a modern meal, there will be considerable variation in the flavour experience over the time it is consumed. This may be more of an issue for savoury foods than for desserts, as the latter may be more uniform in flavour (stressing here that little contemporary research appears to have been done on this issue—so this is 'informed' conjecture). For savoury foods, this probable flavour variation stands in stark contrast to nearly every single study described in this book, which typically employ individual odourants (or combinations), alongside single tastants or other specific components. These experimental conditions are in fact more reminiscent of ancestral dietary patterns—i.e. discrete flavours, 'broadly' continuous over an ingestive episode and thus readily amenable to be learnt about, either immediately (flavour-flavour) or in regards to the food's delayed consequences (flavour–calorie, flavour–aversion, etc.). How then does the flavour system cope (or not) with the complexities of a modern diet?

During development, foods are normally offered in a sequence over an extended period of time, one by one, until they become acceptable to the infant (e.g. rice alone, carrots alone, banana alone, etc.). Children also appear to go about consuming meals in a rather different manner to adults, eating foods sequentially, rather than mixing components as adults typically do (this is based on casual observation of my own three 'experimental participants' and I could find no published data on this topic). One consequence of this is that discrete flavours for different foods may be acquired during childhood, with more complex flavours (combinations) acquired later in development. This might offer some resolution to the problem of variation. When older children (or young adults) start to combine the components of a meal, and thus start to experience flavour variation, these 'new' experiences may be encoded so as to reflect this succession of combinations. Overlap between them (e.g. carrot + gravy and carrot + meat) may allow for the building of a metamemory for the combined flavour of a meal and of its consequences. One caveat here is that this learning may be limited by the similarity of the mixtures to the previously learnt components, with greater similarity retarding further learning (i.e. latent inhibition). Needless to say, this is speculation—and it could be hopelessly incorrect—but understanding olfactory perception has definitely been helped by a careful examination of its natural stimuli and flavour may be no exception. The difference here, of course, is that the flavour system may have evolved to cope with very different stimuli to the ones which we now consume.

One obvious cost associated with a shift to a more varied pattern of food intake is its effect on sensory-specific satiety. As described in the preceding chapter, sensory-specific satiety is delayed if a more varied (in terms of flavour) meal is consumed. Thus one might conclude that any shift to a more complex diet will be associated with an increase in the amount consumed at each meal (more in Chapter 7). A further cost concerns following a savoury dish with a sweet one. Earlier, it was suggested that some form of buffer store must exist, to keep the flavour of recently consumed food available so that it can become associated with later post-ingestional consequences. Are then the post-ingestive consequences of any savoury meal more likely to be associated with the sweet dessert than with the earlier savoury component of the meal? As noted earlier, this will depend upon novelty (or salience) and recency, but there must be general trend (with this ordering of savoury then sweet being common to many Western food-ways) for preferential association of positive post-ingestional qualities to the dessert.

Finally, this section started by raising the question as to whether a food's flavour might be considered as a multimodal object. Using the definition applied earlier, it would appear that if they are objects, they are of a different sort to those defined in the visual, auditory, or olfactory systems. This is because it is highly questionable whether there is a physically present 'ground' for the flavour 'object' to be delineated from. Take orthonasal olfaction, for example. Here multiple volatiles are present in the environment, but the brain/mind can detect one particular combination *against* this physically *present* background (Stevenson and Wilson 2007). This ability to detect and recognize (and then identify) biologically meaningful patterns of stimulation in the environment, whilst competing forms of stimulation are present, is arguably the most important function of all of the exteroceptive senses. For flavour in the mouth, the situation is very different. Here comparisons of the flavour in the mouth are made *against* the *past*, not against other competing and physically present oral-based stimulation. Therefore it would seem, strictly speaking, that flavour in the mouth is never experienced against a physically present 'ground', which would appear to rule it out as being an 'object'. However, when the odourous component of a flavour is experienced in the environment, and the flavour experience is redintegrated, this clearly is an 'object' as under these conditions it can be detected and recognized against competing background odours. On this basis, one could suggest that multimodal flavour objects are constructed in the mouth (the binding process) and utilized by the nose.

The only objection to this account that comes to mind is whether participants have the ability to identify individual 'flavours' in a complex flavour mixture. To take the example of a prototypical English dinner, could a participant, e.g. detect whether a particular mouthful contained a carrot, amongst the gravy and potatoes? Whilst this *may* be possible, it would seem to serve no major functional goal. And perhaps this is a further argument against regarding flavour in the mouth as a multimodal object.

Conclusion

Keeping in mind the functions, which are served by flavour perception appears to be a useful and informative way of thinking about what flavour is and is not. Flavour is not a sense, but it is a sensory system. Flavour is not an object in the mouth, but is an object in the nose. Perhaps most importantly of all, multisensory integration of flavour in the mouth—binding, then learning—provides the basis for detecting and selecting food by the nose, and for recording its immediate and delayed consequences. Of the many questions that remain to be answered in respect to flavour, the nature of the binding process and its relationship to learning and memory would be ones that appear central to further progress. A similar consideration would also apply to the effects of dietary variation on flavour learning. The next chapter identifies some of these important issues that need further enquiry, as well as examining some of the implications that flow from the ideas discussed here and elsewhere in the book.

Chapter 7

Implications

Introduction

The first part of this chapter examines some of the broader theoretical and practical implications that flow from the study of flavour. The six topics discussed here concern: (1) odour-induced tastes and their relationship to the neurodevelopmental synaesthesias; (2) the effect of developments in other areas of affective psychology and neuroscience for the study of flavour hedonics; (3) over-nutrition (i.e. obesity), and the contribution of the flavour system to this epidemic; (4) the ageing of Western populations and the role of the flavour system in under nutrition in this group; (5) maximizing flavour expertise and training; and (6) methodological advances that will likely impact upon flavour research. The second part of this chapter focuses on future directions—namely the outstanding questions that emerge from all of the material discussed in this book. These are organized thematically into five sections: interactions amongst the flavour senses, attention, binding, the orthonasal/retronasal distinction, and hedonics. The chapter concludes with a brief overview of the psychology of flavour and the flavour system.

Synaesthesia

In Chapter 6, there was some preliminary discussion of orthonasally redintegrated flavour as a form of synaesthesia. The aim here is to briefly compare and contrast neurodevelopmental synaesthesias, with the prototypical form of redintegrated flavour—odour-induced tastes—and then examine the implications that flow from this. To recap, synaesthesia occurs when an inducer from one sensory modality (or sub-modality) results in the experience of a concurrent percept from another sensory modality (or sub-modality). The neurodevelopmental synaesthesias are rare. They probably arise, as the name implies, from subtle genetically driven developmental abnormities of the brain. Prevalence estimates vary between 0.05 and 4.4% and the commonest form is letter–colour synaesthesia (Rich and Mattingley 2002), where a letter such as **A** will consistently induce a particular colour, for example, A. Neurodevelopmental synaesthesias involving odour, taste, and flavour have been documented, but they are very rare, and only one contemporary case of word–flavour synaesthesia has been studied in depth (Ward *et al.* 2005). Here, particular words were reported as inducing particular flavours, e.g. the word 'Jail' inducing a concurrent experience of 'cold hard bacon' (Ward and Simner 2003). This word–flavour synaesthesia was found to be highly consistent over time (87% consistency compared to 30% in non-synaesthetic controls), a hallmark of genuine synaesthetic experience. Two further features of this form of synaesthesia are notable and are also common to other forms of neurodevelopmental synaesthesia. First, during eating and drinking, the experience of flavour did not induce verbal experience (i.e. the synaesthesia is asymmetric). Second, the person experiencing the synaesthesia could readily recognize the unusualness of his experience (i.e. the synaesthesia was self-evident).

A comparison of the properties of odour-induced tastes with those of the neurodevelopmental synaesthesias, reveals several parallels as well as some important differences (Stevenson and Boakes 2004). First, the parallels: (1) both are highly consistent over time; (2) both are asymmetric—tastes do not induce odours; (3) in both cases, the inducer and concurrent come from different sensory modalities (or sub-modalities); and (4) the inducer does not activate the receptors normally involved in perceiving the concurrent. Second, the differences: (1) neurodevelopmental synaesthesias appear to require attention to the inducer to obtain a synaesthetic concurrent (i.e. A has to be attended to, to experience A), whilst odour-induced tastes do not appear to require attention to the odour to produce this effect; (2) participants who have been synaesthetic since as early as they can remember, readily recognize the unusual nature of their experiences, but this is not the case with odour-induced tastes (note that this a further potential argument for flavour as a unitary percept); (3) neurodevelopmental synaesthesias are rare, whilst odour-induced taste experiences are common, if not universal; and (4) neurodevelopmental synaesthetes do not misattribute the concurrence to the inducer's perceptual modality (e.g. a concurrent flavour is not felt as being 'seen', it is felt as being 'tasted'), whilst odour-induced tastes appear to be felt as 'smells', not tastes (contrast with flavour in the mouth, where smells are reported to be 'tastes').

A more contentious similarity concerns the role of learning, which is clearly important for odour-induced tastes. It is now becoming apparent that learning must play a role in the neurodevelopmental synaesthesias (Marks and Osgood 2005). Logically, where the inducers are words, numbers, letters, or musical notation, the synaesthete *must* have learned these symbols, and so the synaesthesia could not arguably predate the acquisition of the inducer. More tellingly, instances have now come to light of where coloured fridge magnets or jigsaw puzzles that the synaesthete was exposed to as a child map closely on to the synaesthesia experienced by that person as an adult (Hancock 2006, Witthoft and Winawer 2006). This also appears to be the case for the word–flavour synaesthesia described above, in that the concurrent flavours more closely mirrored foods that the synaesthete ate as a child than those he currently eats as an adult (Ward and Simner 2003).

If odour-induced tastes are a form of synaesthesia, one might expect considerable interest in this phenomenon by students of neurodevelopmental synaesthesia; however, this is not the case. There are at least two reasons for this. The first is definitional. Some would argue that odour-induced tastes cannot be a form of synaesthesia simply because the experience is universal (or seems to be). Such a definitional barrier is a rather weak basis for failing to regard odour-induced tastes as a form of synaesthesia, and as noted in Chapter 6, several accepted types of synaesthesia would also fail this definitional test (e.g. drug-induced synaesthesia). The second reason relates to concerns about the nature of the concurrence and whether it is a perceptual experience, a metaphor, or an explicit semantic recollection (see Marks and Osgood 2005). More recent evidence, reviewed in Chapter 3, strongly suggests that odour induced tastes are perceptual in form.

The apparent similarities between the properties of the neurodevelopmental synaesthesias and those of odour-induced tastes, suggest that the use of the term synaesthesia for the latter is appropriate. What then can the study of odour-induced tastes contribute towards understanding the neurodevelopmental synaesthesias? The principal benefit is in thinking about its neural correlates. Most, if not all studies, suggest that the neurodevelopmental synaesthesias arise as a result of neocortical activity, which is taken to suggest a neocortical abnormality (e.g. Sperling *et al.* 2006). As outlined in Chapter 6, it was suggested that odour-induced tastes may arise via the direct access of olfactory information into the neocortex, followed by activation of primary sensory cortex of other modalities in the *absence* of (normally) associated thalamic processing. This account points to the thalamus, a sub-cortical structure, as having a hitherto unsuspected role in supporting synaesthesia. On this basis, Stevenson and Tomiczek (2007) have argued that thalamic abnormalities could also contribute to the neurodevelopmental synaesthesias.

Looking to what the study of neurodevelopmental synaesthesias might teach students of flavour perception and odour-induced tastes, the role of attention stands out as being important. It was originally believed that neurodevelopmental synaesthesias were principally a pre-attentive phenomenon, just as suggested here for odour-induced tastes. This is now known not to be the case for the neurodevelopmental synaesthesias, at least in many of the forms studied (Ward and Mattingley 2006). The role of attention in odour-induced tastes has been the subject of a lot of conjecture but little experimentation.

The distal cause of odour-induced tastes is the multisensory processing of olfactory, taste, and somatosensory information in the mouth. Just as odour-induced tastes are unusual because of their synaesthesia-like properties, so arguably—and for related reasons—is the function of multisensory processing in this domain. The unique aspect of multisensory processing here is that its functional value lies in the *future*—excepting creaminess perception and auditory–tactile interactions (see Chapter 3). In Chapter 6, it was noted that the general purpose of multisensory processing is to facilitate detection, identification, and appropriate response in the *present*. For flavour in the mouth, these functions appear to be of little immediate value. Identification is best served by the visual and olfactory systems, prior to ingestion, as with detection and location of food. Appropriate response is a possibility. But here, rejection of harmful food is made either on the basis of detecting unimodal parts (bitter, irritation, heat, etc.) or by comparing the flavour with similar prior experiences (flavours past). Thus the primary functional benefit of multisensory processing of flavour is not in its immediate product (as with most studied forms of multisensory processing), but rather in the brain's/mind's ability to use this information at a later point in time.

A further unique component of the flavour system, and one that again relates to the ability of odours to induce tastes, is the distinction between orthonasal and retronasal olfaction. Rozin (1982) was the first contemporary researcher to draw attention to this distinction, which is unique amongst the sensory systems in combining an interoceptive and exteroceptive element within the same modality. Learning and memory appear to provide a bridge between these two components of the flavour system, and the evidence for this claim is quite substantial. However, it would be mistaken to overly stress the retronasal/orthonasal distinction, because the commonalities have to exceed the differences for key functional reasons. For example, there would be little point in learning a food's flavour, if perception of the olfactory component were radically different in each case (i.e. orthonasal vs. retronasal). This would preclude the nose (i.e. orthonasal) from accessing valuable information about a food's likely flavour (i.e. that was gleaned retronasally). Notwithstanding this, identifying the processing differences that exist between these two forms of olfactory perception is important, as it will shed light on both central binding problems discussed in Chapter 6.

Hedonics

Hedonic reactions to stimuli occur in many psychological domains, from facial attractiveness to drug use. It would be surprising if there were not deep similarities in the psychological and biological processes that underpin these various hedonic reactions. For this reason, important conceptual developments in one field of hedonics need to be considered in the light of what they may offer the study of flavour hedonics, and vice versa. The most recent example of this is the distinction between wanting and liking. This has started to spur research in respect to flavour hedonics in both, the psychological and biological, domains. In the psychological domain, this has focussed attention on several issues, including the interaction between homeostatic processes and their relationship with liking and wanting (e.g. Finlayson *et al.* 2008). It has also triggered the exploration of trait differences in motivation, and their relationship to food craving and intake (e.g. Franken and Murris 2005). More interestingly still, are the implications for the conscious control of ingestive behaviour, with the suggestion that implicit forms of liking and wanting may exert significant influences over appetite and possibly food choice (see Finlayson *et al.* 2008, Winkielman *et al.* 2005). Not only is this important because of the increase in average body mass over the last three decades in Western countries and the role of hedonic factors in this, but also because of its theoretical importance in understanding the conscious and unconscious controls of ingestive behaviour, and indeed, more generally, the function of consciousness.

Hand in hand with these psychological investigations, have been explorations of the neural processes that support flavour liking and wanting, as well as trait differences in motivation (most notably, see Chapter 6, and the discussion of Small *et al.* 2005). Some examples should serve to illustrate the direction that this research is going. Rolls and McCabe (2007) explored the neural correlates of seeing and tasting chocolate, between chocolate cravers and non-cravers. They observed differential neural activations between these groups, with differences centred on brain regions suspected of supporting liking (orbitofrontal cortex) and wanting (ventral striatum). In another recent study, Beaver *et al.* (2006) examined the relationship between trait motivation (drive and reward) and neural activation for appetizing food images. They observed that trait differences in drive were more strongly associated with brain regions implicated in wanting (ventral striatum, amygdala, midbrain regions, etc.) whilst trait differences in reward sensitivity were more strongly associated with brain regions implicated in supporting liking (orbitofrontal cortex). These findings raise as many questions as they answer, but one of particular importance concerns the role of the orbitofrontal cortex. Rolls and McCabe (2007) suggest that it is the orbitofrontal cortex that is responsible for driving *both* wanting and liking. Relatedly, it is unclear whether the orbitofrontal cortex actually 'mediates' liking (and wanting) or uses this information in affective decision making. Many neuroimaging studies reviewed here and elsewhere point to the importance of this structure in hedonics, but it is still not clear what its exact role is.

Yeomans (2008) presents an illustration (see his Figure 7.1) of a further problem to which flavour hedonics may contribute, namely whether affective processing is serial or parallel in nature. The issue discussed briefly at several points in this book is perhaps a broader one than Yeomans (2008) implies, including whether affective processing has its own parallel-recognition system, or whether it follows serially from perceptual processing. Whilst it appears that the latter is more likely in humans, a conclusion with which Yeomans (2008) also concurs, the absence of direct empirical evidence in relation to this question remains troubling. Not only is this of significance for how flavour hedonics are conceptualized at both a psychological and neural level, it also has implications for each of the senses that contribute to flavour, and to affective processing in the visual and auditory domains too.

Over-nutrition

There is no doubt that in Western nations there are now more people classified as overweight (i.e. BMI 25–30) and obese (i.e. BMI 30+) than ever before (Bovbjerg 2008). The causes of this increase in average body mass are complex, and involve the interaction of multiple physiological, psychological, and environmental factors. Flavour perception and hedonics contribute in several potential ways to increasing body mass, and it has been argued in a recent and influential review that a deeper understanding of flavour's neural and psychological basis may lead to new ways to tackle the obesity epidemic (Shepherd 2006). In this section, the focus is on what is currently known about the relationship between the flavour system and obesity.

Over the course of a meal, hedonic responses to the same flavour become less positive—sensory-specific satiety (or may be this is a change in wanting—see Chapter 5). This mechanism is one way in which the body can regulate food intake prior to any post-ingestive feedback, as well as acting to promote short-term dietary variety. As reviewed in Chapter 5, more varied meals lead to greater intake, presumably because sensory-specific satiety is, as its name implies, 'specific' for individual flavours. At both an individual and at a population level, one consequence of this is likely to be enhanced intake when a greater variety of flavours (i.e. food types) are available in the environment (McCrory et al. 1999). Clearly, this is the case in many Western nations. For example, in the US in 1978, 400 new snack foods and 380 new bakery products were introduced to market. In 1993, this was 2250 new snack foods and 1500 new bakery products. Relatedly, most supermarkets now stock over 10 000 different product lines. In contrast, hunter–gatherers such as the Hadza had available around 1–200 plant and animal species *overall* and, of course, many of these were restricted to certain times of the year (Woodburn 1966).

A further question is whether sensory-specific satiety is less effective in obese individuals. Any such difference could either be a cause or a consequence of weight gain. It could be a cause, as less efficient sensory-specific satiety might result in heightened consumption of all food types within a meal. It could be a consequence, as metabolic or hormonal changes might affect the neural modulation of appetite, including sensory-specific satiety. Two studies have directly compared sensory-specific satiety between lean and obese individuals. Sensory-specific satiety was observed in both groups and to the same degree (Brondel *et al.* 2007, Snoek *et al.* 2004). Taken at face value, this might suggest that this regulatory mechanism is unrelated to excess body mass. However, obese individuals *must* consume more calories, otherwise they would not be in positive energy balance and it would be surprising if reduced sensory-specific satiety were not a contributory factor. One possibility relates to the more general problem of studying ingestive behaviour in the obese. Remarkably, it has been very difficult to obtain firm evidence that obese individuals do, in fact, consume more food. Indeed, it is only with more recent urinary-metabolite studies that definitive evidence of over-consumption, relative to 'reported' consumption, has come to light (Bingham *et al.* 2007, Zhang *et al.* 2000). It may be that their behaviour under laboratory conditions (or whenever they are observed) may not resemble their behaviour when eating alone or with other obese individuals.

As described in Chapter 5 (see e.g. Figure 5.3), more palatable foods are over-consumed, and typically more palatable foods are also more energy dense (Yeomans 2008). In addition, as humans learn to like flavours associated with positive post-ingestional effects (i.e. foods high in calories) liking for such flavours increases (at least initially), acting as a further spur to over-consumption. One way these processes might be regulated is by learning the satiating effects of the food (learned satiety), and using this as an additional cue to regulate intake. However, the evidence for this form of regulation is surprisingly inconsistent, for reasons that are not well understood.

It has been suggested that our innate preference for energy-dense foods (sweet and fatty) and the relatively weak regulatory mechanisms (in contrast to the relatively strong mechanisms that 'promote' intake) arose from evolutionary pressures to over-consume in times of plenty so as to be prepared for times of famine. In this regard, individuals who become obese may in fact be those who are most suited to survive under ancestral conditions (this widely held view may be wrong as ancestral hunter–gatherers may have had both an adequate and mainly regular supply of nutrients; see e.g. Cohen 2000). One might suspect that obese individuals would also possess differential perceptual and affective responses to such food (more below), as well as having an enhanced capacity to learn about their rewarding aspects. Whilst it is acknowledged that obese individuals are especially sensitive to food-related cues (wanting), it is not yet known whether their flavour-related learning systems are also more sensitive.

Cabanac (1971) demonstrated that the body's state of depletion or repletion could influence whether or not the sight and smell of food are experienced as being pleasant or unpleasant, respectively. Davidson *et al.* (2005) have suggested an interesting variation on this type of homeostatic model in which satiety may act to inhibit the access of pleasant flavour-related memories into consciousness. Thus, feeling full may result in the inhibition of such memories when a food is seen or thought about, thereby reducing the likelihood that such a food will be eaten *in this state*. The hippocampus appears to be the regulatory centre for such inhibition in conceptually similar types of task in both animals and humans (e.g. Anderson *et al.* 2004). Recent animal work indicates that regular consumption of a diet rich in saturated fats and simple carbohydrates, at levels equivalent to those consumed by many Westerners, can selectively damage the hippocampus (Molteni *et al.* 2004). This damage affects both its mnemonic and inhibitory functions (Molteni *et al.* 2002). It has been suggested that such damage may also occur in humans (e.g. Vaynman and Gomez-Pinilla 2006), and there is circumstantial evidence that it does (e.g. Elias *et al.* 2005). Davidson *et al.* (2005) have argued that this type of dietary-induced damage to the hippocampus could lead to a 'vicious circle' model of obesity in which impaired inhibitory processing results in overeating, weight gain, and further hippocampal damage (Davidson *et al.* 2005). The details of this interesting model remain to be tested in humans.

A long history surrounds the investigation of perceptual and hedonic differences in response to flavour, between obese and normal-weight individuals. For taste, the pattern of results has been varied, with some studies obtaining differences in sensitivity (reduced in the obese) and others not detecting such differences (see Bartoshuk *et al.* 2006). Eliminating problems connected with measuring differences in perceived intensity between non-randomly assigned groups (i.e. between obese and lean individuals), reveals that at least for sweet tastes, obese individuals, relative to those of *less*-than-normal body weight (BMI <18.5), perceive it as less intense (Bartoshuk *et al.* 2006). Moreover, obese individuals report liking sweetness more, as its intensity increases, but this relationship is much weaker for overweight and normal-weight individuals. Whilst the sizes of both these effects are not large, small changes in food preferences brought about by a heightened enjoyment of sweet tastes (and the need for sweeter tastes to achieve optimal enjoyment) would be sufficient over a long period of time to add appreciably to a person's body mass.

There are several possible explanations for abnormal responsiveness to sweet taste in obese individuals and the precise cause is not currently known. Widespread metabolic changes accompany weight gain and these may have a direct effect on the chemical senses, including taste. Additionally, Bartoshuk and colleagues (Bartoshuk *et al.* 2006) have detailed two further possibilities. First, that damage to the chorda tympani nerve resulting from ear infections during childhood may result in impaired taste perception as an adult. Presumably, this damage must be bilateral; if not, then one would expect that the undamaged side would show a compensatory increase in activity (and thus no loss of taste sensitivity) due to the release from inhibition of the non-damaged side. Second, several studies (but not all) have identified an association between BMI and PROP sensitivity (recall PROP sensitivity is mediated by the density of fungiform papillae on the front of the tongue). Individuals with such heightened sensitivity—and greater density of papillae—are more sensitive to sweet tastes and tend to dislike them more as well. More interestingly still, they also tend to be leaner.

Although differences in somatosensory perception between lean and obese individuals, especially for fat, are not revealing when tested alone, combinations of sweet tastes and fat together may be important. In a widely cited study, Drewnowski *et al.* (1985) found differences between obese, recovered obese, and normal-weight women when their hedonic ratings for sugar–fat mixtures were compared. Normal-weight women exhibited maximum preference for a mixture of 20.7% fat and 7.7% sugar, in contrast to 34.4% fat and 4.4% sugar for obese individuals. Recovered obese had fat preferences similar to the obese (35.1%), but sweet preferences more akin to normal-weight individuals (10.1% sugar). The ratio of sugar to fat for optimal liking significantly differed between normal-weight and obese women. Response surface modelling clearly indicated that, for obese women, as long as the fat solutions were sweetened, fatty solutions were liked—there being no breakpoint in preference as for normal-weight women.

Conceptually similar findings have been obtained from food-preference surveys of obese women, who report preferring sweet–fatty foods more than obese men. Obese men, however, appear to prefer savoury–fatty foods (Drewnoski 1994). Again, the precise basis of these differences in fat preference (and perception?) is not understood, and it is likely that metabolic differences produced by excess body mass may account for some of the variance. However, Bartoshuk *et al.* (2006) have recently suggested that it may also relate to differences in taste sensitivity, and that reduced ability to perceive sweet tastes may be associated with increased preference for fatty foods.

Differences in olfactory perception are also evident in obese individuals, although these have not received the same attention as taste and somatosensory stimuli. Richardson *et al.* (2004) reported that morbidly obese adults (BMI >45) had significantly impaired odour identification and threshold performance, relative to less obese individuals. Needless to say, such differences may result from other concurrent medical conditions, such as type II diabetes, which are far more common in the morbidly obese. As with earlier taste studies, not all reports find evidence of impairment. Orebowski *et al.* 2000 found that obese children (aged 10–16 years) without complicating medical conditions (i.e. the obesity not being the result of another disorder) were, on average, able to identify target odours at lower concentrations than normal controls. If, as Bartoshuk *et al.* (2006) have recently suggested, individuals with a history of tonsil and middle ear infections during childhood have a heightened risk of obesity later in life, one might also suspect that this would compromise olfactory sensitivity. This is because such a history of infections might be expected to also damage the olfactory system and hence impair odour perception. In this case, a person might compensate by selecting fattier foods, to make up for the loss of taste- and olfactory-driven pleasure. Moreover, many food-based odourants are fat soluble, so increasing the fat content of the food would also potentially increase the amount of detectable volatile chemicals (e.g. Carrapiso 2007). This would provide an additional incentive for choosing fattier food. Alternatively, increasing the size of each mouthful of food, irrespective of fat content, can also result in greater flavour release (Linforth *et al.* 2005) and this too might offer a further compensatory strategy that could promote excess energy intake.

Under-nutrition

The elderly, in Western countries, are prone to malnourishment. In the UK, studies estimate that between 21 and 61% of elderly, hospitalized patients are malnourished, and whilst prevalence estimates are lower in community settings, under-nutrition is still widely observed (Hickson 2005). This is a problem because under-nutrition is known to leave elderly people more vulnerable to infectious disease. Relatedly, it also increases morbidity and mortality in hospital settings. As the population ages, with a growing proportion of elderly people— already 16% of the UK population (65+), finding ways of improving nutritional status will become an evermore pressing problem.

Ageing can affect several aspects of ingestive behaviour, most notably in reducing appetite via illness-related conditions, and through hormonal, immune, and metabolic changes that accompany old age. All of the chemical senses are compromised by ageing. For taste, sensitivity declines with age, such that 11 times as much salt and 3 times as much sugar are required for an elderly person to detect these tastes, relative to a younger person (Hickson 2005). Similar changes are known to occur for other basic tastants as well (Schiffman *et al.* 1993). These changes appear to result from both a loss of taste buds and from impaired receptor functioning.

A compromised sense of smell is also observed in the elderly, with poorer thresholds, reduced identification rate, and impaired discriminative ability, relative to younger controls (Schiffman 1992). Here cumulative damage to the olfactory epithelium changes in release of female sex hormones and impaired memory functioning (required for odour identification and discrimination) can all contribute to poorer performance. Whether changes also occur in somatosensory perception is not currently known, but the tactile qualities of food can be a major issue for the elderly, especially if the person has lost their teeth and/or has problems swallowing.

Improving appetite via flavour enhancement is one strategy that can be successfully adopted to improve the nutritional status of the elderly (Schiffman 2000). Several studies have demonstrated that adding odours to foods to complement natural flavours (e.g. adding roast beef odour to beef) can increase the amount of food consumed. Moreover, the extra amount consumed correlates positively with the degree of olfactory impairment, suggesting that olfactory loss is one factor in reduced appetite (Schiffman 1992). The enhancement strategy can also be extended to adding tastants such as monosodium glutamate, with similar success (Schiffman 2000). Presumably, this approach could be extended to all aspects of flavour—olfactory, taste, and texture—to maximize appeal, increase consumption, and thus improve nutritional status. Although food manufacturers currently target certain age groups with specific products (notably children and adolescents), there appears to be little in the way of elderly specific foods. One could foresee that this might be a very lucrative market in the future.

Perceptual expertise and training

One of the most striking things to arise from Chapter 4 was the lack of published empirical work examining both, the effects of training in applied settings and the optimal parameters needed to produce expertise. As many authors have noted (e.g. Labbe *et al.* 2004) it is important to optimize training, so as to limit expenditure whilst maximizing its impact. A logical starting point is to define what training should result in, thus providing an appropriate goal. This would include the three key features of expertise that were discussed in Chapter 4. First, perceptual experience of the full range of stimuli that compose the 'domain' in which expertise is to be developed. Second, semantic knowledge about the domain and any classification system that operates within it, along with knowledge about scaling and measurement, need to be developed as well. Third, linking parts with names, so that a bridge is formed between the perceptual and semantic domains. Measuring whether training has been successful would then include: (1) demonstrating improved discriminability (i.e. a measure of the first component); (2) demonstrating domain- and skill-relevant knowledge (i.e. a measure of the second component); and (3) demonstrating the ability to accurately and reliably name stimulus parts (i.e. a measure of the third component). Optimizing this process, and determining what skills carry over into other flavour domains, are relevant questions for applied settings and for understanding the characteristics of perceptual learning with flavours.

Training then should, arguably, lead to an improvement in the three components identified above. What are the limits then to these skills? For flavour, it should be possible to identify most of the elements (i.e. discrete conscious experience that corresponds with a particular stimulus) for taste and somatosensory stimuli. However, for the olfactory component, detection of elements is likely to be rather limited (perhaps two or three) and whilst this can be improved by training, there appear to be rather strict perceptual limits imposed by the processing strategy that the brain employs for odour perception. In terms of similarities, the olfactory component of flavour can have a very large number indeed. The capacity to make reliable similarity judgements probably depends upon both, perceptual experience (i.e. having smelled the item to which the olfactory component is to be compared) and being able to link the name to the smell, when making similarity judgements using lists of olfactory referents (e.g. smells like cheddar cheese). The ultimate limits on the ability to make reliable olfactory similarity judgements are not known, but it is likely to exceed the number of elements available for taste and somatosensory stimuli. In addition, whilst most naive participants would be able to identify somatosensory and taste elements, their ability to identify olfactory similarities is likely to be much more limited.

Two issues that are often discussed in the applied literature are whether experts (i.e. trained panels) are necessary for perceptually orientated tasks and whether naive consumers are necessary for hedonic tasks (see e.g. Ishii *et al.* 2007, Moskowitz 1996, and Hough 1998). The discussion above should provide some pointers for the tenor of the answers here. In respect to experts versus novices for perceptual orientated task, the answer will be that *if* the domain is one with which the novice has some experience (e.g. regular wine drinkers) and *if* the tasks are appropriate (e.g. not too much focus on olfactory similarities) then, by and large, novices will perform in a manner similar to experts. Differences between these two groups should emerge in a manner consistent with the discussion above. That is: (1) novices should start to encounter problems if they are asked to detect and scale parts, where the part's 'name' is not known to them or where they are unfamiliar with the part's referent; and (2) where lack of perceptual expertise makes discrimination between one stimulus and another problematic (i.e. lack of perceptual experience).

For the second question, hedonics, a somewhat similar answer would follow—it depends upon the likely difference in domain experience between the prototypical consumer and expert. However, in this case, conventional wisdom (i.e. naive consumers are best for this task) is more likely to be correct because naive participants are *less likely* to attend to specific parts of the stimulus and more likely to judge the whole. Of course, the very task of asking naive participants to make any judgement immediately generates a context (i.e. greater attention to the stimulus) that is different from the one in which normal eating and drinking occur. Indeed, there is still some uncertainty surrounding the exact nature of the relationship between what is eaten and hedonic evaluations. Whilst this relationship is clearly positive and predictive (i.e. the more you like something, the more likely you are to eat it and vice versa), it is far from perfect, and the cause(s) of the unexplained variance are not fully understood.

Methodology

In reading many of the experiments described in this book, one would be hard pressed not to be in open admiration at the imagination and ingenuity that flavour researchers have shown. Notwithstanding this, there are some recent advances that appear to be especially important for shedding light on several topical questions. The first is the use of catheterization to deliver odourants to either the anterior or posterior nares (Heilmann and Hummel 2004). Not only has this technique been used to explore differences in neural processing that appear to correlate with anterior or posterior delivery (Small *et al.* 2005), the technique has also resolved a long running debate about the nature of somato-sensory (viscosity)-olfactory interactions (Bult *et al.* 2002). As the binding problem is of major scientific interest, and a central problem in the psychology of flavour (as multisensory integration; Verhagen and Engelen 2006), this delivery technique is one which may allow important insights into how the brain localizes retronasal odourants to the mouth and orthonasal odourants to the nose.

A second technique is one that has been developed and utilized by Taylor's group at the University of Nottingham (e.g. Davidson *et al.* 1999). Here the idea has been to measure in-breath volatiles and taste-based parameters (e.g. residual sucrose in chewing gum) and then to relate these physical parameters to ratings of odour and taste intensity. This type of technique can explore in great detail temporal parameters of flavour that have not been well studied. Most notable amongst these are adaptation effects, especially to the olfactory components, and the degree to which these affect participants' judgements of flavour over time. This topic of sensory adaptation during eating and drinking is clearly important and how it is avoided or minimized—physiologically or psychologically—is poorly understood. A further issue, and one that may relate to avoiding adaptation, is the pulsatile release of odourants into the nasopharynx during the consumption of solid food (see Chapter 1). This has implications for the study of flavour binding in regards to the apparent simultaneous presence of the component modalities of flavour (see Chapter 6 for some discussion of this issue). This makes understanding the dynamics of odour release during ingestion particularly relevant.

A third technique is the adaptation of Borg's log magnitude scale (originally to assess physical exertion) for use in the chemical senses (Green *et al.* 1993) and its further revision to eliminate problems that arise from comparing non-randomly assigned groups (Bartoshuk *et al.* 2006). As described above, this type of scale has been used to assess both hedonic and perceptual responses to flavour stimuli across participants of different BMI, and appears to offer high sensitivity as well as ease of use. If the promise of this measurement approach holds true, it should allow for meaningful comparison between groups whose perceptual worlds may be quite different—such as that between obese and normal-weight individuals.

Future directions

This section is organized into five parts: interactions between the flavour senses; attention; binding; the orthonasal/retronasal distinction; and hedonics. Each part contains an outline of some of the unresolved questions that have arisen in various sections of this book.

Interactions

A major distinction that continues to attract attention is whether interactions between the visual and the flavour senses are semantically or perceptually mediated. So, e.g. when white wine is coloured red, is the resulting flavour evaluation ('like red wine') a consequence of 'knowing' what red wine should be like (and rating it accordingly) or is it a consequence of 'experiencing' a red wine-flavour percept? This problem is difficult to answer, but it is very important for establishing how flavour perception is influenced both, by visual cues and relatedly when semantic information is provided about the stimulus. This same problem also extends into the hedonic domain (recall, e.g. experiments on labelling and hedonic evaluations of smell) and it may be here that a much more direct influence is exerted (i.e. hedonic reactions alter). This problem also has significant practical implications, namely in the effect of food labelling.

A second issue concerns the limits of similarity between redintegrated flavour parts (e.g. the 'sweet' in sweet smells or the 'fatty' in fatty smells) and their stimulus-driven equivalents (e.g. sweet tastes, fatty sensations, etc.). At a psychological level, this may provide important insights into how these two modes of perception differ (e.g. addressing questions related to the assignment of these qualia to 'smell'). At the neural level, direct comparison of sweet-taste perception and odour-induced sweetness would allow for the identification of overlapping commonalities and differences in processing—as suggested by recent neuropsychological findings.

A third issue concerns the apparently multimodal percept of creaminess. Is this really a multimodal percept as claimed here and elsewhere? Is the claim made here (see Chapter 3) that similar creaminess percepts may be arrived at through manipulating very different stimulus parameters correct? Is the claim that experts and naive participants judge creaminess in largely the same manner valid? Is creaminess something of an exception, e.g. could it be an eliminative emergent property, rather than a preservative one? Finally, and also relating to creaminess, is the mystery of why more viscous stimuli should suppress olfaction (see Chapter 2). Both, the cause of this effect—which is now known to be of central origin—and its functional significance, are not understood.

Attention

The experimental evidence clearly reveals that we have some capacity to selectively attend to stimuli in the mouth, whilst having a more limited capacity (if any) to attend to retronasal olfactory elements. Two questions arise from these findings. The first relates to the observation that participants do not seem to have a problem in evaluating what are clearly olfactory similarities in flavour, which must require selective attention. How this may square with the findings noted above regarding elements seems to warrant study (e.g. could it simply reflect task-based limitations?). A further question here is how prior experience may influence attention to mixtures of odours and tastes (i.e. see Ashkenazi and Marks (2004) and the results of their Experiment 3, in Table 4.3).

The second question concerns whether it is possible to selectively attend to discrete multimodal flavour 'objects' that are concurrently present (object is in quotes because as described in Chapter 6, object *may* not be the appropriate term with which to refer to flavour in the mouth). For example, if a person were (as normal) eating a combination of foods, to what extent is it possible to selectively attend to the'carrot'and then the'meat'? Not only is this of interest from the perspective of attentional capacities, it is also highly relevant to the conceptual use of the term object in respect to flavour perception.

At several points in this book, the argument has been made that flavour learning (i.e. encoding the flavour percept) does not require the participant to consciously attend to the various components that come to be associated. Yet on the other hand, it would appear that the conditions which best support this form of learning—'unfamiliar flavours'—are exactly those that might favour disproportionate attention to what is happening in the mouth. Of course, it may be that attending to the flavour is not the same as attending to the flavour's parts, but, nonetheless, it would seem important to understand what role attention plays in flavour encoding.

In the discussion above on synaesthesia, it was pointed out that attention might be crucial in being able to experience a synaesthetic effect. The role of attention in the experience of odour-induced tastes has not been established, although it has been suggested that it is a pre-attentive phenomenon (Stevenson and Tomiczek 2007). This needs to be tested, because a similar assumption was made about the neurodevelopmental synaesthesias and it was shown to be incorrect for many of the cases where it has been appropriately examined. Not only would such test be important in establishing a further similarity or difference between odour-induced tastes and the neurodevelopmental synaesthesias, it would also be important in understanding how flavour redintegration might occur.

Binding

In Chapter 6, it was suggested that there were two central binding questions that needed to be addressed within the context of the flavour system. The first concerned binding of flavour in the mouth, and the second the binding of redintegrated flavour to the nose. The study of both of these is in its earliest stages. A major question that concerns both types of binding is its neural basis. Neuroimaging provides one approach to this problem, especially as it may lead to the identification of brain areas that can then be used to search for patients who have specific lesions in these areas. This approach may be forced upon us by necessity, because the identification of flavour-related deficits is not typically at the forefront of either a patient's or neurologist's mind. Their focus, naturally, is on major deficits—mnemonic, visual, auditory, or motor, unless the flavour-related problem is grossly apparent (e.g. Gourmand syndrome (Regard and Landis 1997) or Kluver-Bucy syndrome (Lopez *et al.* 1995)). Thus 'casual' identification of interesting patients (with flavour deficits) may not be possible without knowing potentially interesting lesion sites. An additional route would be to develop a quick, reliable, and cheap screening method to identify possible binding-related deficits.

The focus here on the deficit (neuropsychological) approach is quite deliberate, because it has been instrumental in advancing research on binding in other domains (e.g. Revonsuo 1999, Robertson 2003). Arguably, the same should apply to flavour. A related problem concerns the role of experience (learning) in flavour binding—what role does this have in the context of flavour in the mouth? Clearly, experience is the key to redintegrative flavour binding, as the content to be bound is a consequence of learning, but we still know very little about the neural substrates that support this process either.

Finally, whilst there is plenty of circumstantial evidence favouring the idea of 'unitary' flavour perception direct evidence for this mode of flavour perception is sparse, especially given the wide acceptance that this idea has. Neuropsychology may again be one way to resolve this, as binding failures should amount phenomenally to a loss of unitary flavour experience. This is not the only potential approach. The study, e.g. of illusory conjunctions for colour–form binding in normal participants, suggests another. Arguably, there is a need for analogous and novel experimental approaches in normal participants for the study of flavour binding.

The orthonasal/retronasal distinction

Recent work identifying distinctions between irritant and mechanoreceptive sensitivity of the anterior and posterior parts of the nose, and neuroimaging data of differential delivery effects, point towards many of the unknowns surrounding the distinction between orthonasal and retronasal perception. Although psychological evidence points to experience as the bridge between the interoceptive and exteroreceptive components of the olfactory system, there is little in the way of neuroimaging or neuropsychological data. A further question is whether localization of olfactory sensation to the external or internal milieu can be accomplished by the direction of nasal airflow, as apart from anecdotal reports, there is little yet in the way of confirmatory behavioural data. The neural mechanisms responsible for detecting any differences in airflow are also poorly understood, as are the way in which odourants are routed to the olfactory receptors during routine eating and drinking (related problems here arise in respect to the apparently pulsatile nature of delivery—constancy, filling in, and adaptation). The cause of the perceptual and hedonic differences between these two routes of delivery is also not understood. For example, to what extent are they due to peripheral or central effects? Finally, how does olfaction's unique neural architecture contribute/relate to the orthonasal/retronasal distinction?

Whilst we know considerably more now than when Rozin's (1982) article rekindled research on this topic, much remains to be done.

Hedonics

Several important questions need to be addressed in the domain of flavour hedonics. These include the distinction between serial and parallel processing of affect and, relatedly, whether hedonic responses to, say, a sweet-smelling odour rely upon reactivation of affective systems after redintegration of the flavour memory or whether they result from affective memory. Both questions relate to the broader issue of the psychological and neural architecture of hedonic processing. The former concerns whether hedonic processing operates on the 'output' of perceptual processing (serial). The alternative is that independent pathways (to those involved in perceptual processing), from receptors upwards, ultimately result in affective states. Whilst the first-mentioned alternative appears to be favoured in the literature (presumably on the grounds of parsimony), the evidence base is not well developed.

A second question concerns whether learned affective responses arise as a result of redintegration of perceptual experience, which then invokes hedonic processing, or whether hedonic processes are activated by an independent pathway that must involve some form of memory system. For example, in coming to like an odour paired with a sweet taste, is the resultant liking for that odour a consequence of the redintegrated taste? or is it a consequence of the flavour activating a mnemonic process, where what is stored is some code reflecting the 'degree' to which positive or negative affective states should be aroused? The first mentioned might work for flavour–flavour learning, but what of learning involving a delayed consequence?

The brain appears to modulate some hedonic processes based upon state, whilst others appear to be largely independent of state (i.e. needing). This distinction can be made for nearly all of the hedonic processes discussed in Chapter 5, and perhaps it is most stark for that between sensory-specific satiety and alliaesthesia. Is this distinction achieved by regulating the output of common hedonic systems, so that some outputs are affected by bodily state and others are not, or is it achieved by independent hedonic systems? In discussing sensory-specific satiety, a significant focus was upon this as a means for regulating intake. An additional mechanism is conditioned satiety, and the status of this is currently ambiguous. Given the interest in appetite regulation, in light of the obesity epidemic, it would be prudent to determine whether the satiating properties of a food are, in fact, used by the body to regulate intake prior to the onset of gut-based physiological satiety signals.

Three further issues also warrant mention. Many times in Chapter 5 (and 6), it was noted that the study of flavour hedonics needs to grapple more directly with the concepts of wanting and liking (e.g. in the appetizer effect and in sensory-specific satiety as suggested in the General Discussion of Chapter 5). Interesting work on this by several groups suggests that this will be productive, including linking this distinction to that between orthonasal and retronasal perception (see Chapter 6), and to implicit factors in triggering of eating and selecting food (and also perhaps picas; e.g. Reynolds *et al.* 1968). Indeed, this leads to a further major question noted in passing above—the relationship between hedonic evaluations of a food (in a laboratory setting) and actual food choice. As noted before, there is clearly evidence that the two are related, but the relationship is weaker than one might at first assume. A third issue concerns the role of conscious awareness in delayed flavour learning. To what extent does a person need to be consciously aware of nausea or the satiating post-ingestive effects of food, for this type of learning to be acquired? For example, people may differ in their sensitivity to satiation (i.e. their capacity to 'feel' full), would this be independent of their ability to acquire flavour–energy relationships?

Conclusion

In studying the psychology of flavour, the broader context cannot be ignored. Flavour is one part of a larger neurobiobehavioural system devoted to ingestion. Within this larger context, the flavour system accomplishes a number of functions. This starts with the location and appraisal of food prior to ingestion. The visual system has access to a wealth of accumulated semantic information about food and drink. The olfactory system is able to redintegrate a flavour, if the odour being sniffed was once part of that flavour. How this is achieved and how the redintegrated flavour is perceived as 'olfactory' and as an attribute of the external world is a binding problem of considerable complexity. Once food is placed in the mouth, multiple sensory systems—olfaction, taste, and somatosensation—act together to produce a largely preservative emergent property—flavour. The binding processes that supports the emergence of flavour also represents a further complex problem. The taste and somatosensory parts of flavour can be individually perceived, and can attract attention if the stimulus is bitter, burning, or sharp, leading potentially to rejection of the food. The olfactory elements are not readily discriminable, although their similarities to other odours and flavours can be perceived—and especially so after training. The overall flavour in the mouth is compared to memories of flavours past, and where there is a considerable mismatch, this, too, is attention demanding and can lead to rejection. The experience of flavour can be encoded into memory, especially if it is unfamiliar, and the brain possesses an ability to associate this information selectively with subsequent post-ingestive events, such as repletion or sickness. During ingestion, changes in hedonic reactions to flavour result in intake regulation prior to the onset of gut-mediated satiety signals, and reduced hedonic responsiveness to food is maintained whilst the body is replete—for some hours after a meal. Finally, the experience of flavour, and its consequences, are learned and used in subsequent decision making about food. Apart from the multisensory nature of flavour, and the dominance of its hedonic dimension, learning and memory stand out as prominent features in nearly all aspects of the flavour system.

Closing remarks

The study of flavour is of great practical significance to the food industry. Equally, the study of flavour should be of considerable interest to experimental psychologists and neuroscientists because of what it can tell us about several basic psychological and neural processes. Inevitably, these different perspectives lead to different expectations about what we need to know and what one wants to know (i.e. which journals one chooses to read). Hopefully, this book will promote the sort of cross-disciplinary dialogue that is needed to fully understand our experience of flavour.

References

Abdi H (2002). What can cognitive psychology and sensory evaluation learn from each other? *Food Quality and Preference*, **13**, 445–451.

Albin KC, Carstens MI and Carstens E (2008). Modulation of oral heat and cold pain by irritant chemicals. *Chemical Senses*, **33**, 3–15.

Alley RL and Alley TR (1998). The influence of physical state and color on perceived sweetness. *The Journal of Psychology*, **132**, 561–568.

Anderson DB and Pennebaker JW (1980). Pain and pleasure: Alternative interpretations for identical stimulation. *European Journal of Social Psychology*, **10**, 207–212.

Anderson M, Ochsner K, Kuhl B, *et al.* (2004). Neural systems underlying the suppression of unwanted memories. *Science*, **303**, 232–235.

Appleton KM, Gentry RC and Shepherd R (2006). Evidence of a role for conditioning in the development of liking for flavours in humans in everyday life. *Physiology and Behavior*, **87**, 478–486.

Arabie P and Moskowitz HR (1971). The effects of viscosity upon perceived sweetness. *Perception and Psychophysics*, **9**, 410–412.

Ashkenazi A and Marks LE (2004). Effect of endogenous attention on detection of weak gustatory and olfactory flavors. *Perception and Psychophysics*, **66**, 596–608.

Atkinson P (1984). Eating virtue. In (ed.) A Murcott, *The Sociology of Food and Eating*, pp. 9–17. Gower Pub Co, UK.

Auvray M and Spence C (2008). The multisensory perception of flavor. *Consciousness and Cognition*, **17**, 1016–1031.

Ayabe-Kanamura S, Saito S, Distel H, Martinez-Gomez M and Hudson R (1998). Differences and similarities in the perception of everyday odors: A Japanese–German cross-cultural study. *Annals of the New York Academy of Sciences*, **855**, 694–700.

Bacon AW, Miles S and Schiffman SS (1994). Effect of race on perception of fat alone and in combination with sugar. *Physiology and Behavior*, **55**, 603–606.

Baek I, Linforth RST, Blake A and Taylor AJ (1999). Sensory perception is related to the rate of change of volatile concentration in-nose during eating of model gels. *Chemical Senses*, **24**, 155–160.

Baeyens F, Eelen P, Van den Bergh O and Crombez G (1990). Flavor–flavor and color–flavor conditioning in humans. *Learning and Motivation*, **21**, 434–455.

Baeyens F, Crombez G, De Houwer J and Eelen P (1996). No evidence for modulation of evaluative flavor–flavor associations in humans. *Learning and Motivation*, **27**, 200–241.

Baeyens F, Crombez G, Hendrickx H and Eelen P (1995). Parameters of human evaluative flavor–flavor conditioning. *Learning and Motivation*, **26**, 141–160.

Baeyens F, Eelen P, Crombez G and De Houwer J (2001). On the role of beliefs in observational flavor conditioning. *Current Psychology: Developmental, Learning, Personality*, **20**, 183–203.

Baeyens F, Vansteenwegen D, De Houwer J and Crombez G (1996). Observational conditioning of food valence in humans. *Appetite*, **27**, 235–250.

Ballester J, Patris B, Symoneaux R and Valentin D (2008). Conceptual vs. perceptual wine spaces: Does expertise matter? *Food Quality and Preference*, **19**, 267–276.

Barbano MF and Cador M (2007). Opioids for hedonic experience and dopamine to get ready for it. *Psychopharmacology*, **191**, 497–506.

Baron RF and Penfield MP (1996). Capsaicin heat intensity-concentration, carrier, fat level, and serving temperature effects. *Journal of Sensory Studies*, **11**, 295–316.

Bartoshuk, LM (1975). Taste mixtures: Is mixture suppression related to compression? *Physiology and Behavior*, **14**, 643–649.

Bartoshuk, LM (1977). Psychophysical studies of taste mixtures. In (eds) J. Le Magnen and P. Macleod, *Olfaction and Taste VI*, pp. 377–384. IRL, London.

Bartoshuk LM (1993). The biological basis of food perception and acceptance. *Food Quality and Preference*, **4**, 21–32.

Bartoshuk LM, Duffy VB and Miller IJ (1994). PTC/PROP tasting: Anatomy, psychophysics, and sex effects. *Physiology and Behavior*, **56**, 1165–1171.

Bartoshuk LM, Duffy VB, Hayes JE, Moskowitz HR and Snyder DJ (2006). Psychophysics of sweet and fat perception in obesity: Problems, solutions and new perspectives. *Philosophical Transactions of the Royal Society B*, **361**, 1137–1148.

Bartoshuk LM, Rennert K, Rodin J and Stevens JC (1982). Effects of temperature on the perceived sweetness of sucrose. *Physiology and Behavior*, **28**, 905–910.

Batsell WR and Brown AS (1998). Human flavor–aversion learning: A comparison of traditional aversions and cognitive aversions. *Learning and Motivation*, **29**, 383–396.

Batsell WR, Brown AS, Ansfield ME and Paschall GY (2002). "You will eat all of that!" A retrospective analysis of forced consumption episodes. *Appetite*, **38**, 211–219.

Bayarri S, Calvo C, Costell E and Duran L (2001). Influence of color on perception of sweetness and fruit flavor of fruit drinks. *Food Science and Technology International*, **7**, 399–404.

Bayarri S, Taylor AJ and Hort J (2006). The role of fat in flavor perception: Effect of partition and viscosity in model emulsions. *Journal of Agricultural and Food Chemistry*, **54**, 8862–8868.

Beaver JD, Lawrence AD, Van Ditzhuijzen J, Davis MH, Woods A and Calder AJ (2006). Individual differences in reward drive predict neural responses to images of food. *Journal of Neuroscience*, **26**, 5160–5166.

Belasco W (1997). Food, morality, and social reform. In (eds) A Brandt and P Rozin, *Morality and Health*, pp. 185–199. Routledge, New York.

Bell GA, Laing DG and Panhuber H (1987). Odour mixture suppression: Evidence for a peripheral mechanism in human and rat. *Brain Research*, **426**, 8–18.

Bellisle F (1999). Glutamate and the UMAMI taste: Sensory, metabolic, nutritional and behavioural considerations. A review of the literature published in the last 10 years. *Neuroscience and Biobehavioral Reviews*, **23**, 423–438.

Bende M and Nordin S (1997). Perceptual learning in olfaction: Professional wine tasters versus controls. *Physiology and Behavior*, **62**, 1065–1070.

Berg HW, Filipello F, Hinreiner E and Webb AD (1955). Evaluation of thresholds and minimum difference concentrations for various constituents of wines. I. water solutions of pure substances. *Food Technology*, **9**, 23–26.

Berglund B and Olsson MJ (1993). Odor-intensity interaction in binary mixtures. *Journal of Experimental Psychology: Human Perception and Performance*, **19**, 302–314.

Bermudez-Rattoni F (2004). Molecular mechanisms of taste-recognition memory. *Nature Reviews Neuroscience*, **5**, 209–217.

Berridge KC (1996). Food reward: Brain substrates of wanting and liking. *Neuroscience and Biobehavioral Reviews*, **20**, 1–25.

Berridge KC (2000). Measuring hedonic impact in animals and infants: Microstructure of affective taste reactivity patterns. *Neuroscience and Biobehavioral Reviews*, **24**, 173–198.

Berridge KC (2004). Motivation concepts in behavioral neuroscience. *Physiology and Behvaior*, **81**, 179–209.

Berridge KC and Kringelbach ML (2008). Affective neuroscience of pleasure: Reward in humans and animals. *Psychopharmacology*, **199**, 457–480.

Berthoud HR and Morrison C (2008). The brain, appetite, and obesity. *Annual Review of Psychology*, **59**, 55–92.

Biederman I and Shiffrar MM (1987). Sexing day-old chicks: A case study and expert system analysis of a difficult perceptual-learning task. *Journal of Experimental Psychology: Leaning, Memory and Cognition*, **13**, 640–645.

Bingham AF, Birch GG, de Graaf C, Behan JM and Perring KD (1990). Sensory studies with sucrose–maltol mixtures. *Chemical Senses*, **15**, 447–456.

Bingham AF, Hurling R and Stocks J (2005). Acquisition of liking for spinach products. *Food Quality and Preference*, **16**, 461–469.

Bingham S, Luben R, Welch A, Tasevska N, Wareham N and Khaw K (2007). Epidemiologic assessment of sugars consumption using biomarkers: Comparison of obese and non-obese individuals in the European Prospective Investigation of Cancer Norfolk. *Cancer Epidemiology Biomarkers and Prevention*, **16**, 1651–1654.

Birch LL (1986). The acquisition of food acceptance patterns in children. In (eds) R Boakes, D Poplewell and M Burton, *Eating Habits*, pp. 107–129. Wiley, England.

Birch LL (1980). Effects of peer models' food choices and eating behaviors on preschoolers' food preferences. *Child Development*, **51**, 489–496.

Birch LL, Birch D, Marlin DW and Kramer L (1982). Effects of instrumental consumption on children's food preference. *Appetite: Journal for Intake Research*, **3**, 125–134.

Birch LL, Gunder L, Grimm-Thomas K and Laing DG (1998). Infants' consumption of a new food enhances acceptance of similar foods. *Appetite*, **30**, 283–295.

Birch LL and Marlin DW (1982). I don't like it; I never tried it: Effects of exposure on two-year-old children's food preferences. *Appetite: Journal of Intake Research*, **3**, 353–360.

Birch LL, McPhee L, Steinberg L and Sullivan S (1990). Conditioned flavor preferences in young children. *Physiology and Behavior*, **47**, 501–505.

Bitnes J, Rodbotten M, Lea P, Ueland O and Martens M (2007). Effect of product knowledge on profiling performance comparing various sensory laboratories. *Journal of Sensory Studies*, **22**, 66–80.

Blackwell L (1995). Visual cues and their effects on odour assessment. *Nutrition and Food Science*, **5**, 24–28.

Blake AA (2004). Flavour perception and the learning of food preferences. In (eds) A Taylor and D Roberts, *Flavor Perception*, pp. 172–202. Blackwell Publishing Ltd, Oxford.

Blass EM and Shah A (1995). Pain reducing properties of sucrose in human newborns. *Chemical Senses*, **20**, 29–35.

Bodyfelt FW, Tobias J and Trout GM (1988). *Sensory Evaluation of Dairy Products*. Van Nostrand, NY.

Boland AB, Delahunty CM and van Ruth SM (2006). Influence of the texture of gelatin gels and pectin gels on strawberry flavour release and perception. *Food Chemistry*, **96**, 452–460.

Bonnans S and Noble AC (1993). Effect of sweetener type and of sweetener and acid levels on temporal perception of sweetness, sourness and fruitiness. *Chemical Senses*, **18**, 273–283.

Booth DA, Lee M and McAleavey C (1976). Acquired sensory control of satiation in man. *British Journal of Psychology*, **67**, 137–147.

Booth DA, Mather P and Fuller J (1982). Starch content of ordinary foods associatively conditions human appetite and satiation, indexed by intake and eating pleasantness of starch-paired flavours. *Appetite*, **3**, 163–184.

Boring EG (1942). *Sensation and Perception in the History of Experimental Psychology*. Appleton-Century Inc., NY.

Bosman F, van der Bilt A, Abbink JH and van der Glas HW (2004). Neuromuscular control mechanisms in human mastication. *Journal of Texture Studies*, **35**, 201–221.

Bovbjerg VE (2008). The epidemiology of obesity: Causal roots – routes of cause. In (ed.) EM Blass, *Obesity*, pp. 19–63. Sinauer and Associates, MA.

Bowers RL, Doran TP, Edles PA and May K (1994). Paired-associate learning with visual and olfactory cues: Effects of temporal order. *The Psychological Record*, **44**, 501–507.

Brannan GD, Setser CS and Kemp KE (2001). Interaction of astringency and taste characteristics. *Journal of Sensory Studies*, **16**, 179–197.

Brand G (2006). Olfactory/trigeminal interactions in nasal chemoreception. *Neuroscience and Biobehavioral Reviews*, **30**, 908–917.

Breslin PAS, Gilmore MM, Beauchamp GK and Green BG (1993). Psychophysical evidence that oral astringency is a tactile sensation. *Chemical Senses*, **18**, 405–417.

Brondel L, Romer M, Van Wymelbeke V, *et al.* (2007). Sensory-specific satiety with simple foods in humans: No influence of BMI? *International Journal of Obesity*, **31**, 987–995.

Brown WE, Langley KR, Martin A and MacFie HJH (1994). Characterisation of patterns of chewing behaviour in human subjects and their influence on texture perception. *Journal of Texture Studies*, **25**, 455–468.

Brunstrom JM (2004). Does dietary learning occur outside awareness? *Consciousness and Cognition*, **13**, 453–470.

Brunstrom JM, Downes CR and Higgs S (2001). Effects of dietary restraint on flavour–flavour learning. *Appetite*, **37**, 197–206.

Brunstrom JM and Fletcher JM (2008). Flavour-flavour learning occurs automatically and only in hungry participants. *Physiology and Behavior*, **93**, 13–19.

Brunstrom JM and Higgs S (2002). Exploring evaluative conditioning using a working memory task. *Learning and Motivation*, **33**, 433–455.

Brunstrom JM, Higgs S and Mitchell G (2005). Dietary restraint and US devaluation predict evaluative learning. *Physiology and Behavior*, **85**, 524–535.

Brunstrom JM and Mitchell G (2007). Flavor–nutrient learning in restrained and unrestrained eaters. *Physiology and Behavior*, **90**, 133–141.

Buck LB (2000). The molecular architecture of odor and pheromone sensing in mammals. *Cell*, **100**, 611–618.

Buckner RL and Wheeler ME (2001). The cognitive neuroscience of remembering. *Nature Reviews Neuroscience*, **9**, 624–634.

Buettner A, Beer A, Hannig C and Settles M (2001). Observation of the swallowing process by application of videofluoroscopy and real time magnetic resonance imaging – consequences for retronasal stimulation. *Chemical Senses*, **26**, 1211–1219.

Buettner A, Beer A, Hannig C, Settles M and Schieberle P (2002). Physiological and analytical studies on flavor perception dynamics as induced by the eating and swallowing process. *Food Quality and Preference*, **13**, 497–504.

Bujas Z, Ajdukovoc D, Szabo S, Mayer D and Vodanovic M (1995). Central processes in gustatory adaptation. *Physiology and Behavior*, **57**, 875–880.

Bult JHF, de Wijk RA and Hummel T (2007). Investigations on multimodal sensory integration: Texture, taste, and ortho- and retronasal olfactory stimuli in concert. *Neuroscience Letters*, **411**, 6–10.

Bull T (1966). Taste and the chorda tympani. *Journal of Laryngology and Otology*, **79**, 479–493.

Burdach KJ, Kroeze JHA and Koster EP (1984). Nasal, retronasal, and gustatory perception: An experimental comparison. *Perception and Psychophysics*, **36**, 205–208.

Cabanac M (1971). Physiological role of pleasure. *Science*, **173**, 1103–1107.

Cabanac M and Fantino M (1977). Origin of olfacto-gustatory alliesthesia: Intestinal sensitivity to carbohydrate concentration. *Physiology and Behavior*, **18**, 1039–1045.

Cabanac M and Rabe EF (1976). Influence of a monotonous food on body weight regulation in humans. *Physiology and Behavior*, **17**, 675–678.

Cabeza R and Nyberg L (2000). Imaging cognition II: An empirical review of 275 PET and fMRI studies. *Journal of Cognitive Neuroscience*, **12**, 1–47.

Cain WS (1979). To know with the nose: Keys to odor and identification. *Science*, **203**, 468–470.

Cain WS, de Wijk R, Lulejian C, Schiet F and See L-C. (1998). Odor identification: Perceptual and semantic dimensions. *Chemical Senses*, **23**, 309–326.

Cain WS and Drexler M (1974). Scope and evaluation of odor counteraction and masking. *Annals of New York Academy of Sciences*, **237**, 427–439.

Cain WS and Murphy CL (1980). Interaction between chemoreceptive modalities of odour and irritation. *Nature*, **284**, 255–257.

Cain WS, Schiet FT, Olsson MJ and de Wijk RA (1995). Comparison of models of odor interaction. *Chemical Senses*, **20**, 625–637.

Calvert GA (2001). Crossmodal processing in the human brain: Insights from functional neuroimaging studies. *Cerebral Cortex*, **11**, 1110–1123.

Calvert GA, Brammer MJ and Iversen SD (1998). Crossmodal identification. *Trends in Cognitive Sciences*, **2**, 247–253.

Calvert GA, Spence C and Stein B (2004). *The Handbook of Multisensory Processes*. MIT Press, MA.

Calvino AM, Garcia-Medina MR, Comette-Muniz JE (1990). Interactions in caffeine- sucrose and coffee–sucrose mixtures: Evidence of taste and flavor suppression. *Chemical Senses*, **13**, 505–519.

Calvino AM, Garcia-Medina MR, Comette-Muniz JE and Rodriguez MB (1993). Perception of sweetness and bitterness in different vehicles. *Perception and Psychophysics*, **54**, 751–758.

Calvo C, Salvador A and Fiszman SM (2001). Influence of the colour intensity on the perception of colour and sweetness in various fruit-flavored yoghurts. *European Food Research and Technology*, **213**, 99–103.

Cannon DS, Best MR, Batson JD and Feldman M (1983). Taste familiarity and apomorphine-induced taste aversions in humans. *Behavior Research and Therapy*, **21**, 669–673.

Capaldi ED and Privitera GJ (2007). Flavor–nutrient learning independent of flavor–taste learning with college students. *Appetite*, **49**, 712–715.

Caporale G, Policastro S and Monteleone E (2004). Bitterness enhancement induced by cut grass odorant (cis-3-hexen-1-ol) in a model olive oil. *Food Quality and Preference*, **15**, 219–227.

Cardello AV, Maller O, Bloom D, Masor HB, Dubose C and Edelman B. (1985). Role of consumer expectations in the acceptance of novel foods. *Journal of Food Science*, **50**, 1707–1714.

Cardello AV, Maller O, Kapsalis JG, *et al.* (1982). Perception of texture by trained and consumer panellists. *Journal of Food Science*, **47**, 1186–1197.

Cardello AV and Sawyer FM (1992). Effects of disconfirmed consumer expectations on food acceptability. *Journal of Sensory Studies*, **7**, 253–277.

Cardello AV, Schutz H, Snow C and Lesher L (2000). Predictions of food acceptance, consumption and satisfaction in specific eating situations. *Food Quality and Preference*, **11**, 201–216.

Carrapiso AI (2007). Effect of fat content on flavour release from sausages. *Food Chemistry*, **103**, 396–403.

Case TI, Stevenson RJ and Dempsey RA (2004). Reduced discriminability following perceptual learning with odours. *Perception*, **33**, 113–119.

Caul JF (1957). The profile method of flavor analysis. *Advances in Food Research*, **7**, 1–40.

Cereda C, Ghika J, Maeder P and Bogousslavsky J (2002). Strokes restricted to the insular cortex. *Neurology*, **59**, 1950–1955.

Chale-Rush A, Burgess JR and Mattes RD (2007). Multiple routes of chemosensitivity to free fatty acids in humans. *American Journal of Physiology - Gastrointestinal and Liver Physiology*, **292**, G1206–G1212.

Chambers DH, Allison AA and Chambers E (2004). Training effects on performance of descriptive panellists. *Journal of Sensory Studies*, **19**, 486–499.

Chambers E and Smith EA (1993). Effects of testing experience on performance of trained sensory panellists. *Journal of Sensory Studies*, **8**, 155–166.

Chan MM and Kane-Martinelli C (1997). The effect of color on perceived flavor intensity and acceptance of foods by young adults and elderly adults. *Journal of American Dietetic Association*, **97**, 657–659.

Changizi MA and Hall WG (2001). Thirst modulates a perception. *Perception*, **30**, 1489–1497.

Chapuis J, Messaoudi B, Ferreira G and Ravel N (2007). Importance of retronasal and orthonasal olfaction for odor aversion memory in rats. *Behavioral Neuroscience*, **121**, 1383–1392.

Chen V and Halpern BP (2008). Retronasal but not oral-cavity-only identification of "purely olfactory" odorants. *Chemical Senses*, **33**, 107–118.

Chernin A (2008). The effects of food marketing on children's preferences: Testing the moderating roles of age and gender. *Annals of the American Academy of Political and Social Science*, **615**, 102–118.

Chollet S and Valentin D (2001). Impact of training on beer flavor perception and description: Are trained and untrained subjects really different? *Journal of Sensory Studies*, **12**, 601–618.

Chollet S, Valentin D and Abdi H (2005). Do trained assessors generalize their knowledge to new stimuli? *Food Quality and Preference*, **16**, 13–23.

Christensen CM (1980a). Effects of solution viscosity on perceived saltiness and sweetness. *Perception and Psychophysics*, **28**, 347–353.

Christensen CM (1980b). Effects of taste quality and intensity on oral perception of viscosity. *Perception and Psychophysics*, **28**, 315–320.

Christensen CM (1983). Effects of color on aroma, flavor and texture judgements of foods. *Journal of Food Science*, **48**, 787–790.

Christensen CM (1984). Food texture perception. In (ed.) E Mark, *Advances in Food Research*, pp. 159–199. Academic Press, New York.

Christensen CM (1985). Effect of color on judgements of food aroma and flavor intensity in young and elderly adults. *Perception*, **14**, 755–762.

Civille GV and Szcesniak AS (1973). Guidelines to training a texture profile panel. *Journal of Texture Studies*, **4**, 204–223.

Clark CC and Lawless HT (1994). Limiting response alternatives in time-intensity scaling: An examination of the halo-dumping effect. *Chemical Senses*, **19**, 583–594.

Classen C (1992). The odor of the other: Olfactory symbolism and cultural categories. *Ethos*, **20**, 133–166.

Clegg S, Kilcast D and Arazi S (2003). The structural and compositional basis of creaminess in food emulsion gels. *Proceedings of the Third International Symposium on Food Rheology and Structure* (pp. 373–377). Swiss Federal Institute of Technology, Zurich.

Cliff M and Noble AC (1990). Time-intensity evaluation of sweetness and fruitiness and their interaction in a model solution. *Journal of Food Science*, **55**, 450–455.

Cohen MN (2000). History, diet and hunter-gatherers. In (eds) KF Kiple and KC Ornelas, *The Cambridge World History of Food*, pp. 63–74. CUP, Cambridge.

Cometto-Muniz JE, Cain WS and Hudnell HK (1997). Agonistic sensory effects of airborne chemicals in mixtures: Odor, nasal pungency, and eye irritation. *Perception and Psychophysics*, **59**, 665–674.

Cometto-Muniz JE, Garcia-Medina MR and Calvino AM (1989). Perception of pungent odorants alone and in binary mixtures. *Chemical Senses*, **14**, 163–173.

Cometto-Muniz JE, Garcia-Medina MR, Calvino AM and Noriega G (1987). Interactions between CO_2 oral pungency and taste. *Perception*, **16**, 629–640.

Cometto-Muniz JE and Hernandez SM (1990). Odorous and pungent attributes of mixed and unmixed odorants. *Perception and Psychophysics*, **47**, 391–399.

Conner MT, Haddon AV, Pickering ES and Booth DA (1988). Sweet tooth demonstrated: Individual differences in preference for both sweet foods and foods highly sweetened. *Journal of Applied Psychology*, **73**, 275–280.

Cook DJ, Hollowood TA, Linforth RST and Taylor AJ (2002). Perception of taste intensity in solution of random-coil polysaccharides above and below C. *Food Quality and Preference*, **13**, 473–480.

Cook DJ, Hollowood TA, Linforth RST and Taylor AJ (2003). Oral shear stress predicts flavour perception in viscous solutions. *Chemical Senses*, **28**, 11–23.

Coppens E, Vansteenwegen D, Baeyens F, Vandenbulcke M, Van Paesschen W and Eelen P (2006). Evaluative conditioning is intact after unilateral resection of the anterior temporal lobe in humans. *Neuropsychologia*, **44**, 840–843.

Cowart BJ (1987). Oral chemical irritation: Does it reduce perceived taste intensity? *Chemical Senses*, **12**, 467–479.

Cowart BJ (1998). The addition of CO2 to traditional taste solutions alters taste quality. *Chemical Senses*, **23**, 397–402.

Cox SML, Andrade A and Johnsrude IS (2005). Learning to like: A role for human orbitofrontal cortex in conditioned reward. *Journal of Neuroscience*, **25**, 2733–2740.

Crandall CS (1984). The liking of foods as a result of exposure: Eating doughnuts in Alaska. *The Journal of Social Psychology*, **125**, 187–194.

Cruz A and Green BG (2000). Thermal stimulation of taste. *Nature*, **403**, 889–892.

Daget N and Joerg M (1991). Creamy perception in model soups. *Journal of Texture Studies*, **22**, 168–189.

Daget N, Joerg M and Bourne M (1988). Creamy perception in model desert creams. *Journal of Texture Studies*, **18**, 367–388.

Dalton P, Doolittle N, Nagata H and Breslin PAS (2000). The merging of the senses: Integration of subthreshold taste and smell. *Nature Neuroscience*, **3**, 431–432.

Davidson JM, Linforth RST, Hollowood TA and Taylor AJ (1999). Effect of Sucrose on the Perceived Flavor Intensity of Chewing Gum. *Journal of Agricultural and Food Chemistry*, **47**, 4336–4340.

Davidson T, Kanoski S, Walls E and Jarrard L (2005). Memory inhibition and energy regulation. *Physiology and Behavior*, **86**, 731–746.

Davis RG (1977). Acquisition and retention of verbal associations to olfactory and abstract visual stimuli of varying similarity. *Journal of Experimental Psychology: Human Learning and Memory*, **3**, 37–51.

Davis RG (1981). The role of nonolfactory context cues in odor identification. *Perception and Psychophysics*, **30**, 83–89.

Davis RG and Pangborn RM (1985). Odor pleasantness judgments compared among samples from 20 nations using microfragrances. *Chemical Senses*, **30**, 413.

de Araujo, Rolls ET, Kringelbach ML, McGlone F and Phillips N (2003). Taste–olfactory convergence, and the representation of the pleasantness of flavour, in the human brain. *European Journal of Neuroscience*, **18**, 2059–2068.

De Castro, JM (1996) How can eating behavior be regulated in the complex environments of free living humans. *Neuroscience and Biobehavioral Reviews*, **20**, 119–131.

Deems DA, Doty RL, Settle RG, *et al.* (1991). Smell and taste disorders, a study of 750 patients from the university of Pennsylvania smell and taste center. *Archives of Otolaryngology Head and Neck Surgery*, **117**, 519–528.

De Gelder B and Bertelson P (2003). Multisensory integration, perception and ecological validity. *Trends in Cognitive Sciences*, **7**, 460–467.

De Houwer J, Thomas S and Baeyens F (2001). Associative learning of likes and dislikes: A review of 25 years of research on human evaluative conditioning. *Psychological Bulletin*, **127**, 853–869.

Delamatar AR (2007). Extinction of conditioned flavor preferences. *Journal of Experimental Psychology*, **33**, 160–171.

De Liver Y, van der Pligt J and Wigboldus D (2005). Unpacking attitudes towards genetically modified food. *Appetite*, **45**, 242–249.

Delwiche J (2004). The impact of perceptual interactions on perceived flavor. *Food Quality and Preference*, **15**, 137–146.

Delwiche J and Heffelfinger AL (2005). Cross-modal additivity of taste and smell. *Journal of Sensory Studies*, **20**, 512–525.

Dematte ML, Sanabria D and Spence C (2006). Cross-modal associations between odors and colors. *Chemical Senses*, **31**, 531–538.

de Roos KB (2003). Effect of texture and microstructure on flavour retention and release. *International Dairy Journal*, **13**, 593–605.

Desor JA and Beauchamp GK (1974). The human capacity to transmit olfactory information. *Perception and Psychophysics*, **16**, 551–556.

de Wijk RA, Polet IA, Engelen L, van Doorn RM and Prinz JF (2004). Amount of ingested custard dessert as affected by its color, odor, and texture. *Physiology and Behavior*, **82**, 397–403.

de Wijk RA and Prinz JF (2005). The role of friction in perceived oral texture. *Food Quality and Preference*, **16**, 121–129.

de Wijk RA, Prinz JF, Polet IA and van Doorn RM (2004). Amount of ingested custard as affected by its colour, smell, and texture. *Physiology and Behavior*, **82**, 397–403.

de Wijk RA, Rasing F and Wilkinson CL (2003). Texture of semi-solids: Sensory flavor–texture interactions for custard desserts. *Journal of Texture Studies*, **34**, 131–146.

de Wijk RA, Terpstra MEJ, Janssen AM and Prinz JF (2006). Perceived creaminess of semi-solid foods. *Trends in Food Science and Technology*, **17**, 412–422.

de Wijk RA, van Gemert LJ, Terpstra MEJ and Wilkinson C (2003). Texture of semi-solids: Sensory and instrumental measurements on vanilla custard deserts. *Food Quality and Preference*, **14**, 315–317.

Diaz ME (2004). Comparison between orthonasal and retronasal flavour perception at different concentrations. *Flavour and Fragrance Journal*, **19**, 499–504.

Djordjevic J, Zatorre RJ and Jones-Gotman M (2004). Odor-induced changes in taste perception. *Experimental Brain Research*, **159**, 405–408.

Dobraszczyk BJ and Vincent JFV (1999). Measurement of mechanical properties of food materials in relation to texture: the materials approach. In (ed.) A Rosenthal, *Food Texture: Measurement and Perception*, pp. 99–151. Aspen Publishers, Gaithersburg.

Dodds WJ (1989). The physiology of swallowing. *Dysphagia*, **3**, 171–178.

Dravnieks A (1985). *Atlas of Odor Character Profiles*. American Society for Testing and Materials, PA.

Drewnowski A (1992). Sensory preferences and fat consumption in obesity and eating disorders. In (ed.) D Mela, *Dietary Fats: Determinants of Preference Selection and Consumption*, pp. 59–77. Elsevier Applied Science, London.

Drewnowski A (1994). Human preferences for sugar and fat. In (ed.) J Fernstorm and G Miller, *Appetite and Body Weight Regulation: Sugar, Fat, and Macronutrient Substitutes*, pp. 99–112. CRC Press, London.

Drewnowski A, Brunzell JD, Sande K, Iverius PH and Greenwood MRC (1985). Sweet tooth reconsidered: Taste responsiveness in human obesity. *Physiology and Behavior*, **35**, 617–622.

DuBose CN, Cardello AV and Maller O (1980). Effects of colorants and flavorants on identification, perceived intensity, and hedonic quality of fruit-flavored beverages and cake. *Journal of Food Science*, **45**, 1393–1415.

Duchamp-Viret P, Duchamp A and Chaput MA (2003). Single olfactory sensory neurons simultaneously integrate the components of an odour mixture. *European Journal of Neuroscience*, **18**, 2690–2696.

Duclaux R, Feisthauer J and Cabanac JFEM (1973). Effets du repas sur l'agrement d'odeurs alimentaires et nonalimentaires chez l'homme. *Physiology and Behavior*, **10**, 1029–1033.

Duffy VB, Hayes JE and Dinehart ME (2006). Genetic differences in sweet taste perception. In (ed.) W Spillane, *Optimising Sweet Taste in Foods*, pp. 30–53, CRC Press, Boston.

Dufour DL and Sander JB (2000). Insects. In (eds) KF Kiple and KC Ornelas, *The Cambridge World History of Food*, pp. 555–558. CUP, Cambridge.

Dwyer DM (2005). Reinforcer devaluation in palatability-based learned flavor preferences. *Journal of Experimental Psychology: Animal Behavior Processes*, **31**, 487–492.

Dykens EM (2000). Contaminated and unusual food combinations: What do people with Prader-Willi syndrome choose? *Mental Retardation*, **38**, 163–171.

Elias M, Elias P, Sullivan L, Wolf P and Agostino R (2005). Obesity, diabetes and cognitive deficit: The Framingham heart study. *Neurobiology of Ageing*, **26**, S11–16.

Elgart BZ and Marks LE (2006). Detection of weak gustatory–olfactory flavor mixtures. *Chemical Senses*, **31**, A49.

Engelen L, de Wijk RA, van der Bilt A, Prinz JF, Janssen AM and Bosman F (2005). Relating particles and texture perception. *Physiology and Behavior*, **86**, 111–117.

Engelen L, de Wijk RA, Prinz JF, Janssen AM, Weenen H and Bosman F (2003). The effect of oral and product temperature on perception of flavor and texture attributes of semi solid. *Appetite*, **41**, 273–281.

Engen T (1972). The effect of expectation on judgements of odor. *Acta Psychologica*, **36**, 450–458.

Engen T (1974). Method and theory in the study of odor preferences. In (eds) JW Johnston, DG Moulton and A Turk, *Human Responses to Environmental Odors*, pp. 121–141). Academic Press, NY.

Engen T (1982). *The Perception of Odors*. Academic Press, NY.

Enns MP and Hornung DE (1985). Contributions of smell and taste to overall intensity. *Chemical Senses*, **10**, 357–366.

Fallon AE and Rozin P (1983). The psychological bases of food rejections by humans. *Ecology of Food and Nutrition*, **13**, 15–26.

Farah MJ (1990). *Visual Agnosia*. MIT Press, MA.

Faurion A, Cerf B, Van de Moortele P-F, Lobel E, Macleod P and Le Bihan D (1999). Human taste cortical areas studied with functional magnetic resonance imaging: Evidence of functional lateralization related to handedness. *Neuroscience Letters*, **277**, 189–192.

Faurion A, Cerf B, Pillias A-M and Boireau N (2005). Increased taste sensitivity by familiarization to novel stimuli: psychophysics, fMRI and electrophysiological techniques suggest modulations at peripheral and central levels. In (eds) C Rouby, B Schaal, DI Dubois, R Gervais and A Holley, *Olfaction, Taste and Cognition*, pp. 350–366. CUP, Cambridge.

Faust J (1974). A twin study of personal preferences. *Journal of Biosocial Science*, **6**, 75–91.

Ferry AL, Hort J, Mitchell JR, Cook DJ, Lagarridue S and Pamies BV (2006). Viscosity and flavour perception: Why is starch different from hydrocolloids? *Food Hydrocolloids*, **20**, 855–862.

Fields, AP (2006). I don't like it because it eat sprouts: Conditioning preferences in children. *Behaviour Research and Therapy*, **44**, 439–455.

Finlayson G, King N and Blundell J (2007). Liking vs. wanting food: Importance for human appetite control and weight regulation. *Neuroscience and Biobehavioral Reviews*, **31**, 987–1002.

Finlayson G, King N and Blundell J (2008). The role of implicit wanting in relation to explicit liking and wanting for food: Implications for appetite control. *Appetite*, **50**, 120–127.

Fischer R, Griffin F, England S and Garn SM (1961). Taste thresholds and food dislikes. *Nature*, **191**, 1328.

Fogel RW (2004). *The Escape from Hunger and Premature Death*. CUP, Cambridge.

Forde CG and Delahunty CM (2002). Examination of chemical irritation and textual influence on food preferences in two age cohorts using complex food systems. *Food Quality and Preference*, **13**, 571–581.

Frandsen LW, Dijksterhuis GB, Brockhoff PB, Nielsen JH and Martens M (2007). Feelings as a basis for discrimination: Comparison of a modified authenticity test with the same–different for slightly different types of milk. *Food Quality and Preference*, **18**, 97–105.

Frank ME (1989). Processing of mixtures of stimuli with different tastes by primary mammalian taste neurons. In (eds) DG Laing, WS Cain, RL McBride and BW Ache, *Perception of complex smells and tastes*, pp. 127–147. Academic Press, Sydney.

Frank RA and Byram J (1988). Taste–smell interactions are tastant and odorant dependent. *Chemical Senses*, **13**, 445–455.

Frank RA, Ducheny K and Mize SJS (1989). Strawberry odor, but not red color, enhances the sweetness of sucrose solutions. *Chemical Senses*, **14**, 371–377.

Frank RA, van der Klaauw NJ and Schifferstein HNJ (1993). Both perceptual and conceptual factors influence taste–odor and taste–taste interactions. *Perception and Psychophysics*, **54**, 343–354.

Franken IHA and Muris P (2005). Individual differences in reward sensitivity are related to food craving and relative body weight in healthy women. *Appetite*, **45**, 198–201.

Frasnelli J, Heilmann S and Hummel T (2004). Responsiveness of human nasal mucosa to trigeminal stimuli depends on the site of stimulation. *Neuroscience Letters*, **362**, 65–69.

Frost MB, Dijksterhuis GB and Martens M (2001). Sensory perception of fat in milk. *Food Quality and Preference*, **12**, 327–336.

Frost MB and Janhoj T (2007). Understanding creaminess. *International Dairy Journal*, **17**, 1298–1311.

Frost MB and Noble AC (2002). Preliminary study of the effect of knowledge and sensory expertise on liking for red wines. *American Journal of Oenology and Viticulture*, **53**, 275–284.

Furnham A and Walker J (2001). The influence of personality traits, previous experience of art, and demographic variables on artistic performance. *Personality and Individual Differences*, **31**, 997–1017.

Galef BG (1991). A contrarian view of the wisdom of the body as it relates to dietary self-selection. *Psychological Review*, **98**, 218–223.

Galef BG and Stein M (1985). Demonstrator influence on observer diet preference: Analysis of critical social interactions and olfactory signals. *Animal Learning and Behavior*, **13**, 31–38.

Galst JP and White MA (1976). The unhealthy persuader: The reinforcing value of television and children's purchase-influencing attempts at the supermarket. *Child Development*, **47**, 1089–1096.

Galloway JH (2000). Sugar. In (eds) KF Kiple and KC Ornelas, *The Cambridge World History of Food*, pp. 437–449. CUP, Cambridge.

Ganchrow JR, Steiner JE and Daher M (1983). Neonatal facial expressions in response to different qualities and intensities of gustatory stimuli. *Infant Behavior and Development*, **6**, 473–484.

Garb JL and Stunkard AJ (1974). Taste aversions in man. *American Journal of Psychiatry*, **131**, 1204–1207.

Garner WR (1974). Attention: The processing of multiple sources of information. In (eds) EC Carterette and MP Friedman, *Handbook of Perception, Volume 2*, pp. 23–59. Academic Press, NY.

Gawel R (1997). The use of language by trained and untrained experienced wine tasters. *Journal of Sensory Studies*, **12**, 267–284.

Gent JF, Goodspeed RB, Zagraniski RT and Catalanotto FA (1987). Taste and smell problems: Validation of questions for the clinical history. *Yale Journal of Biology and Medicine*, **60**, 27–35.

Gerber JC, Small D, Heilmann S and Hummel T. (2003). Comparison of orthonasal and retronasal perception of non-food odors: A functional MR imaging study. *Chemical Senses*, **28**, A34.

Gibson EL, Wainwright CJ and Booth DA (1995). Disguised protein in lunch after low-protein breakfast conditions food–flavor preferences dependent on recent lack of protein intake. *Physiology and Behavior*, **58**, 363–371.

Gibson JJ (1966). *The Senses Considered as Perceptual Systems*. Allen & Unwin, London.

Gilbert AN, Martin R and Kemp SE (1996). Cross-modal correspondence between vision and olfaction: The color of smells. *American Journal of Psychology*, **109**, 335–351.

Gillan DJ (1982). Mixture suppression: The effect of spatial separation between sucrose and NaCl. *Perception and Psychophysics*, **32**, 504–510.

Giraudet P, Berthommier F and Chaput M (2001). Mitral cell temporal response patterns evoked by odor mixtures in rat olfactory bulb. *Journal of Neurophysiology*, **88**, 829–838.

Glanville EV and Kaplan AR (1965). Food preference and sensitivity of taste for bitter compounds. *Nature*, **205**, 851–853.

Glanz K, Basil M, Maibach E, Goldberg J and Snyder D (1998). Why Americans eat what they do: Taste, nutrition, cost, convenience, and weight control concerns as influences of food consumption. *Journal of the American Dietetic Association*, **98**, 1118–1126.

Glautier S, Bankart J and Williams A (2000). Flavour conditioning and alcohol: A multilevel model of individual differences. *Biological Psychology*, **52**, 17–36.

Glendinning JI (1994). Is the bitter rejection response always adaptive. *Physiology and Behavior*, **56**, 1217–1227.

Goldberg ME, Gorn GJ and Gibson W (1978). TV messages for snack and breakfast foods: Do they influence children's preferences? *Journal of Consumer Research*, **5**, 73–81.

Gonzalez J, Barros-Loscertales A, Pulvermuller F, *et al.* (2006). Reading *cinnamon* activates olfactory brain regions. *Neuroimage*, **32**, 906–912.

Gonzalez R, Benedito J, Carcel JA and Mulet A (2001). Cheese hardness assessment by experts and untrained judges. *Journal of Sensory Studies*, **16**, 277–285.

Gottfried JA and Dolan RJ (2003). The nose smells what the eye sees: Crossmodal visual facilitation of human olfactory perception. *Neuron*, **39**, 375–386.

Gottfried JA, O'Doherty J and Dolan RJ (2002). Appetitive and aversive olfactory learning in humans studied using event-related functional magnetic resonance imaging. *Journal of Neuroscience*, **15**, 10829–10837.

Grabenhorst F, Rolls ET and Bilderbeck A (2007). How cognition modulates affective responses to taste and flavour: Top-down influences on the orbitofrontal and pregenual cingulate cortices. *Cerebral Cortex*, **18**, 1549–1559.

Graillon A, Barr RG, Young SN, Wright JH and Hendricks LA (1997). Differential response to intraoral sucrose, quinine and corn oil in crying human newborns. *Physiology and Behavior*, **62**, 317–325.

Gratzer W (2005). *Terrors of the Table*. OUP, Oxford.

Gray DE (1972). *American Institute of Physics Handbook* (3rd Edition). McGraw Hill, New York.

Green BG (1985). Menthol modulates oral sensations of warmth and cold. *Physiology and Behavior*, **35**, 427–434.

Green BG (1986b). Sensory interactions between capsaicin temperature in oral cavity. *Chemical Senses*, **11**, 371–382.

Green BG (1987). The effect of cooling on the vibrotactile sensitivity of the tongue. *Perception and Psychophysics*, **42**, 423–430.

Green BG (1990). Effects of thermal, mechanical, and chemical stimulation on the perception of oral irritation. In (eds), BG Green, JR Mason and MR Kare, *Chemical Senses: Irritation, Volume 2*, pp. 171–192. Marcel Dekker, New York.

Green BG (1992). The effects of temperature and concentration on the perceived intensity and quality of carbonation. *Chemical Senses*, **17**, 435–450.

Green BG (1993). Oral astringency: A tactile component of flavor. *Acta Psychologica*, **84**, 119–125.

Green BG (2002). Studying taste as a cutaneous sense. *Food Quality and Preference*, **14**, 99–109.

Green BG (2005). Lingual heat and cold sensitivity following exposure to capsaicin or menthol. *Chemical Senses*, **30**, i201–i202.

Green BG, Alvarez-Reeves M, George P and Akirav C (2005). Chemesthesis and taste: Evidence of independent processing of sensation intensity. *Physiology and Behavior*, **86**, 526–537.

Green BG and Frankman SP (1987). The effects of cooling the tongue on the perceived intensity of taste. *Chemical Senses*, **12**, 609–619.

Green BG and Frankman SP (1988). The effect of cooling on the perception of carbohydrate and intensive sweeteners. *Physiology and Behavior*, **43**, 515–519.

Green BG, Shaffer GS and Gilmore M (1993). Derivation and evaluation of a semantic scale of oral sensation magnitude with apparent ratio properties. *Chemical Senses*, **18**, 683–702.

Greene LS, Desor JA and Maller O (1975). Heredity and experience: Their relative importance in the development of taste preference in man. *Physiology and Behavior*, **89**, 279–284.

Guinard JX and Marty C (1995). Time-intensity measurement of flavor release from a model gel system: Effect of gelling agent type and concentration. *Journal of Food Science and Technology*, **60**, 727–730.

Guinard JX and Mazzucchelli R (1996). The sensory perception of texture and mouthfeel. *Journal of Food Science and Technology*, **7**, 213–219.

Guinard JX, Pangborn RM and Lewis MJ (1985). Preliminary studies on acidity–astringency interactions in model solutions and wines. *Journal of the Science of Food and Agriculture*, **37**, 811–817.

Haberly LB (2001). Parallel-distributed processing in olfactory cortex: New insights from morphological and physiological analysis of neuronal circuitry. *Chemical Senses*, **26**, 551–576.

Haider H and Frensch PA (1996). The role of information reduction in skill acquisition. *Cognitive Psychology*, **30**, 304–337.

Hall IS and Hall CS (1939). A study of disliked and unfamiliar foods. *Journal of the American Dietetic Association*, **15**, 540–548.

Hancock P (2006). Monozygotic twins' colour-number association: A case study. *Cortex*, **42**, 147–150.

Harper LV and Sanders KM (1975). The effect of adults' eating on young children's acceptance of unfamiliar foods. *Journal of Experimental Child Psychology*, **20**, 206–214.

Harper R, Land DG, Griffiths NM and Bate-Smith EC (1968). Odour qualities: A glossary of usage. *British Journal of Psychology*, **59**, 231–252.

Harper SJ and McDaniel MR (1993). Carbonated water lexicon: Temperature and CO_2 level influence on descriptive ratings. *Journal of Food Science*, **58**, 893–898.

Harris JA and Thein T (2005). Interactions between conditioned and unconditioned flavor preferences. *Journal of Experimental Psychology: Animal Behavior Processes*, **31**, 407–417.

Havermans RC and Jansen A (2007). Increasing children's liking of vegetables through flavour-flavour learning. *Appetite*, **48**, 259–262.

Heath MR and Prinz JF (1999). Oral processing of foods and the sensory evaluation of texture. In (ed.) A Rosenthal, *Food Texture: Measurement and Perception*, pp. 18–29. Aspen Publishers, Gaithersburg.

Heilmann S and Hummel T (2004). A new method for comparing orthonasal and retronasal olfaction. *Behavioral Neuroscience*, **118**, 412–419.

Hendy HM, Williams KE and Camise TS (2005). "Kids choice" school lunch program increases children's fruit and vegetable acceptance. *Appetite*, **45**, 250–263.

Herman CP and Polivy J (1984). A boundary model for the regulation of eating. In (eds) AJ Stunkard and E Stellar, *Eating and its Disorders*, pp. 141–156. Raven Press, NY.

Hersleth M, Berggren R, Westad F and Martens M (2007). Perception of bread: A comparison of consumers and trained assessors. *Journal of Food Science*, **70**, S95–S101.

Herz RS (2003). The effect of verbal context on olfactory perception. *Journal of Experimental Psychology: General*, **132**, 595–606.

Herz RS and von Clef J (2001). The influence of verbal labelling on the perception of odors: Evidence for olfactory illusions? *Perception*, **30**, 381–391.

Hetherington MM (1996). Sensory-specific satiety and its importance in meal termination. *Neuroscience and Biobehavioral Reviews*, **20**, 113–117.

Hickson M (2005). Malnutrition and ageing. *Postgraduate Medical Journal*, **82**, 2–8.

Higgs, S, Williamson AM, Rotshstein P and Humphreys GW (2008). Sensory-specific satiety is intact in amnesiacs who eat multiple meals. *Psychological Science*, **19**, 623–628.

Hill JM and Radimer KL (1996). Health and nutrition messages in food advertisements: A comparative content analysis of young and mature Australian women's magazines. *Journal of Nutrition Education*, **28**, 313–320.

Hinton PB and Henley TB (1993). Cognitive and affective components of stimuli presented in three modes. *Bulletin of the Psychonomic Society*, **31**, 595–598.

Hirsch AR (1990). Smell and taste: How the culinary experts compare to the rest of us. *Food Technology*, **September Issue**, 96–101.

Hobden K and Pliner P (1995). Effects of a model on food neophobia in humans. *Appetite*, **25**, 101–114.

Hodgson M, Linforth RST and Taylor A (2003). Simultaneous real-time measurements of mastication, swallowing, nasal airflow and aroma release. *Journal of Agricultural Food Chemistry*, **51**, 5052–5057.

Hodzic A, Veit R, Karim AA, Erb M and Godde B (2004). Improvement and decline in tactile discrimination behavior after cortical plasticity induced by passive tactile coactivation. *The Journal of Neuroscience*, **24**, 442–446.

Hollins M, Faldowski R, Rao S and Young F (1993). Perceptual dimensions of tactile surface texture: A multidimensional scaling analysis. *Perception and Psychophysics*, **54**, 697–705.

Hollowood TA, Linforth RST and Taylor AJ (2002). The effect of viscosity on the perception of flavour. *Chemical Senses*, **27**, 583–591.

Honey RC and Hall G (1989). Acquired equivalence and distinctiveness of cues. *Journal of Experimental Psychology: Animal Behavior Processes*, **15**, 338–346.

Hornung DE and Enns MP (1986). The contributions of smell and taste to overall intensity: A model. *Perception & Psychophysics*, **39**, 385–391.

Hough G (1998). Experts versus consumers: A critique. *Journal of Sensory Studies*, **13**, 285–289.

Hughson AL and Boakes RA (2002). The knowing nose: The role of knowledge in wine expertise. *Food Quality and Preference*, **13**, 463–472.

Hutchinson SE, Trantow LA and Vickers ZM (1990). The effectiveness of common foods for reduction of capsaicin burn. *Journal of Sensory Studies*, **4**, 157–164.

Hummel T, Heilmann S, Landis BN, *et al.* (2006). Perceptual differences between chemical stimuli presented through the orth- or retronasal route. *Flavour and Fragrance Journal*, **21**, 42–47.

Humphreys GW and Riddoch MJ (2006). Features, objects, action: The cognitive neuropsychology of visual object processing, 1984–2004. *Cognitive Neuropsychology*, **23**, 156–183.

Hvastja L and Zanuttini L (1989). Odour memory and odour hedonics in children. *Perception*, **18**, 391–396.

Hyman A (1983). The influence of color on the taste perception of carbonated water preparations. *Bulletin of the Psychonomic Society*, **21**, 145–148.

Ishii R, Kawaguchi H, O'Mahony M and Rousseau B (2007). Relating consumer and trained panels' discriminative sensitivities using vanilla flavored ice cream as a medium. *Food Quality and Preference*, **18**, 89–96.

Ishii R, Yamaguchi S and O'Mahony M (1992). Measures of taste discriminability for sweet, salty and umami stimuli: Japanese versus Americans. *Chemical Senses*, **17**, 365–380.

Jacquot L, Mannin J and Brand G (2004). Influence of nasal trigeminal stimuli on olfactory sensitivity. *Comptes Rendus Biologies*, **327**, 305–311.

Jamie I, Mela DJ and Bratchell N (1993). A study of texture–flavor interactions using free-choice profiling. *Journal of Sensory Studies*, **8**, 177–188.

Jellinek JS and Koster EP (1979). Perceived fragrance complexity and its relation to familiarity and pleasantness. *Journal of the Society of Cosmetic Chemists*, **30**, 253–262.

John T and Keen SL (1985). Determinants of taste perception and classification among the Aymara of Bolivia. *Ecology of Food and Nutrition*, **16**, 253–271.

Johnson JL and Clydesdale FM (1982). Perceived Sweetness and redness in colored sucrose solutions. *Journal of Food Science*, **47**, 747–752.

Johnson JL, Dzendolet E and Clydesdale FM (1983). Psychophysical relationship between sweetness and redness in strawberry-flavored drinks. *Journal of Food Protection*, **46**, 21–25.

Johnson JL, Dzendolet E, Damon P, Sawyer M and Clydesdale FM (1982). Psychophysical relationship between perceived sweetness and color in cherry-flavored beverages. *Journal of Food Protection*, **45**, 601–606.

Johnson JL and Vickers Z (1992). Factors influencing sensory-specific satiety. *Appetite*, **19**, 15–31.

Johnson JL and Vickers Z (1993). Effects of flavor and macronutrient composition of food servings on liking, hunger and subsequent intake. *Appetite*, **21**, 25–39.

Johnsrude IS, Owen AM, White NM, Zhao WV and Bohbot V (2000). Impaired preference conditioning after anterior temporal lobe resection in humans. *Journal of Neuroscience*, **20**, 2649–2656.

Jones MO (2000). What's disgusting, why and what does it matter? *Journal of Folklore Research*, **37**, 53–72.

Jordt S, McKemy DD and Julius D (2003). Lessons from peppers and peppermint: The molecular logic of thermosensation. *Current Opinion in Neurobiology*, **13**, 487–492.

Juteau A, Tournier C and Guichard E (2004). Influence of type and amount of gelling agent on flavour perception: Physicochemical effect or interaction between senses? *Flavour and Fragrance Journal*, **19**, 483–490.

Kadohisa M and Wilson DA (2006). Olfactory cortical adaptation facilitates detection of odors against background. *Journal of Neurophysiology*, **95**, 1888–1896.

Kajiura H, Cowart BJ and Beauchamp GK (1992). Early developmental change in bitter taste responses in human infants. *Developmental Psychology*, **25**, 375–386.

Kappes SM, Schmidt SJ and Lee SY (2006). Color halo/horns and halo-attribute dumping effects within descriptive analysis of carbonated beverages. *Journal of Food Science*, **71**, S590–S595.

Karrer T and Bartoshuk L (1995). Effects of capsaicin desensitization on taste in humans. *Physiology and Behavior*, **57**, 421–429.

Keast RSJ and Breslin PAS (2002). An overview of binary taste-taste interactions. *Food Quality and Preference*, **14**, 111–124.

Keast RSJ, Dalton PH and Breslin PAS (2004). Flavor interactions at the sensory level. In (eds) A Taylor and D Roberts, *Flavor Perception*, pp. 228–255. Blackwell Publishing Ltd, Oxford.

Kemp SE and Gilbert AN (1997). Odor intensity and color lightness are correlated sensory dimensions. *American Journal of Psychology*, **110**, 35–46.

Kern DL, McPhee L, Fisher J, Johnson S and Birch LL (1993). The postingestive consequences of fat conditioned preferences for flavours associated with high dietary fat. *Physiology and Behavior*, **54**, 71–76.

King BM, Arents P, Bouter N, *et al.* (2006). Sweetner/sweetness-induced changes in flavor perception and flavor release of fruity and green character in beverages. *Journal of Agricultural and Food Chemistry*, **54**, 2671–2677.

Kobayashi C, Kennedy LM and Halpern BP (2006). Experience-induced changes in taste identification of monosodium glutamate (MSG) are reversible. *Chemical Senses*, **31**, 301–306.

Kokini JL (1985). Fluid and semi-solid food texture and texture–taste interactions. *Food Technology*, **39**, 86–94.

Kokini JL (1987). The physical basis of liquid food texture and texture-taste interactions. *Journal of Food Engineering*, **6**, 51–81.

Kokini JL, Bistany K, Poole M and Stier E (1982). Use of mass transfer theory to predict viscosity-sweetness interactions of fructose and sucrose solutions containing tomato solids. *Journal of Texture Studies*, **13**, 187–200.

Kokini JL and Cussler El (1984). Predicting the texture of liquid and melting semi-solid foods. *Journal of Food Science*, **48**, 1221–1225.

Kora EP, Latrille E, Souchon I and Martin N (2003). Texture-flavor interactions in low fat stirred yoghurt: How mechanical treatment, thickener concentration and aroma concentration affect perceived texture and flavor. *Journal of Sensory Studies*, **18**, 367–390.

Koster MA, Prescott J and Koster EP (2004). Incidental learning and memory for three basic tastes in food. *Chemical Senses*, **29**, 441–453.

Koza BJ, Cilmi A, Dolese M and Zellner DA (2005). Color enhances orthonasal olfactory intensity and reduces retronasal olfactory intensity. *Chemical Senses*, **30**, 643–649.

Kringelbach ML, O'Doherty J, Rolls ET and Andrews C (2000). Sensory-specific satiety for the flavour of food is represented in the orbitofrontal cortex. *NeuroImage*, **11**, S767.

Kringelbach ML, O'Doherty J, Rolls ET and Andrews C (2003). Activation of the human orbitofrontal cortex to a liquid food stimulus is correlated with its subjective pleasantness. *Central Cortex*, **13**, 1064–1071.

Krondl M, Coleman P, Wade J and Milner J (1983). A twin study examining the genetic influence on food selection. *Human Nutrition: Applied Nutrition*, **37A**, 189–198.

Kroeze JHA and Bartoshuk LM (1985). Bitterness suppression as revealed by split-tongue taste stimulation in humans. *Physiology and Behavior*, **35**, 779–783.

Kubovy M and Van Valkenburg D (2001). Auditory and visual objects. *Cognition*, **80**, 97–126.

Kuznicki JT and Ashbaugh N (1982). Space and time separation of taste mixture components. *Chemical Senses*, **7**, 39–62.

Kuznicki JT and Turner LS (1988). Temporal dissociation of taste mixture components. *Chemical Senses*, **13**, 45–62.

Kuznicki JT, Hayward T and Schultz J (1983). Perceptual processing of taste quality. *Chemical Senses*, **7**, 273–292.

LaBar KS, Gitelman DR, Parrish TB, Kim YH, Nobre AC and Mesulam MM (2001). Hunger selectively modulates corticolimbic activation to food stimuli in humans. *Behavioral Neuroscience*, **115**, 493–500.

Labbe D, Damevin L, Vaccher C, Morgenegg C and Martin N (2006). Modulation of perceived taste by olfaction in familiar and unfamiliar beverages. *Food Quality and Preference*, **17**, 582–589.

Labbe D, Rytz A and Hugi A (2004). Training is a critical step to obtain reliable product profiles in a real food industry context. *Food Quality and Preference*, **15**, 341–348.

Laeng B, Berridge KC and Butter CM (1993). Pleasantness of a sweet taste during hunger and satiety: effects of gender and "sweet tooth." *Appetite*, **21**, 247–254.

Laing DG, Eddy A and Best J (1994).Perceptual characteristics of binary, trinary, and quaternary odor mixtures consisting of unpleasant constituents. *Physiology and Behavior*, **56**, 81–93.

Laing DG and Francis GW (1989). The capacity of humans to identify odors in mixtures. *Physiology and Behavior*, **46**, 809–814.

Laing DG and Glemarec A (1987). Selective attention and the perceptual analysis of odor mixtures. *Physiology and Behavior*, **52**, 1047–1053.

Laing DG, Link C, Jinks AL and Hutchinson I (2002). The limited capacity of humans to identify the components of taste mixtures and taste-odour mixtures. *Perception*, **31**, 617–635.

Laing DG and Willcox ME (1987). An investigation of the mechanisms of odor suppression using physical and dichorhinic mixtures. *Behavioural Brain Research*, **26**, 79–87.

Lanier SA, Hayes JE and Duffy VB (2005). Sweet and bitter tastes of alcoholic beverages mediate alcohol intake in of-age undergraduates. *Physiology and Behavior*, **83**, 821–831.

Larsen CS (2000). Dietary reconstruction and nutritional assessment of past peoples: the bioanthropological record. In (eds) KF Kiple and KC Ornelas, *The Cambridge World History of Food*, pp. 13–33. CUP, Cambridge.

Laska M and Hudson R (1991). A comparison of the detection thresholds of odour mixtures and their components. *Chemical Senses*, **16**, 651–662.

Laska M and Hudson R (1992). Ability to discriminate between related odor mixtures. *Chemical Senses*, **17**, 403–415.

Lavin JG and Lawless HT (1998). Effects of color and odor on judgements of sweetness among children and adults. *Food quality and Preference*, **9**, 283–289.

Lawless HT (1984). Flavor description of white wine by "expert" and nonexpert wine consumers. *Journal of Food Science*, **49**, 120–123.

Lawless HT (1995). Flavor. In (eds) M Friedman and E Carterette, *Handbook of Perception and Cognition. Volume 16, Cognitive Ecology*, pp. 325–380. Academic Press, SanDiego.

Lawless HT, Corrigan CJ and Lee CB (1994). Interactions of astringent substances. *Chemical Senses*, **19**, 141–154.

Lawless HT and Heymann H (1998). *Sensory Evaluation of Food Principles and Practices.* Chapman and Hall, New York.

Lawless HT, Hartono C and Hernandez S (2000). Thresholds and suprathreshold intensity functions for capsaicin in oil and aqueous based carriers. *Journal of Sensory Studies*, **15**, 437–447.

Lawless HT and Stevens DA (1984). Effects of oral chemical irritation on taste. *Physiology and Behavior*, **32**, 995–998.

Lawless HT and Stevens DA (1988).Responses by humans to oral chemical irritants as a function of locus of stimulation. *Perception and Psychophysics*, **43**, 72–78.

Lawless HT and Stevens DA (1989).Mixtures of oral chemical irritants. In (eds) D Laing, W Cain, R McBride and B Ache, *Perception of Complex Smells and Tastes*, pp. 297–309. Academic Press, Sydney.

Lawless HT, Stevens DA, Chapman KW and Kurtz A (2005). Metallic taste from electrical and chemical stimulation. *Chemical Senses*, **30**, 185–194.

Le Berre E, Thomas-Danguin T, Beno N, Coureaud G, Etievant P and Prescott J (2008). Perceptual processing strategy and exposure influence the perception of odor mixtures. *Chemical Senses*, **33**, 193–199.

Lee K (1989). Food neophobia: Major causes and treatments. *Food Technology*, **43**, 62–72.

Leger GC, Hummel T, Conley D, Mak YE, Simmons KB and Small DM (2003). Retronasal presentation of a food odor preferentially activates cortical chemosensory areas compared to orthonasal presentation of the same odor and retronasal presentation of a nonfood odor. *Chemical Senses*, **28**, 554.

Lepper MR, Greene D and Nisbett RE (1973). Understanding children's intrinsic interest with extrinsic reward: A test of the 'overjustification' hypothesis. *Journal of Personality and Social Psychology*, **28**, 129–137.

Leshem M, Abutbul A, Eilon R (1999). Exercise increases the preference for salt in humans. *Appetite*, **32**, 251–260.

Leshem M, Saadi A, Alem N and Hendi K (2008). Enhanced salt appetite, diet and drinking in traditional Bedouin women in the Negev. *Appetite*, **50**, 71–82.

Lesschaeve I and Issanchou S (1996). Effects of panel experience on olfactory memory performance: Influence of stimuli familiarity and labelling ability of subjects. *Chemical Senses*, **21**, 699–709.

Levine AS and Billington CJ (2004). Opioids as agents of reward-related feeding: A consideration of the evidence. *Physiology and Behavior*, **82**, 57–61.

Levy CM, MacRae A and Koster EP (2006). Perceived stimulus complexity and food preference development. *Acta Psychologica*, **123**, 394–413.

Lewkowski MD, Ditto B, Roussos M and Young SN (2003). Sweet taste and blood pressure related analgesia. *Pain*, **106**, 181–186.

Li W, Luxenberg E, Parrish T and Gottfried JA (2006). Learning to smell the roses: Experience-dependent neural plasticity in human piriform and orbitofrontal cortices. *Neuron*, **52**, 1097–1108.

Liem DG and Mennella JA (2003). Heightened sour preferences during childhood. *Chemical Senses*, **28**, 173–180.

Linforth RST, Baek I and Taylor AJ (1999). Simultaneous instrumental and sensory analysis of volatile release from gelatine and pectin/gelatine gels. *Food Chemistry*, **65**, 77–83.

Linforth RST, Blisset A and Taylor AJ (2005). Differences in the effect of bolus weight on flavor release into the breath between low-fat and high-fat products. *Journal of Agricultural and Food Chemistry*, **53**, 7217–7221.

Livermore A and Laing DG (1996). Influence of training and experience on the perception of multicomponent odor mixtures. *Journal of Experimental Psychology: Human Perception and Performance*, **22**, 267–277.

Livermore A and Laing DG (1998a). The influence of odor type on the discrimination and identification of odorants in multicomponent odor mixtures. *Physiology and Behavior*, **65**, 311–320.

Livermore A and Laing DG (1998b). The influence of chemical complexity on the perception of multicomponent odor mixtures. *Perception and Psychophysics*, **60**, 650–661.

Logue AW, Ophir I and Strauss KE (1981). The acquisition of taste aversions in humans. *Behaviour Research and Therapy*, **19**, 319–333.

Looy H and Weingarten HP (1992). Facial expressions and genetic sensitivity to 6-n-Propylthiouracil predict hedonic response to sweet. *Physiology and Behavior*, **52**, 75–82.

Looy H, Callaghan S and Weingarten HP (1992). Hedonic response of sucrose likers and dislikers to other gustatory stimuli. *Physiology and Behavior*, **52**, 219–225.

London RM, Snowdon CT and Smithana JM (1979). Early experiences with sour and bitter solutions increases subsequent ingestion. *Physiology and Behavior*, **22**, 1149–1155.

Lopez OL, Becker JT, Klunk W and DeKosky ST (1995). The nature of behavioral disorders in human Kluver-Bucy syndrome. *Neuropsychiatry, Neuropsychology and Behavioral Neurology*, **8**, 215–221.

Lovibond PW and Shanks DR (2002). The role of awareness in Pavlovian conditioning: Empirical evidence and theoretical implications. *Journal of Experimental Psychology: Animal Behavior Processes*, **28**, 3–26.

Lucas PW, Prinz JF, Agrawal KR and Bruce IC (2002). Food physics and oral physiology. *Food Quality and Preference*, **13**, 203–213.

Lundgren B, Pangborn RM, Daget N, *et al.* (1986). An interlaboratory study of firmness, aroma and taste. *Lebensmittel-Wissenschaft und Technologie*, **19**, 66–76.

Lyman BJ and Green BG (1990). Oral astringency: Effects of repeated exposure and interactions with sweeteners. *Chemical Senses*, **15**, 151–164.

Lyman BJ and McDaniel MA (1986). Effects of encoding strategy on long-term memory for odours. *Quarterly Journal of Experimental Psychology*, **38A**, 753–765.

Lynch J, Liu YH, Mela DJ and MacFie HJH (1993). A time-intensity study of the effect of oil mouthcoatings on taste perception. *Chemical Senses*, **18**, 121–129.

Maarse H (1991). *Volatile Compounds in Foods and Beverages*. Marcel Dekker, NY.

Maga JA (1974). Influence of color on taste thresholds. *Chemical Senses and Flavor*, **1**, 115–119.

Maga JA (1994). Glycoalkaloids in Solanaceae. *Food Reviews International*, **10**, 385–418.

Mak YE, Simmons KB, Gitelman DR and Small DM (2005). Taste and olfactory intensity perception changes following left insular stroke. *Behavioral Neuroscience*, **119**, 1693–1700.

Manes F, Springer J, Jorge R and Robinson RG (1999). Verbal memory impairment after left insular cortex infarction. *Journal of Neurology, Neurosurgery and Psychiatry*, **67**, 532–534.

Marciani L, Pfeiffer JC, Hort J, *et al.* (2006). Improved methods for fMRI studies of combined taste and aroma stimuli. *Journal of Neuroscience Methods*, **158**, 186–194.

Marinho H (1942). Social influence in the formation of enduring preferences. *Journal of Abnormal and Social Psychology*, **37**, 448–468.

Marks LE and Osgood EC (2005). Developmental constraints on theories of synesthesia. In (eds) LC Robertson and N Sagiv, *Synesthesia: Perspectives from cognitive neurosciences*, pp. 215–236. OUP, NY.

Marks LE and Wheeler ME (1998). Attention and the detectability of weak tastes. *Chemical Senses*, **23**, 19–29.

Marsh KB, Friel EN, Gunson A, Lund C and MacRae E (2006). Perception of flavour in standardised fruit pulps with additions of acids or sugars. *Food Quality and Preference*, **17**, 376–386.

Marshall SG and Vaisey M (1972). Sweetness perception in relation to some textural characteristics of hydrocolloid gels. *Journal of Texture Studies*, **3**, 173–185.

Marshall K, Laing DG, Jinks AL, Effendy J and Hutchinson I (2005). Perception of temporal order and the identification of components in taste mixtures. *Physiology and Behavior*, **83**, 673–681.

Marshall K, Laing DG, Jinks AL and Hutchinson I (2006). The capacity of humans to identify components in complex odor–taste mixtures. *Chemical Senses*, **31**, 539–545.

Martins Y and Pliner P (2005). Human food choices: An examination of the factors underlying acceptance/rejection of novel and familiar animal and nonanimal foods. *Appetite*, **45**, 214–224.

Mattes RD (1997). The taste for salt in humans. *The American Journal of Clinical Nutrition*, **65**, 692S–697S.

McBride RL and Finlay DC (1989). Perception of taste mixtures by experienced and novice assessors. *Journal of Sensory Studies*, **3**, 237–248.

McBurney DH, Collings VB and Glanz LM (1973). Temperature dependence of human taste responses. *Physiology and Behavior*, **11**, 89–94.

McBurney DH and Gent JF (1979). On the nature of taste qualities. *Psychological Bulletin*, **86**, 151–167.

McCormick DA and Bal T (1994). Sensory gating mechanisms of the thalamus. *Current Opinion in Neurobiology*, **4**, 550–556.

McCrory MA, Fuss PJ, McCallum JE, Yao M, Vinken, AG, Hays NP and Roberts SB (1999). Dietary variety within food groups: Association with energy intake and body fatness in men and women. *American Journal of Clinical Nutrition*, **69**, 440–447.

McDermott L, O'Sullivan T, Stead M and Hastings G (2006). International food advertising, pester power and its effects. *International Journal of Advertising*, **25**, 513–539.

McFarlane T and Pliner P (1997). Increasing willingness to taste novel foods: Effects of nutrition and taste information. *Appetite*, **28**, 227–238.

Mead S, Stumpf MPH, Whitfield J, *et al.* (2003). Balancing selection at the prion protein gene consistent with prehistoric kurulike epidemics. *Science*, **300**, 640–643.

Mehiel R and Bolles RC (1988). Learned flavor preferences based on calories are independent of initial hedonic value. *Animal Learning and Behavior*, **16**, 383–387.

Meilgaard M, Civille CV and Carr BT (1991). *Sensory Evaluation Techniques*. CRC, FL.

Mela DJ (1988). Sensory assessment of fat content in fluid dairy products. *Appetite*, **10**, 37–44.

Mela DJ and Marshall RJ (1992). Sensory properties and perceptions of fats. In (ed.) D Mela, *Dietary Fats: Determinants of Preference Selection and Consumption*, pp. 43–57. Elsevier Applied Science, London.

Melcher JM and Schooler JW (1996). The misremembrance of wines past: Verbal and perceptual expertise differentially mediate verbal overshadowing of taste memory. *Journal of Memory and Language*, **35**, 231–245.

Mesulam M-M (2000). *Principles of Behavioral and Cognitive Neurology*. OUP, Oxford.

Meullenet JF, Lyon BG, Carpenter JA and Lyon CE (1998). Relationships between sensory and instrumental texture profile attributes. *Journal of Sensory Studies*, **13**, 77–93.

Michener W and Rozin P (1994). Pharmacological versus sensory factors in the satiation of chocolate craving. *Physiology and Behavior*, **56**, 419–422.

Mingo S and Stevenson RJ (2007). Phenomenological differences between familiar and unfamiliar odours. *Perception*, **36**, 931–947.

Miyaoka Y and Pritchard TC (1996). Responses of primate cortical neurons to unitary and binary tastes. *Journal of Neurophysiology*, **75**, 396–411.

Mobini S, Chambers LC and Yeomans MR (2007). Effects of hunger state on flavour pleasantness conditioning at home: Flavour–nutrient learning vs. flavour–flavour learning. *Appetite*, **48**, 20–28.

Mojet J and Koster EP (2002). Texture and flavour memory in foods: An incredible learning experiment. *Appetite*, **28**, 110–117.

Mojet J and Koster EP (2005). Sensory memory and food texture. *Food Quality and Preference*, **16**, 251–266.

Mojet J, Koster EP and Prinz JF (2005). Do tastants have a smell? *Chemical Senses*, **30**, 9–21.

Molteni R, Barnard Z, Ying Z, Roberts C and Gomez-Pinilla F (2002). A high-fat, refined sugar diet reduces hippocampal brain-derived neurotrophic factor, neuronal plasticity, and learning. *Neuroscience*, **112**, 803–814.

Molteni R, Wu A, Vaynman S, Ying Z, Barnard R and Gomez-Pinilla F (2004). Exercise reverses the harmful effects of consumption of a high fat diet on synaptic and behavioral plasticity associated to the action of brain-derived neurotrophic factor. *Neuroscience*, **123**, 429–440.

Moncrieff RW (1951). *The Chemical Senses*. Leonard Hill, London.

Moncrieff RW (1966). *Odour preferences*. Leonard Hill, London.

Mook DG and Votaw MC (1992). How important is hedonism? Reasons given by college students for ending a meal. *Appetite*, **18**, 69–75.

Moore FW (1970). Food habits in non-industrial societies. In (ed.) J Dupont, *Dimensions of nutrition*, pp. 181–221. Associated University Press, CO.

Morran J and Marchesan M (2004). Taste and odour testing: How valuable is training? *Water Science and Technology*, **49**, 69–74.

Morris JS and Dolan RJ (2001). Involvement of human amygdala and orbitofrontal cortex in hunger-enhanced memory for food stimuli. *The Journal of Neuroscience*, **21**, 5304–5310.

Morrot G, Brochet F and Dubourdieu D (2001). The color of odors. *Brain and Language*, **79**, 309–320.

Moskowitz HR (1971). The sweetness and pleasantness of sugars. *American Journal of Psychology*, **84**, 387–405.

Moskowitz HR (1996). Experts versus consumers: A comparison. *Journal of Sensory Studies*, **11**, 19–37.

Moskowitz HR and Arabie P (1970). Taste intensity as a function of stimulus concentration and solvent viscosity. *Journal of Texture Studies*, **1**, 502–510.

Moskowitz HR and Barbe CD (1977). Profiling of odor components and their mixtures. *Sensory Processes*, **1**, 212–226.

Moskowitz HR, Kapsalis JG, Cardello AV, Fishken D, Maller O and Segars RA (1979). Determining relationships among objective, expert, and consumer measures of texture. *Food Technology*, **October Issue**, 84–88.

Moskowitz HR, Kumaraiah V, Sharma KN, Jacobs HL and Sharma SD (1975). Cross-cultural differences in simple taste preferences. *Science*, **190**, 1217–1218.

Mower GD, Mair RG and Engen T (1977). Influence of internal factors on the perceived intensity and pleasantness of gustatory and olfactory stimuli. In (eds)M Kare and O Maller, *The Chemical Senses and Nutrition*, pp. 104–118. American Press, New York.

Munoz AM and Civille GV (1987). Factors affecting perception and acceptance of food texture by American consumers. *Food Reviews International*, **3**, 285–322.

Murakami M, Kashiwadani H, Kirino Y and Mori K (2005). State-dependent sensory gating in olfactory cortex. *Neuron*, **46**, 285–296.

Murphy C and Cain WS (1980). Taste and olfaction: Independence vs. interaction. *Physiology and Behavior*, **24**, 601–605.

Murphy C, Cain WS and Bartoshuk LM (1977). Mutual action of taste and olfaction. *Sensory Processes*, **1**, 204–211.

Myles-Worsley M, Johnston WA and Simons MA (1988). The influence of expertise on X-ray image processing. *Journal of Experimental Psychology: Learning, Memory and Cognition*, **14**, 553–557.

Nasrawi CW and Pangborn RM (1989). The influence of tastants on oral irritation by capsaicin. *Journal of Sensory Studies*, **3**, 287–294.

Nasrawi CW and Pangborn RM (1990). Temporal gustatory and salivary responses to capsaicin upon repeated stimulation. *Physiology and Behavior*, **47**, 611–615.

Neta ER, Johanningsmeier SD and McFeeters RF (2007). The chemistry and physiology of sour taste – A review. *Journal of Food Science*, **72**, R33–38.

Noble AC (1996). Taste–aroma interactions. *Trends in Food Science and Technology*, **7**, 439–444

Nosofsky RM (1986). Attention, similarity and the identification–categorization relationship. *Journal of Experimental Psychology: General*, **115**, 39–57.

Obrebowski A, Obrebowska-Karsznia Z and Gawlinski M (2000). Smell and taste in children with simple obesity. *International Journal of Pediatric Otorhinolaryngology*, **55**, 191–196.

O'Doherty J, Rolls ET, Francis S, *et al.* (2000). Sensory-specific satiety-related olfactory activation of the human orbitofrontal cortex. *Neuroreport*, **11**, 399–403.

Ohloff G, Winter B and Fehr C (1991). Chemical classifications and structure odour relationships. In (eds) PM Muller and D Lamparsky, *Perfumes: Art, Science and Technology*, pp. 287–330. Elsevier, London.

Olsen SJ (2000). Dogs. In (eds) KF Kiple and KC Ornelas, *The Cambridge World History of Food*, pp. 508–516. CUP, Cambridge.

Olson DG, Caporaso F and Mandigo RW (1980). Effects of serving temperature on sensory evaluation of beef steaks from different muscles and carcass maturities. *Journal of Food Science*, **45**, 627–631.

Oram N, Laing DG, Hutchinson I, *et al.* (1995). The influence of flavor and color on drink identification by children and adults. *Developmental Psychobiology*, **28**, 239–246.

O'Regan JK and Noe A (2001). A sensorimotor account of vision and visual consciousness. *Behavioral and Brain Sciences*, **24**, 939–1031.

Ortner DJ and Theobald G (2000). Paleopathological evidence of malnutrition. In (eds) KF Kiple and KC Ornelas, *The Cambridge World History of Food*, pp. 34–43. CUP, Cambridge.

Osterbauer RA, Matthews PM, Jenkinson M, Beckmann CF, Hansen PC and Calvert GA (2005). Color of scents: Chromatic stimuli modulate odor responses in the human brain. *Journal of Neurophysiology*, **93**, 3434–3441.

Owen DH and Machamer PK (1979). Bias-free improvement in wine discrimination. *Perception*, **8**, 199–209.

Paivio A (1986). *Mental Representations: A Dual Coding Approach*. OUP, NY.

Pangborn RM (1959). Influence of hunger on sweetness preferences and taste thresholds. *The American Journal of Clinical Nutrition*, **7**, 280–287.

Pangborn RM (1960). Influence of color on the discrimination of sweetness. *The American Journal of Psychology*, **73**, 229–238.

Pangborn RM (1975). Cross-cultural aspects of flavour preferences. *Food Technology*, **29**, 34–36.

Pangborn RM, Chrisp RB and Bertolero LL (1970). Gustatory, salivary, and oral thermal responses to solutions of sodium chloride at four temperatures. *Perception and Psychophysics*, **8**, 69–75.

Pangborn RM, Gibbs ZM and Tassan C (1978). Effect of hydrocolloids on apparent viscosity and sensory properties of selected beverages. *Journal of Texture Studies*, **9**, 415–436.

Pangborn RM and Hansen B (1963). The influence of color on discrimination of sweetness and sourness in pear-nectar. *The American Journal of Psychology*, **76**, 315–317.

Pangborn RM and Koyasako A (1981). Time-course of viscosity, sweetness and flavor in chocolate desserts. *Journal of Texture Studies*, **12**, 141–150.

Pangborn RM, Trabue IM and Szczesniak AS (1973). Effect of hydrocolloids on oral viscosity and basic taste intensities. *Journal of Texture Studies*, **4**, 224–241.

Pangborn RM and Szczesniak AS (1974). Effect of hydrocolloids and viscosity on flavor and odor intensities of aromatic flavor compounds. *Journal of Texture Studies*, **4**, 467–482.

Parr WV, Heatherbell D and White GK (2004). Demystifying wine expertise: Olfactory threshold, perceptual skill and semantic memory in expert and novice wine judges. *Chemical Senses*, **27**, 747–755.

Parr WV, White GK and Heatherbell D (2002). Exploring the nature of wine expertise: What underlies wine experts' olfactory recognition memory advantage? *Food Quality and Preference*, **15**, 411–420.

Parry CM, Erkner A and le Coutre J (2004). Divergence of TR2 chemosensory receptor families in humans, bonobos and chimpanzees. *Proceedings of the National Academy of Sciences*, **101**, 14830–14834.

Patel KA and Schlundt DG (2001). Impact of moods and social context on eating behaviour. *Appetite*, **36**, 111–118.

Paulus K and Reisch AM (1980). The influence of temperature on the threshold values of primary tastes. *Chemical Senses*, **5**, 11–21.

Pearce JM (2002). Evaluation and development of a connectionist theory of configural learning. *Animal Learning and Behavior*, **30**, 73–95.

Pelchat ML and Pliner P (1995). "Try it. You'll like it." Effects of information on willingness to try novel foods. *Appetite*, **24**, 153–166.

Pelletier CA, Lawless HT and Horne J (2004). Sweet–sour suppression in older and young adults. *Food Quality and Preference*, **15**, 105–116.

Pepino MY and Mennella JA (2006). Children's liking of sweet tastes and its biological basis. In (ed.) W Spillane, *Optimising sweet taste in foods*, pp. 54–65, CRC Press, Boston.

Peron RM and Allen GL (1988). Attempts to train novices for beer flavor discrimination: A matter of taste. *The Journal of General Psychology*, **115**, 403–418.

Perl E, Shay U, Hamburger R and Steiner JE (1992). Taste and odor-reactivity in elderly demented patients. *Chemical Senses*, **17**, 779–794.

Peryam DR (1963). The acceptance of novel foods. *Food Technology*, **17**, 33–39.

Peto E (1935). Contribution to the development of smell feeling. *British Journal of Medical Psychology*, **15**, 314–320.

Pfeiffer JC, Hollowood TA, Hort J and Taylor AJ (2005). Temporal synchrony and integration of sub-threshold taste and smell signals. *Chemical Senses*, **30**, 539–545.

Pfeiffer JC, Hort J, Hollowood TA and Taylor AJ (2006). Taste-aroma interactions in a ternary system: A model of fruitiness perception in sucrose/acid solutions. *Perception and Psychophysics*, **68**, 216–227.

Philipsen DH, Clydesdale FM, Griffin RW and Stern P (1995). Consumer age affects response to sensory characteristics of a cherry flavored beverage. *Journal of Food Science*, **60**, 364–368.

Pierce J and Halpern BP (1996). Orthonasal and retronasal odorant identification based upon vapor phase input from common substances. *Chemical Senses*, **21**, 529–543.

Plata-Salaman CR, Smith-Swintosky R and Scott TR (1996). Gustatory neural coding in the monkey cortex: Mixtures. *Journal of Neurophysiology*, **75**, 2369–2379.

Pliner P (1982). The effects of mere exposure on liking for edible substances. *Appetite: Journal for Intake Research*, **3**, 283–290.

Pliner P and Loewen RE (1997). Temperament and food neophobia in children and their mothers. *Appetite*, **28**, 239–254.

Pliner P and Pelchat ML (1991). Neophobia in humans and the special status of foods of animal origin. *Appetite*, **16**, 205–218.

Pliner P and Pelchat M and Grabski M (1993). Reduction of neophobia in humans by exposure to novel foods. *Appetite*, **20**, 111–123.

Porubska K, Veit R, Preissl H, Fritsche A and Birbaumer N (2006). Subjective feeling of appetite modulates brain activity: An fMRI study. *NeuroImage*, **32**, 1273–1280.

Powell LM, Szczypka G and Chaloupka FJ (2007). Adolescent exposure to food advertising on television. *American Journal of Preventative Medicine*, **33**, S251–256.

Prescott J (1999). Flavour as a psychological construct: Implications for perceiving and measuring the sensory qualities of foods. *Food Quality and Preference*, **10**, 349–356.

Prescott J, Allen S and Stephens L (1994). Interactions between oral chemical irritation, taste and temperature. *Chemical Senses*, **18**, 389–404.

Prescott J, Johnstone V and Francis J (2004). Odor–taste interactions: Effects of attentional strategies during exposure. *Chemical Senses*, **29**, 331–340.

Prescott J and Stevenson RJ (1995). Effects of oral chemical irritation on tastes and flavors in frequent and infrequent users of chili. *Physiology and Behavior*, **58**, 1117–1127.

Prescott J and Wilkie J (2007). Pain tolerance selectively increased by a sweet-smelling odor. *Psychological Science*, **18**, 308–311.

Pritchard TC, Hamilton RB, Morse JR and Norgren R (1986). Projections of thalamic gustatory and lingual areas in the monkey. *Journal of Comparative Neurology*, **244**, 213–228.

Pritchard TC, Macaluso DA and Eslinger PJ (1999). Taste perception in patients with insular cortex lesions. *Behavioral Neuroscience*, **113**, 663–671.

Rabe S, Krings U and Berger RG (2003). Dynamic flavor release from sucrose solutions. *Journal of Agricultural and Food Chemistry*, **51**, 5058–5066.

Rabin MD (1988). Experience facilitates olfactory quality discrimination. *Perception and Psychophysics*, **44**, 532–540.

Randall E and Sanjur D (1981). Food preferences-their conceptualization and relationship to consumption. *Ecology of Food and Nutrition*, **11**, 151–161.

Rankin KM and Marks LE (2000). Chemosensory context effects: Role of perceived similarity and neural commonality. *Chemical Senses*, **25**, 747–759.

Raudenbush B, Schroth F, Reilley S and Frank RA (1998). Food neophobia, odor evaluation and exploratory sniffing behavior. *Appetite*, **31**, 171–183.

Rawson NE and Li X (2004). The cellular basis of flavour perception: Taste and aroma. In (eds) AJ Taylor and DD Roberts, *Flavor Perception*, pp. 57–85. Blackwell, Oxford.

Ray JP and Price JL (1992). The organization of the thalamocortical connections of the mediodorsal thalamic nucleus in the rat, related to the ventral forebrain–prefrontal cortex topography. *Journal of Comparative Neurology*, **323**, 167–197.

Regard M and Landis T (1997). "Gourmand syndrome": Eating passion associated with right anterior lesions. *Neurology*, **48**, 1185–1190.

Reilly S and Bornovalova MA (2005). Conditioned taste aversion and amygdala lesions in the rat: A critical review. *Neuroscience and Biobehavioral Reviews*, **29**, 1067–1088.

Revonsuo A (1999). Binding and the phenomenal unity of consciousness. *Consciousness and Cognition*, **8**, 173–185.

Reynolds RD, Binder HJ, Miller MB, Chang WWY and Horan S (1968). Pagophagia and iron deficiency anemia. *Annals of Internal Medicine*, **69**, 435–440.

Rich AN and Mattingley J (2002). Anomalous perception in synaethesia: A cognitive neuroscience perspective. *Nature Reviews Neuroscience*, **3**, 43–52.

Richardson BE, Vander Woude EA, Sudan R, Thompson JS and Leopold DA (2004). Altered olfactory acuity in the morbidly obese. *Obesity Surgery*, **14**, 967–969.

Richardson JTE and Zucco GM (1989). Cognition and olfaction: A review. *Psychological Bulletin*, **105**, 352–360.

Richardson NJ, Booth DA and Stanley NL (1993). Effect of homogenization and fat content on oral perception of low and high viscosity model creams. *Journal of Sensory Studies*, **8**, 133–143.

Roberts AK and Vickers ZM (1994). A comparison of trained and untrained judges evaluation of sensory attribute intensities and liking of cheddar cheeses. *Journal of Sensory Studies*, **9**, 1–20.

Robertson L (2003). Binding, spatial awareness and perceptual awareness. *Nature Reviews Neuroscience*, **4**, 93–102.

Robinson JO (1970). The misuse of taste names by untrained observers. *British Journal of Psychology*, **61**, 375–378.

Rolls BJ (1988). Food beliefs and food choices in adolescents. *The Medical Journal of Australia*, **148**, S9–S13.

Rolls ET (2006). Brain mechanisms underlying flavour and appetite. *Philosophical Transactions of the Royal Society*, **doi:10.1098/rstb.2006.1852**.

Rolls ET and Baylis LL (1994). Gustatory, olfactory and visual convergence within the primate orbitofrontal cortex. *Journal of Neuroscience*, **14**, 5437–5452.

Rolls ET, Critchely HD, Browning AS, Hernadi I and Lenard L (1999). Responses to the sensory properties of fat of neurons in the primate orbitofrontal cortex. *The Journal of Neuroscience*, **19**, 1532–1540.

Rolls BJ, Hetherington M and Burley VJ (1988). Sensory stimulation and energy density in the development of satiety. *Physiology and Behavior*, **44**, 727–733.

Rolls ET and McCabe C (2007). Enhanced affective brain representations of chocolate in cravers vs. non-cravers. *European Journal of Neuroscience*, **26**, 1067–1076.

Rolls ET and Rolls JH (1997). Olfactory sensory-specific satiety in humans. *Physiology and Behavior*, **61**, 461–473.

Rolls BJ, Rowe EA, Rolls ET, Kingston B, Megson A and Gunary R (1981). Variety in a meal enhances food intake in man. *Physiology and Behavior*, **26**, 215–221.

Rolls ET, Verhagen JV and Kadohisa M (2003). Representations of the texture of the food in the primate orbitofrontal cortex: Neurons responding to viscosity, grittiness and capsaicin. *Journal of Neurophysiology*, **90**, 3711–3724.

Romer M, Lehrner J, Wymelbeke VV, Jiang T, Deecke L and Brondel L (2006). Does modification of olfacto-gustatory stimulation diminish sensory-specific satiety in humans? *Physiology and Behavior*, **87**, 469–477.

Rosenstein D and Oster H (1988). Differential facial responses to four basic tastes in newborns. *Child Development*, **59**, 1555–1568.

Roth HA, Radle LJ, Gifford SR and Clydesdale FM (1988). Psychophysical relationships between perceived sweetness and color in lemon- and lime-flavored drinks. *Journal of Food Science*, **53**, 1116–1119.

Rozin E (1992). *Flavour Principle Cook Book*. Penguin, NJ.

Rozin P (1976). The selection of food by rats, humans and other animals. In (eds), A Hinde, C Beer and E Shaw, *Advances in the study of behavior, Volume 6*, pp. 21–76. Academic Press, NY.

Rozin P (1978). The use of characteristic flavorings in human culinary practice. In (ed.) M Apt, *Flavour: Its Chemical Behavioural and Commercial Aspects*, pp. 101–127. Westview Press, Colorado.

Rozin P (1982). "Taste–smell confusions" and the duality of the olfactory sense. *Perception and Psychophysics*, **31**, 397–401.

Rozin P (1990). Getting to like the burn of chili pepper. In (eds) B Green, R Mason and M Kare, *Chemical Senses Volume 2 Irritation*, pp. 231–269. Marcel Dekker, New York.

Rozin P (1999). The process of moralization. *Psychological Science*, **10**, 218–221.

Rozin P, Dow S, Moscovitch M and Rajaram S (1998). What causes humans to begin and end a meal? A role for memory for what has been eaten, as evidenced by a study of multiple meal eating in amnesic patients. *Psychological Science*, **9**, 392–396.

Rozin P, Fallon A and Augustoni-Ziskind M (1985). The child's conception of food: The development of contamination sensitivity to "disgusting" substances. *Developmental Psychology*, **21**, 1075–1079.

Rozin P, Fallon A and Mandell R (1984). Family resemblance in attitudes to foods. *Developmental Psychology*, **20**, 309–314.

Rozin P, Haidt J and McCauley C (2000). Disgust. In (eds) M Lewis and JM Haviland-Jones, *Handbook of Emotions*, pp. 637–653. Guilford Press, NY.

Rozin P, Hammer L, Oster H, Horowitz T and Marmora V (1986). The child's conception of food: Differentiation of categories of rejected substances in the 16 months to 5 year of age range. *Appetite*, **7**, 141–151.

Rozin P, Markwith M and Stoess C (1997). Moralization and becoming a vegetarian: The transformation of preferences into values and the recruitment of disgust. *Psychological Science*, **8**, 67–73.

Rozin P and Millman L (1987). Family environment, not heredity, accounts for family resemblances in food preferences and attitudes: A twin study. *Appetite*, **8**, 125–134.

Rozin P and Schiller D (1980). The nature and acquisition of a preference for chilli pepper by humans. *Motivation and Emotion*, **4**, 77–101.

Rozin P and Shenker J (1989). Liking oral cold and hot irritant sensations: Specificity to type of irritant and locus of stimulation. *Chemical Senses*, **14**, 771–779.

Saint-Eve A, Kora EP and Martin N (2004). Impact of the olfactory quality and chemical complexity of the flavouring agent on the texture of low fat stirred yoghurts assessed by three different sensory methodologies. *Food Quality and Preference*, **15**, 655–668.

Saint-Eve A, Martin N, Guillemin H, Semon E, Guitchard E and Souchon I (2006). Flavored yoghurt complex viscosity influences real-time aroma release in the mouth and sensory properties. *Journal of Agricultural and Food Chemistry*, **54**, 7794–7803.

Sakai N and Imada S (2003). Bilateral lesions of the insular cortex or the prefrontal cortex block the association between taste and odor in the rat. *Neurobiology of Learning and Memory*, **80**, 24–31.

Sakai N, Kobayakawa T, Gotow N, Saito S and Imada S (2001). Enhancement of sweetness ratings of aspartame by a vanilla odor presented either by orthonasal or retronasal routes. *Perception and Motor Skills*, **92**, 1002–1008.

Salkovskis PM and Clark DM (1990). Affective responses to hyperventilation: A test of the cognitive model of panic. *Behaviour Research and Therapy*, **28**, 51–61.

Saper CB, Chou TC and Elmquist JK (2002). The need to feed: Homeostatic and hedonic control of eating. *Neuron*, **36**, 199–211.

Sauvageot F, Urdapilleta I and Peyron D (2006). Within and between variations of texts elicited from nine wine experts. *Food Quality and Preference*, **17**, 429–444.

Savic I (2001). Processing of odorous signals in humans. *Brain Research Bulletin*, **54**, 307–312.

Savic I, Gulyas B, Larsson M and Roland PE (2000). Olfactory pathways are organized in parallel and hierarchical manner. *Neuron*, **26**, 735–745.

Scalera G (2002). Effects of conditioned food aversions on nutritional behavior in humans. *Nutritional Neuroscience*, **5**, 159–188.

Schaal B, Soussignan R, Marlier L, Kontar F, Karima IS and Tremblay RE (1997). Variability and invariability in early odour preferences: Comparative data from children belonging to three cultures. *Chemical Senses*, **22**, 212.

Schifferstein HNJ and Frijters JER (1990). Sensory integration in citric acid/sucrose mixtures. *Chemical Senses*,**15**, 87–109.

Schifferstein HNJ, Kole PW and Mojet J (1999). Asymmetry in the disconfirmation of expectations for natural yoghurt. *Appetite*, **32**, 307–329.

Schifferstein HNJ and Verlegh PWJ (1996). The role of congruency and pleasantness in odor-induced taste enhancement. *Acta Psychologica*, **94**, 87–105.

Schiffman SS (1992). Olfaction in aging and medical disorders. In (eds) MJ Serby and KL Chobor, *Science of olfaction*, pp. 500–525. Springer-Verlag, NY.

Schiffman SS (2002). Taste quality and neural coding: Implications from psychophysics and neurophysiology. *Physiology and Behavior*, **69**, 147–159.

Schiffman SS and Erickson RP (1971). A psychophysical model for gustatory quality. *Physiology and Behavior*, **7**, 617–633.

Schiffman SS, Robinson DE and Erickson RP (1977). Multidimensional scaling of odorants: Examination of psychological and physiochemical dimensions. *Chemical Senses and Flavor*, **2**, 375–390.

Schiffman SS, Sattely-Miller EA, Graham BG, *et al*. (2000). Effect of temperature pH, and ions on sweet taste. *Physiology and Behavior*, **68**, 469–481.

Schiffman SS, Suggs MS and Simon SA (1992). Astringent compounds suppress taste responses in gerbil. *Brain Research*, **595**, 1–11.

Schiffman SS, Warwick ZS and Mackey M (1994). Sweetness and appetite in normal, overweight, and elderly persons. In (eds) J Fernstorm and G Miller, *Appetite and Body Weight Regulation: Sugar, Fat, and Macronutrient Substitutes*, pp. 99–112, CRC Press, London.

Schlundt DG, Virts KL, Sbrocco T, Pope-Cordle J and Hill JO (1993). A sequential behavioral analysis of craving sweets in obese women. *Addictive Behaviors*, **18**, 67–80.

Schmidt HJ and Beauchamp GK (1988). Adult-like odor preferences and aversions in three-year old children. *Child Development*, **59**, 1136–1143.

Schoenbaum G and Eichenbaum H (1995). Information coding in the rodent prefrontal cortex. I: Single neuron activity in orbitofrontal cortex compared with that in pyriform cortex. *Journal of Neurophysiology*, **74**, 733–762.

Schultz HG (1964). A matching-standards method for characterizing odor qualities. *Annals of the New York Academy of Sciences*, **116**, 517–526.

Scott JW, Acevedo HP, Sherrill L and Phan M (2007). Responses of the rat olfactory epithelium to retronasal air flow. *Journal of Neurophysiology*, **97**, 1941–1950.

Scott TR and Mark GP (1987). The taste system encodes stimulus toxicity. *Brain Research*, **414**, 197–203.

Shaffer SE and Tipper BJ (1994). Effects of learned flavor cues on single meal and daily food intake in humans. *Physiology and Behavior*, **55**, 979–986.

Shepherd GM (2006). Smell images and the flavour system in the human brain. *Nature*, **444**, 316–321.

Simon SA, de Araujo IE, Gutierrez R and Nicolelis MAL (2006). The neural mechanisms of gustation: A distributed processing code. *Nature Reviews Neuroscience*, **7**, 890–901.

Simons CT, O'Mahony M and Carstens E (2002). Taste suppression following lingual capsaicin pre-treatment in humans. *Chemical Senses*, **27**, 353–365.

Simpson J, Anthony SH, Schmeer S and Overton PG (2007). Food-related contextual factors substantially modify the disgust response. *Food Quality and Preference*, **18**, 183–189.

Singer W (1996). Neuronal synchronization: A solution to the binding problem? In (eds) R Llinas and PS Churchland, *The Mind–Brain Continuum*, pp.101–130. MIT Press, MA.

Sizer F and Harris N (1985). The influence of common food additives and temperature on threshold perception of capsaicin. *Chemical Senses*, **10**, 279–286.

Small DM, Gerber JC, Mak YE and Hummel T (2005). Differential neural responses evoked by orthonasal versus retronasal odorant perception in humans. *Neuron*, **47**, 593–605.

Small DM, Jones-Gotman M and Dagher A (2003). Feeding-induced dopamine release in dorsal striatum correlates with meal pleasantness ratings in healthy human volunteers. *NeuroImage*, **19**, 1709–1715.

Small DM, Jones-Gotman M, Zatorre RJ, Petrides M and Evans AC (1997a). A role for the right anterior temporal lobe in taste quality recognition. *The Journal of Neuroscience*, **17**, 5136–5142.

Small DM, Jones-Gotman M, Zatorre RJ, Petrides M and Evans AC (1997b). Flavor processing: More than the sum of its parts. *NeuroReport*, **8**, 3913–3917.

Small DM and Prescott J (2005). Odor/taste integration and the perception of flavor. *Experimental Brain Research*, **166**, 345–357.

Small DM, Voss J, Mak YE, Simmons KB, Parrish T and Gitelman D (2004). Experience-dependent neural integration of taste and smell in the human brain. *Journal of Neurophysiology*, **92**, 1892–1903.

Small DM, Zatorre RJ, Dagher A, Evans AC and Jones-Gotman M (2001). Changes in brain activity related to eating chocolate. *Brain*, **124**, 1720–1733.

Smit HJ and Blackburn RJ (2005). Reinforcing effects of caffeine and theobromine as found in chocolate. *Psychopharmacology*, **181**, 101–106.

Smith DV (1989). Neural and behavioral mechanisms of taste mixture perception in mammals. In (eds) DG Laing, WS Cain, RL McBride and BW Ache, *Perception of complex smells and tastes*, pp. 149–170. Academic Press, Sydney.

Smith DV and Margolskee RF (2001). Making sense of taste. *Scientific American*, **March**, 26–33.

Snoek HM, Huntjens L, van Gemart LJ, de Graaf C and Weenen H (2004). Sensory-specific satiety in obese and normal-weight women. *American Journal of Clinical Nutrition*, **80**, 823–831.

Sobel N, Prabhakaran V, Zhao Z, Desmond JE, Glover GH, Sullivan EV and Gabrieli JDE (2000). Time course of odorant-induced activation in the human primary olfactory cortex. *Journal of Neurophysiology*, **83**, 537–551.

Solomon GEA (1997). Conceptual change and wine expertise. *The Journal of the Learning Sciences*, **6**, 41–60.

Solomon GEA (1990). Psychology of novice and expert wine talk. *American Journal of Psychology*, **103**, 495–517.

Sorensen LB, Moller P, Flint A, Martens M and Raben A (2003). Effect of sensory perception of foods on appetite and food intake: A review of studies on humans. *International Journal of Obesity*, **27**, 1152–1166.

Soussignan R, Schaal B and Marlier L (1999). Olfactory alliesthesia in human neonates: Prandial state and stimulus familiarity modulate facial and autonomic responses to milk odors. *Developmental Psychobiology*, **35**, 3–14.

Soussignan R, Schaal B, Marlier L and Jiang T (1997). Facial and autonomic responses to biological and artificial olfactory stimuli in human neonates: Re-examining early hedonic discrimination of odors. *Physiology and Behavior*, **62**, 745–758.

Spence C, McGlone FP, Kettenmann B and Kobal G (2001). Attention to olfaction: A psychophysical investigation. *Experimental Brain Research*, **138**, 432–437.

Spence C and Zampini M (2006). Auditory contributions to multisensory product perception. *Acta Acustica United With Acustica*, **92**, 1009–1025.

Sperling JM, Prvulovic D, Linden DEJ, Singer W and Stirnm A (2006). Neuronal correlates of colour-graphemic synaesthesia: A fMRI study. *Cortex*, **42**, 295–303.

Stanek EJ, Calabrese EJ, Mundt K, Pekow P and Yeatts KB (1998). Prevalence of soil mouthing/ingestion among healthy children aged 1 to 6. *Journal of Soil Contamination*, **7**, 227–242.

Stein BE, Wallace MT and Stanford TR (2001). Brain mechanisms for synthesizing information from different sensory modalities. In (ed.) B Goldstein, *Blackwell Handbook of Perception*, pp. 709–736. Blackwell, MA.

Steiner JE (1979). Human facial expressions in response to taste and smell stimulation. In (eds) H Reese and L Lipsitt, *Advances in Child Development and Behavior Volume 13*, pp. 257–295, Academic Press, New York.

Steiner JE, Glaser D, Hawilo ME and Berridge KC (2001). Comparative expression of hedonic impact: Affective reactions to taste by human infants and other primates. *Neuroscience and Biobehavioral Reviews*, **25**, 53–74.

Stevens DA and Lawless HT (1987). Enhancement of responses to sequential presentation of oral chemical irritants. *Physiology and Behavior*, **39**, 63–-65.

Stevenson RJ (2001). Is sweetness taste enhancement cognitively impenetrable? Effects of exposure, training and knowledge. *Appetite*, **36**, 241–242.

Stevenson RJ and Boakes RA (2003). A mnemonic theory of odor perception. *Psychological Review*, **110**, 340–364.

Stevenson RJ and Boakes RA (2004). Sweet and sour smells: Learned synesthesia between the senses of taste and smell. In (eds) G. Calvert, C. Spence and B. Stein, *The Handbook of Multisensory Processes*, pp. 69–83. MIT Press, MA.

Stevenson RJ, Boakes RA and Prescott J (1998). Changes in odor sweetness resulting from implicit learning of a simultaneous odor–sweetness association: An example of learned synesthesia. *Learning and Motivation*, **29**, 113–132.

Stevenson RJ, Boakes RA and Wilson JP (2000a). Resistance to extinction of conditioned odor perceptions: Evaluative conditioning is not unique. *Journal of Experimental Psychology: Leaning, Memory and Cognition*, **26**, 423–440.

Stevenson RJ, Boakes RA and Wilson JP (2000b). Counterconditioning following human odor–taste and color–taste learning. *Learning and Motivation*, **31**, 114–127.

Stevenson RJ and Case TI (2003). Preexposure to the stimulus elements, but not training to detect them, retards human odour-taste learning. *Behavioural Processes*, **61**, 13–25.

Stevenson RJ, Mahmut M and Sundqvist N (2007). Age-related changes in odor discrimination. *Developmental Psychology*, **43**, 253–260.

Stevenson RJ, Miller LA and Thayer ZC (2008). Impairments in the perception of odor-induced tastes and their relationship to impairments in taste perception. *Journal of Experimental Psychology: Human Perception and Performance*, **34**, 1183–1197.

Stevenson RJ and Oaten M (2008). The effect of appropriate and inappropriate stimulus color on odor discrimination. *Perception and Psychophysics*, **70**, 640–646.

Stevenson RJ, Prescott J and Boakes RA (1995). The acquisition of taste properties by odors. *Learning and Motivation*, **26**, 433–455.

Stevenson RJ, Prescott J and Boakes RA (1999). Confusing taste and smells: How odours can influence the perception of sweet and sour tastes. *Chemical Senses*, **24**, 627–635.

Stevenson RJ and Repacholi BM (2003). Age-related changes in children's hedonic response to male body odor. *Developmental Psychology*, **39**, 670–679.

Stevenson RJ and Tomiczek C (2007). Olfactory-induced synesthesias: A review and model. *Psychological Bulletin*, **133**, 294–309.

Stevenson RJ, Tomiczek C and Oaten M (2007). Olfactory hedonic context affects both self-report and behavioural indices of palatability. *Perception*, **36**, 1698–1708.

Stevenson RJ and Wilson DA (2007). Olfactory perception: An object recognition approach. *Perception*, **36**, 1821–1833.

Stevenson RJ and Yeomans MR (1993). Differences in ratings of intensity and pleasantness for the capsaicin burn between chilli likers and non-likers: Implications for liking development. *Chemical Senses*, **18**, 471–482.

Stillman JA (1993). Color influences flavor identification in fruit-flavored beverages. *Journal of Food Science*, **58**, 810–812.

Stoffregen TA and Bardy BG (2001). On specification and the senses. *Behavioral and Brain Sciences*, **24**, 195–261.

Stone H and Oliver S (1966). Effect of viscosity on the detection of relative sweetness and intensity of sucrose solutions. *Journal of Food Science*, **31**, 129–134.

Stone H and Sidel JL (1993). *Sensory Evaluation Practices*. Academic, FL.

Sullivan SA and Birch LL (1994). Infant dietary experience and acceptance of solid foods. *Pediatrics*, **93**, 271–277.

Sun BC and Halpern BP (2005). Identification of air phase retronasal and orthonasal odorant pairs. *Chemical Senses*, **30**, 693–706.

Sundqvist NC, Stevenson RJ and Bishop IRJ (2006). Can odours acquire fat-like properties? *Appetite*, **47**, 91–99.

Szczesniak AS (2002). Texture is a sensory property. *Food Quality and Preference*, **13**, 215–225.

Szczesniak AS, Brandt MA and Friedman HH (1963). Development of standard rating scales for mechanical parameters of texture and correlation between the objective and the sensory methods of texture evaluation. *Journal of Food Science*, **28**, 397–403.

Szczesniak AS and Kleyn DH (1963). Consumer awareness of texture and other food attributes. *Food Technology*, **17**, 74–77.

Tannahill R. (1988). *Food in History*. Penguin, London.

Teerling A (1992). The colour of taste. *Chemical Senses*, **17**, 886.

Tepper BJ and Kuang T (1996). Perception of fat in milk model system using mutlidimensional scaling. *Journal of Sensory Studies*, **11**, 175–190.

Terasaki M and Imada S (1988). Sensation seeking and food preferences. *Personality and Individual Differences*, **9**, 87–93.

Theunissen MJM and Kroeze JHA (1995). The effect of sweeteners on perceived viscosity. *Chemical Senses*, **20**, 441–450.

Tinley EM, Durlach PJ and Yeomans MR (2004). How habitual caffeine consumption and does influence flavour preference conditioning with caffeine. *Physiology and Behavior*, **82**, 317–324.

Todrank J and Bartoshuk LM (1991). A taste illusion: Taste sensation localized by touch. *Physiology and Behavior*, **50**, 1027–1031.

Tournier C, Martin C, Guichard E, Issanchou S and Sulmont-Rosse C (2007). Contribution to the understanding of consumers' creaminess concept: A sensory and a verbal approach. *International Dairy Journal*, **17**, 555–564.

Treisman AM and Gelade G (1980). A feature-integration theory of attention. *Cognitive Psychology*, **12**, 97–136.

Trelea IC, Atlan S, Deleris I, Saint-Eve A, Marin M and Souchon I (2008). Mechanistic mathematical model for in vivo aroma release during eating of semiliquid foods. *Chemical Senses*, **33**, 181–192.

Tuorila H (1990). The role of attitudes and preferences in food choice. In (eds) J Somogyi and E Koskinen, *Nutritional Adaptation to New Life-Styles*, pp. 125–132, Karger, Basel.

Tuorila H, Meiselman HL, Bell R, Cardello AV and Johnson W (1994). Role of sensory and cognitive information in the enhancement of certainty and liking for novel and familiar foods. *Appetite*, **23**, 231–246.

Valentin D, Chollet S, Beal S and Patris B (2007). Expertise and memory for beers and beer olfactory compounds. *Food Quality and Preference*, **18**, 776–785.

Valentin D, Chrea C and Nguyen DH (2006). Taste–odour interactions in sweet taste perception. In (ed.) W Spillane, *Optimising Sweet Taste in Foods*, pp. 66–84. Woodhead Publishing Limited, Cambridge.

Van der Gaag C, Minderaa RB and Keysers C (2007). Facial expressions: What the mirror neuron system can and cannot tell us. *Social Neuroscience*, **2**, 179–222.

Van der Klaauw NJ and Frank RA (1996). Scaling component intensities of complex stimuli: The influence of response alternatives. *Environment International*, **22**, 21–31.

Van Ruth SM and Roozen JP (2002). Delivery of flavours from food matrices. In (ed.) A Taylor, *Food Flavour Technology*, pp 167–184. Sheffield Academic Press, UK.

Van Vliet T (2002). On the relation between texture perception and fundamental mechanical parameters for liquids and time dependent solids. *Food Quality and Preference*, **13**, 227–236.

Vaisey M, Brunon R and Cooper J (1969). Some sensory effects of hydrocolloid sols on sweetness. *Journal of Food Science*, **34**, 397–400.

Vaynman S and Gomez-Pinilla F (2006). Revenge of the "Sit": How lifestyle impacts neuronal and cognitive health through molecular systems that interface energy metabolism with neuronal plasticity. *Journal of Neuroscience Research*, **84**, 699–715.

Velmans M (1991). Is human information processing conscious? *Behavioral and Brain Sciences*, **14**, 651–726.

Verhagen JV and Engelen L (2006). The neurocognitive bases of human multimodal food perception: Sensory integration. *Neuroscience and Biobehavioral Reviews*, **30**, 613–650.

Verhagen JV, Rolls ET and Kadohisa M (2003). Neurons in the primate orbitofrontal cortex respond to fat texture independently of viscosity. *Journal of Neurophysiology*, **90**, 1514–1525.

Vickers ZM (1984). Crispness and crunchiness – A difference in pitch. *Journal of Texture Studies*, **15**, 157–163.

Vickers ZM (1987). Sensory, acoustical, and force-deformation measurements of potato chip crispness. *Journal of Food Science*, **52**, 138–140.

Vickers ZM and Bourne MC (1976a). Crispness in foods – A review. *Journal of Food Science*, **41**, 1153–1157.

Vickers ZM and Bourne MC (1976b). A psychoacoustical theory of crispness. *Journal of Food Science*, **41**, 1158–1164.

Vickers ZM and Christensen CM (1980). Relationship between sensory crispness and other sensory and instrumental parameters. *Journal of Texture Studies*, **11**, 291–307.

Villa P, Bouville C, Courtin J, *et al.* (1986). Cannibalism in the Neolithic. *Science*, **233**, 431–437.

Visschers RW, Jacobs MA, Frasnelli J, Hummel T, Burgering M and Boelrijk AEM (2006). Cross-modality of texture and aroma perception is independent of orthonasal or retronasal stimulation. *Journal of Agricultural and Food Chemistry*, **54**, 5509–5515.

Voirol E and Daget N (1989). Direct nasal and oronasal profiling of a meat flavouring: Influence of temperature, concentration and additives. *Lebensmittel-Wissenschaft und Technologie*, **22**, 399–405.

von Bekesy G (1964). Olfactory analogue to directional hearing. *Journal of Applied Physiology*, **19**, 363–373.

von Sydow E, Moskowitz H, Jacobs H and Meiselman H (1974). Odor–taste interaction in fruit juices. *Lebensmittel-Wissenschaft und Technologie*, **7**, 18–24.

Wagner AR (1981). SOP: A model of automatic memory processing in animal behavior. In (eds) NE Spear and RR Miller, *Information Processing in Animals: Memory Mechanisms*, pp. 5–47. Erlbaum, NJ.

Walk RD (1966). Perceptual learning and discrimination of wine. *Psychonomic Science*, **5**, 57–58.

Wang GJ, Volkow ND, Telang F, *et al.* (2004). Exposure to appetite food stimuli markedly activates the human brain. *NeuroImage*, **21**, 1790–1797.

Ward J and Mattingley J (2006). Synesthesia: An overview of contemporary findings and controversies. *Cortex*, **42**, 129–136.

Ward J and Simner J (2005). Is synaesthesia an X-linked dominant trait with lethality in males? *Perception*, **34**, 611–623.

Ward J, Simner J and Auyeung V (2005). A comparison of lexical-gustatory and grapheme-colour synaesthesia. *Cognitive Neuropsychology*, **22**, 28–41.

Watson WL, Laing DG, Hutchinson I and Jinks AL (2001). Identification of the components of taste mixtures by adults and children. *Developmental Psychobiology*, **39**, 137–145.

Weel KGC, Boelrijk AEM, Alting AC, *et al.* (2002). Flavor release and perception of flavored whey protein gels: Perception is determined by texture rather than release. *Journal of Agricultural and Food Chemistry*, **50**, 5149–5155.

Weenen H, Jellema RH and de Wijk RA (2005). Sensory sub-attributes of creamy mouthfeel in commercial mayonnaises, custard desserts and sauces. *Food Quality and Preference*, **16**, 163–170.

Welch RB and Warren DH (1980). Immediate perceptual response to intersensory discrepancy. *Psychological Bulletin*, **88**, 638–667.

Wheeler ME, Petersen SE and Buckner RL (2000). Memory's echo: Vivid remembering reactivates sensory-specific cortex. *Proceedings of the National Academy of Sciences*, **97**, 11125–11129.

Wheelock JV (1990). Consumer attitudes towards processed foods. In (eds) J Somogyi and E Koskinen, *Nutritional Adaptation to New Life-Styles*, pp. 125–132, Karger, Basel.

White TL and Prescott J (2007). Chemosensory cross-modal stroop effects: Congruent odors facilitate taste identification. *Chemical Senses*, **32**, 337–341.

Wicker B, Keysers C, Plailly J, Royet J-P, Gallese V and Rizzolatti G (2003). Both of us disgusted in *my* insula: The common neural basis of seeing and feeling disgust. *Neuron*, **40**, 655–664.

Wilkinson C, Dijksterhuis GB and Minekus M (2000).From food structure to texture. *Trends in Food Science and Technology*, **11**, 442–450.

Wilson CE and Brown WE (1997). Influence of food matrix structure and oral breakdown during mastication on temporal perception of flavor. *Journal of Sensory Studies*, **21**, 69–86.

Wilson TD and Klaaren KJ (1992). "Expectation whirls me around": the role of affective expectations in affective experience. In (ed.) MS Clark, *Emotion and Social Behavior. Review of Personality and Social Psychology*, pp. 1–31. Sage, CA.

Wilson DA and Stevenson RJ (2003). Olfactory perceptual learning: The critical role of memory in odor discrimination. *Neuroscience and Biobehavioral Reviews*, **27**, 307–328.

Wilson DA and Stevenson RJ (2006). *Learning to Smell: Olfactory Perception from Neurobiology to Behavior*. John Hopkins University Press, Baltimore.

Winkielman P, Berridge KC and Wilbarger JL (2005). Unconscious affective reactions to masked happy versus angry faces influence consumption behavior and judgments of value. *Personality and Social Psychology Bulletin*, **31**, 121–135.

Witthoft N and Winawer J. (2006). Synesthetic colors determined by having colored refrigerator magnets in childhood. *Cortex*, **42**, 175–183.

Wolters CJ and Allchurch EM (1994). Effect of training procedure on the performance of descriptive panels. *Food Quality and Preference*, **5**, 203–214.

Woodburn J (1968). An introduction to Hadza ecology. In (eds) RB Lee and I DeVore, *Man the hunter*, pp. 49–55. Aldine Publishing Company, Chicago.

Woolley JD, Lee BS, Taha SA and Fields HL (2007). Nucleus accumbens opioid signalling conditions short-term flavour preferences. *Neuroscience*, **146**, 19–30.

Wysocki CJ, Pierce JD and Gilbert AN (1991). Geographic, cross-cultural, and individual variation in human olfaction. In (eds) TV Getchell, LM Bartoshuk, RL Doty and JB Snow, *Smell and Taste in Health and Disease*, pp. 287–314. Raven Press, NY.

Yackinous C and Guinard JX (2000). Flavor manipulation can enhance the impression of fat in some foods. *Journal of Food Science*, **65**, 909–915.

Yau NJN and McDaniel MR (1991a). The effect of temperature on carbonation perception. *Chemical Senses*, **16**, 337–348.

Yau NJN and McDaniel MR (1991b).Carbonation interaction with sweetness and sourness. *Journal of Food Science*, **57**, 1412–1416.

Yeo MA, Treloar SA, Marks GC, Heath AC and Martin NG (1997). What are the causes of individual differences in food consumption and are they modified by personality. *Personality and Individual Differences*, **23**, 535–542.

Yeomans MR (1996). Palatability and the micro-structure of feeding in humans: The appetizer effect. *Appetite*, **27**, 119–133.

Yeomans MR (2000). Rating changes over the course of meals: What do they tell us about motivation to eat. *Neuroscience and Biobehavioral Reviews*, **24**, 249–259.

Yeomans MR (2008). Learning and hedonic contributions to human obesity. In (ed.) EM Blass, *Obesity*, pp. 211–236. Sinauer and Associates, MA.

Yeomans MR, Chambers L, Blumenthal H, Blake A (2008). The role of expectancy in sensory and hedonic evaluation: The case of smoked salmon ice-cream. *Food Quality and Preference*, **19**, 565–573.

Yeomans MR, Gould NJ, Mobini S and Prescott J (2008). Acquired flavor acceptance and intake facilitated by MSG in humans. *Physiology and Behavior*, **93**, 958–966.

Yeomans MR and Gray RW (1997). Effects of naltrexone on food intake and changes in subjective appetite during eating: Evidence for opioid involvement in the appetizer effect. *Physiology and Behavior*, **62**, 15–21.

Yeomans MR and Mobini S (2006). Hunger alters the expression of acquired hedonic but not sensory qualities of food-paired odors in humans. *Journal of Experimental Psychology: Animal Behavior Processes*, **32**, 460–466.

Yeomans MR, Mobini S and Chambers L (2007). Additive effects of flavour–caffeine and flavour–flavour pairings on liking for the smell and flavour of a novel drink. *Physiology and Behavior*, **92**, 831–839.

Yeomans MR, Mobini S, Elliman TD, Walker HC and Stevenson RJ (2006). Hedonic and sensory characteristics of odors conditioned by pairing with tastants in humans. *Journal of Experimental Psychology: Animal Behavior Processes*, **32**, 215–228.

Yeomans MR, Weinberg L and James S (2005). Effects of palatability and learned satiety on energy density influences on breakfast intake in humans. *Physiology and Behavior*, **86**, 487–499.

Zajonc RB (1968). Attitudinal effects of mere exposure. *Journal of Personality and Social Psychology*, **9**, 1–27.

Zald DH (2003). The human amygdala and the emotional evaluation of sensory stimuli. *Brain Research Reviews*, **41**, 88–123.

Zald DH, Lee JT, Fluegel KW and Pardo JV (1998). Aversive gustatory stimulation activates limbic circuits in humans. *Brain*, **121**, 1143–1154.

Zald DH and Pardo JV (2000). Functional neuroimaging of the olfactory system in humans. *International Journal of Psychophysiology*, **36**, 165–181.

Zajonc RB (1980). Feeling and thinking preferences need no inferences. *American Psychologist*, **35**, 151–175.

Zampini M, Sanabria D, Phillips N and Spence C (2007). The multisensory perception of flavor: Assessing the influence of color cues on flavor discrimination responses. *Food Quality and Preference*, **18**, 975–984.

Zampini M and Spence C (2004). The role of auditory cues in modulating the perceived crispness and staleness of potato chips. *Journal of Sensory Studies*, **19**, 347–363.

Zampini M and Spence C (2005). Modifying the multisensory perception of a carbonated beverage using auditory cues. *Food Quality and Preference*, **16**, 632–641.

Zellner DA, Bartoli AM and Eckard R (1991). Influence of color on odor identification and liking ratings. *American Journal of Psychology*, **104**, 547–561.

Zellner DA and Kautz MA (1990). Color affects perceived odor intensity. *Journal of Experimental Psychology: Human Perception and Performance*, **16**, 391–397.

Zellner DA, Rozin P, Aron P and Kulish C (1983). Conditioned enhancement of human's liking for flavor by pairing with sweetness. *Learning and Motivation*, **14**, 338–350.

Zellner DA, Stewart WF, Rozin P and Brown JM (1988). Effect of temperature and expectations on liking for beverages. *Physiology and Behavior*, **44**, 61–68.

Zellner DA, Strickhouser D and Tornow CE (2004). Disconfirmed hedonic expectations produce perceptual contrast, not assimilation. *American Journal of Psychology*, **117**, 363–387.

Zellner DA and Whitten LA (1999). The effect of color intensity and appropriateness on color-induced odor enhancement. *American Journal of Psychology*, **112**, 585–604.

Zhang J, Temme E, Sasaki S and Kesteloot H (2000). Under and overreporting of energy intake using urinary cations as biomarkers: Relation to BMI. *American Journal of Epidemiology*, **152**, 453–462.

Index